Aging and Life

AN INTRODUCTION TO GERONTOLOGY

second edition

Aging and Life

An Introduction to Gerontology

second edition

Arthur N. Schwartz

University of Southern California School of Medicine
California Lutheran Homes

Cherie L. Snyder

Presbyterian Intercommunity Hospital, Family Practice Center
University of Redlands

James A. Peterson

University of Southern California Ethel Percy Andrus Gerontology Center

with Appendix by Jean Mueller

Holt, Rinehart and Winston
New York   Chicago   San Francisco   Philadelphia
Montreal   Toronto   London   Sydney
Tokyo   Mexico City   Rio de Janeiro   Madrid

Publisher: John Michel
Acquisitions Editor: Nedah Abbott
Developmental Editor: Alison Podel
Project Editor: Melanie Miller
Production Manager: Annette Mayeski
Design Supervisor: Louis Scardino
Text Design: Caliber Design Planning, Inc.
Cover Design: Ben Santora

Photograph Credits (by page number): American Forest Industries: 173; Andrus
Gerontology Center: 29; R. Bennett: 307, 315, 327; Follett Publishing Co.: 218; John
King: 138; Monkmeyer Press Photo/Sybil Shelton: 27; Photo Researchers/© Vinnie
Fish: 187; A. Schwartz: 1, 168(l), 282, 325, 334, 336, 337, 351; © Jean Shapiro: 209;
Hal Smith: 16, 20, 22, 35, 39, 63, 69, 73, 83, 97, 109, 119, 131, 150, 155, 168(r), 183,
190, 191, 196, 198, 203, 220, 231, 238, 245, 252, 278, 291, 294, 342, 345, 354, 359

Library of Congress Cataloging in Publication Data

Schwartz, Arthur N.
  Aging & life.

  Rev. ed. of: Introduction to gerontology. © 1979.
  Includes bibliographies and index.
  1. Gerontology. I. Snyder, Cherie L. II. Peterson, James Alfred. III. Schwartz,
Arthur N. Introduction to gerontology. IV. Title. V. Title: Aging and life. [DNLM:
1. Geriatrics. WT 100 S399i]
HQ1061.S3469 1984   362.6′042   83-22685

ISBN 0-03-063678-7

CBS COLLEGE PUBLISHING
Holt, Rinehart and Winston
The Dryden Press
Saunders College Publishing

This Book Is Dedicated . . .

To my wife—matchless collaborator, creative colleague, confidante, and best friend. ANS

To the memory of Louisa Frances Heath, my maternal grandmother, and to Fannie Mae Snyder, my paternal grandmother—dear, thoughtful, remarkable women of great inner strength whose actions in service to others have always spoken louder than words ever could, and to whom I am indebted for their contributions to this book and my life—and to their children, Florence and Darl, who lovingly attest to the fact that the apple doesn't fall far from the tree;

To John and Louise Zebrowski, and to Joan Dietrich, Joanne Allison, Sandra Silva, and Judi Earley, whose constant friendship continues to overcome the obstacles of geography and time; and

To my husband—it takes one to know one! CLS

To my loving wife, Audrey. JAP

Foreword

When the University of Southern California first formed an organizing committee in 1964 to develop a comprehensive program of research and education about aging, there were barely a half-dozen institutions in the country that had pioneered the field and could serve as models. Research in the field was sparse and training almost nonexistent. In the past twenty years the field has grown exponentially. Today over fifteen hundred institutions of higher learning have courses in aging. Gerontology has become a major focus of a great many schools. Because of this the need for textbooks that can integrate the findings of the various disciplines in both introductory and advanced treatments has become imperative. *Aging and Life* has just such a purpose as its goal.

No single text can adequately treat in depth all of the research or all the programs for aging that are now available. The authors have wisely included after each section a selection of further readings that have been carefully chosen to enable students to read more comprehensively about various aspects of aging. Rather than treating the many theories of aging as an abstract conglomerate, the authors have combined theoretical with practical issues in each chapter. Case illustrations and critical discussions have been included to underscore the often controversial problems that face not only the older members of our society today, but also those who attempt to learn more about aging through research and those who provide services to their older constituents.

It is essential that gerontologists develop increasing insight into the many facets of aging, but it is equally important that the focus be always on the aging of individual persons. *Aging and Life* tries to maintain that essential balance between accurate reporting and awareness of persons, so that the uniqueness of the older individual is not lost in statistics. On the other hand, generalizations from statistics enable us to deal more adequately with the life of each older person.

Legislative programs, new research findings, and political changes are making an impact in the field of gerontology every day. It is interesting that changes in the Social Security law and other legislative reforms have come about just as this text was completed, an illustration of how important it is for any teacher to update his or her materials month by month. For writers this means that books on gerontology must be constantly revised; for instructors it means a creative use of new research reports, changes in governmental programs and policies, and economic indices if they are to deal adequately with their field.

This text is a "first" in that it is the first book specially designed and written to provide a general introduction to the field of gerontology for students in a broad range of disciplines. Drs. Schwartz, Snyder, and Peterson have accomplished this remarkably well and as a "plus" have succeeded in producing a substantive, information-packed text that is eminently readable. It will fill a gap in the gerontological literature.

James E. Birren
Director and Dean
Andrus Gerontology Center
The University of Southern California

Preface

This text is an interdisciplinary introduction to the major concepts and issues pertinent to the study of the aging process—gerontology. *Gerontology* is a broad field of inquiry and service into every aspect of human functioning in the later years of life. It is distinguished from *geriatrics,* which denotes the field of medicine devoted to the diseases of old age.

Written for those who are entering the health fields, the behavioral sciences, and policy-making fields, this book is intended to aid them in making decisions and providing services. Such individuals will be far more effective if they base their professional decisions on tested knowledge and accurate information rather than on stereotypes, myths, and "guesses" about the aged and the aging process.

We believe that the study of aging will help improve the circumstances and lives of older persons, and have emphasized pragmatic applications of gerontological knowledge to the problems of the aged. This special attention to practical applications does not minimize our view of the importance of research and scientific inquiry. On the contrary, our goal is to present information about aging to underscore its heuristic value for those who work with elders in direct clinical fashion as well as for those who develop research studies derived from theoretical models.

Many different kinds of information fall within gerontology's purview. Traditionally, the study of aging has been divided into discrete categories and topics. Such an approach is impossible to avoid completely, and this text, in general, is organized in this way. The study of gerontology is not a static or fixed body of facts or findings; rather it is a dynamic, complex field which must, like medicine or psychology or social work, continuously relate itself to the fluid, ever-changing, variable characteristics of the population under consideration.

To approach gerontologists with the question "What causes aging?" would be as inappropriate as it would be to ask "What causes adolescence?" Gerontology and geriatrics have made an excellent beginning in uncovering many salient facts about normal aging. Even so, we are still not entirely clear as to what extent normal aging involves loss and pathology as functions of the passage of time itself, or to what extent multiple loss or malfunction can be attributed to causal factors distinct from and extraneous to the addition of extra years.

In an earlier time attitudes toward long-lived individuals were colored by magic and superstition. Views of aging were based on anecdote and opinion. This is not to say that such speculations in all instances were necessarily invalid or incorrect. Yet, many such perceptions have been shown to be inaccurate or so limited in scope as to have fed myths or stereotypes about aging that continue to persist today.

Later, with the advent of the scientific method (in the 1600s), a marked shift took place. Systematic observation of naturally occurring events led to the discovery of underlying principles and laws governing those events. This basic scientific mode of thought has come to be generally used in the study of underlying processes of aging, especially within the last half-dozen decades. In this respect the relatively young field of gerontology parallels the more extensive history of medicine. The early practice of medicine can be characterized essentially as a practitioner's art. Only later did it add scientific methodology and the resources of a growing technological base. Throughout the recent history of medicine we can trace the consistent interplay between scientific/technological methodology and the experience and requirements of the direct service practitioner/clinician.

The field of gerontology has been developing in a similar fashion: earlier mystical speculations and superstitious responses to the aged were followed in due course by application of scientific/technological methods. These in turn generated information utilized in services to older people. Thus the base of systematic observation and organized information about aging has been extended.

A substantial amount of information about aging is now available to our society. Much of this information is derived from systematic research, much from rich experience in working with the elderly. An urgent task for gerontologists, therefore, is to synthesize data for maximum utility. But there are still far too many gaps in our knowledge and understanding of aging. Because multiple causation (Birren & Clayton, 1975) enjoys the preferred explanatory role in the study of aging, cross-disciplinary cooperation between scientific inquiry and direct service professionalism serves an obvious and useful purpose in providing the richest context for the study of aging. The fact that the full potential of this interaction between research and service has not always been fully realized in no way diminishes its merit as an ideal toward which gerontology can and should strive (Carp, 1974).

As will become apparent, we have tried hard to build some of the bridges between research, practice, and planning by integrating concepts and themes. This ought to provide both guidance and challenge. We realize that no text can presume to be all things to all readers. Our goal, therefore, has been to present a fair and well-balanced overview of gerontology. In so doing, we have tried to emphasize the interdisciplinary nature of gerontology that is characteristic of the field. We hope this text will provide the "generalists" with what they need and want to know; and at the same time offer the "specialists" choices and leads for further detailed exploration and study.

Acknowledgments

The authors wish to gratefully acknowledge the substantial amounts of time and energy so patiently expended by so many in the development and production of this book.

We would like to thank James Birren for providing the foreword to *Aging and Life*. Dr. Birren has devoted the larger part of his own life to the study of the aging process, and we are indebted to him, not only for his addition to our book, but for his lifelong efforts to shape and define the field of gerontology.

We are likewise indebted to Jean Mueller for her outstanding contribution of the Appendix, "Information Retrieval in Gerontology: The Literature Search." Ms. Mueller's many years of service as chief librarian of the Andrus Gerontology Center, University of Southern California, are reflected in her invaluable documentation of the processes through which students and professionals alike must go to keep abreast of the increasing volume of information in the field.

We would like to acknowledge the fine work of our photographer, Hal Smith, who went far beyond the call of duty to provide us with many excellent photographs as well as useful suggestions which we are pleased to have incorporated into the book.

We would also like to commend Lisa Smith for her labors in compiling the subject index for our book. Ms. Smith truly went the extra mile for us, and we thank her for performing this task so very well.

We are grateful to Florence Lynch for her kind efforts in diligent pursuit of information leading to the granting of permission by other authors to cite or include their work in our text. Mrs. Lynch's involvement in this project has been great, and we applaud her efforts in our behalf.

And we would like to express our appreciation to our publishing staff at Holt, Rinehart and Winston. The helpful suggestions and able assistance of our Publisher, John Michel, our Assistant Editor, Alison Podel, and especially our Production Editor, Melanie Miller, throughout the various stages of writing and production have contributed significantly to the quality of the finished product. We count ourselves fortunate to have been able to work with these individuals.

Last, but not least, we wish to thank the following individuals who read through our manuscript in its earlier stages and who provided many valuable comments and criticisms: Peter J. Murk, *Ball State University;* Joann F. Maslin, *Union College;* Suzanne Prescott, *Governors State University;* David Karnos, *Eastern Montana University;* Vern L. Bengston, *Ethel Percy Andrus Gerontology Center*; and L. Robert Martin, *University of Southern California School of Medicine.* In addition, the second author would like to thank her many students from the University of Redlands classes on aging, for whom the manuscript served as their primary text, for their good-natured willingness to put up with the many typo-ridden, unbound pages of the draft and for their many recommendations that helped us tailor the final version to better suit the needs of our future readers.

ANS

CLS

JAP

Contents

Gerontology: A New Look at the Old

Chapter 1

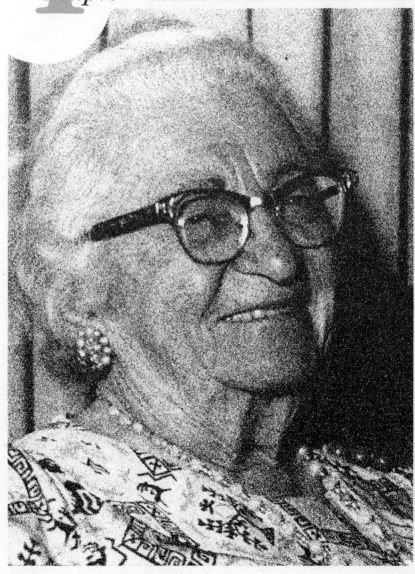

I like Spring, but it is too young
I like Summer, but it is too proud
So I like best of all Autumn

Because its leaves are a little yellow
Its tone mellower
Its colors richer

And it is tinged a little with sorrow
Its golden richness speaks
　　　not of the innocence of spring
　　　nor of the power of summer

But of the mellowness and kindly wisdom
　　　of approaching age

It knows the limitations of life
　　　and is content.
　　　Lin Yutang

Many may discover in this text a fresh perspective on aging: *a new look at the old.* Whether one examines the aging process in terms of its continuities or discontinuities across the lifespan; from a broad, historical perspective or as an urgent contemporary issue; in terms of the **commonalities**[1] of experience among aged **cohorts**[2] or the personal, unique experience of the aged individual—any and all such perspectives provide the serious student of **gerontology**[3] with a remarkably rich array of information.

In the last analysis, gerontology aims at producing new data, broadening the spectrum of knowledge, and deepening our understanding and appreciation of the complex variety of discrete, specific, yet interrelated factors that influence the process of aging.

The multiple dimensions of the aging process are best understood within a matrix that illustrates and illuminates their interrelationships and interactions in the context of the fluid, dynamic processes of adaptation and growth.

---

[1] *commonality:* similarity based on shared characteristics or experience
[2] *cohorts:* group of persons born during a given time period
[3] *gerontology:* the study of the aging process (cf. *geriatrics,* the study of illness in old age)

From Individual Perspective to General Issues

At the very outset of any serious study of gerontology, it must be acknowledged that no adequate definition of aging has as yet been proposed. In spite of many common experiences and events observed across large groups of aged persons from varied cultural backgrounds, only one basic truism emerges: that each individual perceives and thus experiences the process of growing older in a truly personal and **idiosyncratic**[1] way.

The following case illustration is offered to exemplify this point. It is drawn from an interview with an elderly woman that took place in a park located near the center of a large city. While this woman need not be considered typical of all elderly persons, her responses reflect a number of very personal yet commonly shared concerns of the elderly, in an articulate confirmation of **nomothetic**[2] and **idiographic**[3] laws of behavior. This interview further illustrates a number of major issues to which gerontology devotes considerable attention and around which much of this text is organized. The diversity of issues also argues for the necessity of an integrated multidisciplinary approach to the study of aging.

CASE ILLUSTRATION
The Individual Perspective

Mrs. B. is a widow in her mid-seventies, residing near the central city in a congested urban environment. She is a small woman with thinning gray-white hair, and is clean and neatly groomed though plainly dressed. She displays a few pieces of bright jewelry on her gnarled, blue-veined hands and arms. She lives in a tiny, shabby house not far from a city park. That small greenbelt serves as a "living room" for her and her peers. She goes there to visit with acquaintances who happen by, to get a breath of fresh air, and to watch the comings and goings of ducks in the pond and people in the park.

Her first reaction when approached was to wave off the interviewer with her hands, saying, "No, no!" while shaking her head. After some explanations were offered she was drawn into conversation, in which she then engaged with obvious interest and enthusiasm. At the conclusion of the conversation she complimented the interviewer for not having accepted her initial brush-off. "You have to ease in with older people" was her wry comment.

Mrs. B.'s husband died six years ago. The months following his death were the most difficult time for her. The couple had no children, a fact about which she insists she has no regrets. After her husband's death, several neighbors she had known for years also died within a

---

[1] *idiosyncratic:* uniquely characteristic of the individual
[2] *nomothetic:* applicable to or representative of a general group or universe
[3] *idiographic:* applicable to or representative of an individual case or person

short period of time. She presently has no deep or intimate relationships and talked about periodic bouts of loneliness and severe depression. She says a close relationship with others is now impossible for her.

"You can't really trust old people," she says. "They'll be friends with you for awhile and then they'll turn on you—or leave you." Yet at another point in the conversation she confessed that she wished she had a group of friends.

She has kin but has lost track of them. Anyway, she doesn't see relatives as a resource in old age because "you only cause friction if you move in."

She considers her health as good as that of anyone else her own age because she "gets around pretty good." She believes that if she were to become really sick, she would have to hire a nurse or someone else to come in and care for her. The more frightening prospect for her is that if she were to suffer a prolonged illness she might be compelled to dispose of her belongings and move into a nursing home.

She says her life has been "just fine" until recently. Mrs. B. has plenty of energy and goes to dances for entertainment, but only if someone will take her. She still would like to go to "musical events" but is apprehensive about public transportation: "it costs so much," it's "confusing," and she's afraid "something might happen." She does her own marketing and visits a local bank to deposit her Social Security check, but finds these excursions emotionally draining and physically exhausting. Some of her acquaintances tell her she can get "help from the community," but she's not clear how this works or where or how to inquire.

A few months ago she caught the flu and still feels its debilitating effects. Her appetite dropped off; even now she is not eating well. Also, "it's a lot of bother cooking for yourself," she says. She hasn't seen a physician, but plans to do so soon. She adds, "You can't go into old age gracefully. One day you feel just fine and the next day you'll be feeling bad."

She owns her home in a run-down, high-crime neighborhood. People frequently tell her how dangerous it is, but she still insists she isn't afraid to live alone. "If they want to come in and kill me, it's all right with me." So far she feels financially secure and doesn't have to "rely on anyone for anything." She planned and saved for her "retirement," and thinks all young people should do the same. But she is worried about the possibility of having to give up her house "sometime, because of the taxes."

Mrs. B. says the old men in the park and at the dances are "just looking for someone to take care of them." She says this more in disappointment than disgust. "They can be a burden on a woman," she explains. She seems very positive in her insistence that she would never marry again—not even a very rich man.

To reiterate, the experience of aging is highly colored by personal expectations and attitudes. Some of the most fundamental issues that demand the attention of research scientists and service providers alike originate from a growing theoretical base. Other issues derive from patterns of life circumstances and everyday experiences such as those described in the preceding case illustration.

Increasing familiarity with the field will make it evident that gerontology is not preoccupied solely with the systematic search for mere facts about adult development and the aging process. Equally influential is a strong tradition of **pragmatism**[1] which more often than not leads the scientific study of aging to practical outcomes and applications in the service of elderly persons.

General Issues

The concerns of gerontology, therefore, arise from everyday problems of the elderly as much as they do from theoretical perspectives. The list of issues that follows reflects areas of primary service afforded the aged as well as directions taken by biological, social, and other behavioral scientists in their continuing search for knowledge. This list is not intended to be all-inclusive, but is designed to help the student develop something in the way of a **cognitive map**[2] of the field of gerontology. Such constructs indicate not only some of the "discovered territory" in the field of aging but also some of the current and important directions toward which gerontology is moving. The issues are addressed in the form of questions commonly asked by gerontologists in their studies of aging.

1. Health maintenance, nutrition (diet), and exercise What is the desirable balance between health and other high-priority needs of the aged? How is health care to be paid for, and how is cost affected by differential concepts of treatment, cure, and prevention? How is "health" to be defined, and what factors contribute in what significant ways to physical as well as emotional well-being in old age?

2. Family and marital relations What are the marital difficulties and the potential obstacles to sensual and sexual satisfaction for the old? What are the particular and unique problems faced by elderly parents of mature children? Is **role reversal**[3] necessary or inevitable? To what extent are age changes and generation differences responsible for family conflicts? Can feelings of guilt on the part of the **sandwich generation**[4] and manipulative behavior on the part of their elders be dealt with constructively? What is the nature of grandparent-grandchild interactions?

3. Personality variables and adaptive coping mechanisms What are the significant changes that occur in later life and to what extent are

---

[1]*pragmatism:* practicality

[2]*cognitive map:* visual image or representation of objects and/or events as they exist in a specific time and place

[3]*role reversal:* descriptive of the adult child taking on a parental role and the aging parent assuming a child role

[4]*sandwich generation:* middle-aged people who have dependent children and, at the same time, increasingly dependent aging parents

these affected by physical or social factors? How stable are personality, intelligence factors, and learning ability throughout the lifespan? Are there different dimensions of stress in old age? What kinds of adaptation and coping strategies do the elderly use, and how can these be measured and evaluated?

4. Behavioral and cognitive competence   Are there appropriate norms for competence in old age? What is the special significance of memory lapses and confusion? Is senile behavior a fact or an artifact, and are behaviors associated with brain damage reversible? Is compensation for losses an effective intervention for healthy elderly as well as for elderly with multiple disabilities?

5. Migration and mobility   How are the life satisfactions and morale of the aged affected by a mobile society? To what extent are the quality and cost of services to the elderly affected by transportation factors? What impact does migration have upon housing, education, health services, and family and friendship networks with respect to the aged?

6. Attitudes, religious beliefs, and norms (expectations)   Are the expectations of the aged different from or similar to those of other age groups? How important is religion and its practice to the elderly? Do we have adequate relevant norms for old age or are these yet to be established? Are these positive or negative norms?

7. Environmental planning, design, and impact   Which environmental factors affect the aging process and how can these be measured? What should be the priorities when considering prosthetic environmental design versus cost? Should the environment be designed to "fit" the elderly, or the elderly helped to fit the environment? What is the most useful design perspective for long-term-care facilities?

8. Dying, bereavement, and grief   What kinds of services and care do the dying need? How do we help the elderly deal with bereavement and grief? What problems arise from the preponderance of elderly widows, and what are their special needs? What emotional supports are needed for the dying and their families, and who should be trained to provide these supports?

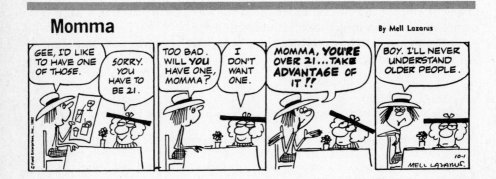

9. Economics and the elderly, work and productivity   Is there an optimal age for retirement, or should retirement be based on other criteria (e.g., productivity, interest, functional capability)? Are there alternative definitions of productivity which are more appropriate for the aged? How does inflation affect the elderly, and should they be given greater opportunities for work? Do work opportunities exploit the elderly?

10. Public policy, planning, and administration   Which decision makers most affect the lives of the elderly? How are policy decisions affecting the old made and implemented? On what basis is planning done, and what must administrators and service providers know to run effective and relevant programs for the elderly?

11. Housing, congregate living, and long-term care   How do individual preferences and life-style affect congregate living? What are the social implications and consequences of housing design and location for the elderly? Is long-term care a first alternative or a last resort? Which models of congregate living are most appropriate and relevant to elderly persons?

12. Legal protection, crime, and safety   How do the aged become special victims of crime? Are there special legal services needed by the old, and how are these to be provided? When and where is advocacy for the old appropriate, and who should provide it?

We recognize that other terms and formulations can be (and often are) used to denote these as well as other relevant issues in gerontology. Possible additions, for example, might include such important and pressing issues as education and training in gerontology, the appropriate utilization of the communications media to represent and serve the needs of the aged, the role of the expressive arts with respect to aging, the proper training and appropriate use of volunteer services, cultivation of a larger and more integrated role of family members within the context of the long-term-care (nursing home) enterprise, and funding resources for research, practice, and information exchange on aging.

How Old Is Gerontology?

The individual experience and personal perspective of aging are intriguing particularly because of their insistent demonstration of individual differences. The major source of fascination lies, of course, in comparisons of one's own experiences with the personal experiences described by others. Increasing awareness of these variations has given rise to growing interest in an autobiographical approach to the study of the later years of life (cf. Butler, 1974; Lauer & Goldfield, 1970; Likorish, 1975; Reedy & Birren, 1980).

The unending cycle of human birth, maturation, and death continues to generate seemingly endless curiosity. Human interest in every detail of the constantly evolving drama of human existence dates back to ancient times.

From the beginning, the name of the game seems to have been survival.

Until recently, relatively few individuals survived much beyond what we now consider to be the middle years. Early seers like Cicero (Copely, 1967) who recorded observations about the characteristics of the old nevertheless indicated that the average lifespan during early recorded history barely exceeded twenty-five years. Perhaps that is why old age, this relatively little-studied phase of the life cycle, came to be colored so much by superstitious thinking and attitudes.

For example, the Trobriand Islanders and the Sinu of Japan believed the secret of long life among their forebears lay in their ancestors' ability to shed their skins like snakes. This same notion of rejuvenation as the secret of long life is embedded in the more familiar story of the Spanish explorer Ponce de León's legendary search for the "fountain of youth," primarily in that territory now known as Florida.

This yearning for longer life has dominated the fantasies and searching of people in all ages. People will travel great distances in the hope of discovering some special climate or chemical that might prove to be the key to long life. Dr. Paul Niehaus in Switzerland has attracted people from all over the world who come to try his injections of ground-up, homogenized sheep embryos. If those fail, they may travel to Rumania, where Dr. Ana Aslan offers to all comers an elixir called Gerovital which promises to retard the aging process. Long life is so precious that pseudo- and quasi-scientific prescriptions lure hundreds of thousands of men and women into spending millions of dollars on dubious nostrums.

Until less than a half century ago, mystical, magical, and superstitious approaches dominated much thinking about aging and long life. Those who did survive into their seventies and eighties were usually heralded as wise and accorded special status. As the natural purveyors of family, clan, or tribal history and wisdom, they lived relatively good lives—as good as many elderly today, if not better. The ancient tradition in the Far East (Japan and China, in particular) of referring to the old as "respected elders" has been maintained there until recent times. In the United States, with the gradual transition to and emphasis upon industrialization, urbanization, individual productivity, "progress," and youth, many long-livers—especially those who became infirm and destitute—were sent off to the "poor farm," and a poor answer for them it certainly was. Whatever deference may have been accorded the old in our own society in the past has largely vanished, as witnessed by the fact that few designations of special status given to age *qua* age now exist (with the exception of limited instances, such as the title "emeritus" given to a few distinguished academics, scientists, and clergy).

Early Study of Old Age

Prior to this century certain individuals anticipated the systematic and scientific study of aging as we know it today. Roger Bacon, Francis Galton, and Francis Bacon are counted among the early investigators and writers in this field. Already in the thirteenth century Roger Bacon suggested that the organism becomes increasingly vulnerable over time because of the interaction of inherited factors and physical health (Hendricks & Hendricks, 1977). Francis Bacon was one of the first to suggest that improved hygiene could increase life expectancy (Freeman, 1965). In the nineteenth century Francis Galton collected data on some dozen-and-a-half physical measures from a sample of visitors to the International Health Exhibition in London as the result of his interest in variations in physical characteristics across age groups. A Belgian scientist, Lambert Quètelet, was one of the first to apply the concept of measures of central tendency in his inquiries about aging, birth rates, and death rates in the early 1800s (Birren & Clayton, 1975). During the latter part of the nineteenth century a Russian scientist by the name of S. P. Botkin studied a large sample of persons over age sixty-five living in St. Petersburg (Hendricks & Hendricks, 1977). Botkin was attempting to differentiate "pathological" from "normal" aging; an interesting finding is the distinction he drew between biological and chronological age.

Modern Gerontology

Early concerns about aging were characterized by a great deal of philosophical reflection, serious as well as idle speculation, and not a little intuitive guessing. This is not to say that ruminations of this sort always prove to be invalid. On the contrary, early as well as more contemporary historians, philosophers, novelists, playwrights, and other observers of the human condition have produced insights of a high order.

What must be recognized is that systematic, reliable, empirical evidence that leads us closer to facts about aging is essential if we are to have any confidence whatsoever that we are indeed approaching what can be called the truth with respect to what that process is all about. The scientific method, in addition to uncovering new information, will appear at times to discover things about aging we have "always known" by virtue of common sense, but it will also invalidate other commonsense notions by demonstrating them to be myths or stereotypes.

The advent of the twentieth century marked the beginning of the systematic study of aging. In 1908 two significant books appeared, Minto's *The Problems of Age, Growth, and Death,* and Metchnikoff's *The Prolongation of Life.* These were followed by two widely cited classics in gerontology, G. Stanley Hall's *Senescence, the Second Half of Life* in 1922, and E. V. Cowdry's *Problems of Aging* in 1939. Hall, a specialist in child and adolescent psychology, was president of Clark University when he wrote *Senescence,* a monograph that grew from his own concern about his anticipated retirement. Cowdry is considered by some to be the "founding father" of modern gerontology, a judgment based on Cowdry's seminal volume, his early recognition of the interdisciplinary nature of gerontology, his synthesizing skills in bringing together a variety of interests in this field, and the significant contribution of his organizational work, particularly in establishing the International Association of Gerontology (IAG).

Following these pioneer beginnings, the truly scientific study of aging seems to have begun to burgeon by the late 1930s through the 1940s. The study of aging began to attract national attention and support thanks to a series of crucial, well-timed conferences. Particularly instrumental in this regard was the Josiah Macy Foundation, whose interest and activities led to the convening of a scientific meeting at Woods Hole, Massachusetts, in 1937, sponsored by the National Research Council and the Union of American Biological Societies. In the following year the National Research Council's committee on the biological processes of aging sponsored another conference.

The mobilizing of national conferences gained momentum during 1940–41, when such influential groups as the American Orthopsychiatric Association, the Medical Clinics of North America, the American Chemical Society, the Public Health Service, and the National Institutes of Health (NIH) sponsored conferences on topics related to aging. The issues ranged from aging as a public health problem, industrial aspects of aging workers, and intellectual changes with age to the mental health of and psychotherapy for those in the later years of life. Many of the concerns about aging raised in those conferences anticipated some of the contemporary issues in gerontology.

Scientific inquiry into these questions about aging was interrupted by the involvement of the United States in World War II from 1941 to 1945. Following the war years, the resurgence of activity by gerontologists of every description was marked by the founding of the Gerontological Society of America, Inc., in 1945, with headquarters in Washington, D.C.

The National Advisory Committee, appointed by the Surgeon General in 1940, developed a unit on gerontology within the National Institute of Health. This led to legislation that culminated in the establishment of the National Institute on Aging (NIA). Legislation authorizing this unit was signed into law in 1974. Robert Butler, a psychiatrist and gerontologist, became its first director in 1976.

The worldwide scope of the scientific study of aging was signaled by the organization of the International Association of Gerontology (IAG) in 1948. Its organizational meeting was held in Liege, Belgium. Gerontologists representing a variety of disciplines and gerontological interests throughout the world have attended subsequent triennial meetings of the International Congress in such diverse locations as London, St. Louis, Copenhagen, Washington, D.C., Vienna, Kiev (Russia), Jerusalem, Tokyo, and Hamburg, Republic of West Germany.

Today the scientific study of aging is receiving more attention than ever, and in particular, there is worldwide interest in professional planning and practice (delivery of services) in the field. There is a continuing debate as to whether gerontology has reached the stage of development at which it ought to be recognized as a unique and formal discipline in its own right, as is the case with psychology, biology, astronomy, medicine, theology, and law.

What Is Old?

In the twentieth century an entirely new phenomenon has appeared. Since 1900 the segment of the population aged sixty-five years and older has increased much more rapidly than the rest of the population in the United States. At the turn of the century approximately 3 million Americans were sixty-five or older. Today, approximately 25.8 million Americans (11.3 percent) are sixty-five or older, 8.6 times as many as in 1900. The number and proportion of individuals aged seventy-five or older have increased even more dramatically. Four out of every ten older persons, or about 10 million, are seventy-five or older. The percentage of increase for different cohorts from 1960 to 1970 and the number, percent distribution, and percent change in number of population by broad age groups in 1970 and 1975, with projections to 1985 and 2000, are shown in Tables 1–1 and 1–2, respectively. Data presented in Table 1–2 are graphically represented in Figure 1–1.

Additionally, there are approximately 2 million people eighty-five years of age or older in the United States. These figures not only indicate the truly dramatic increase in the number of persons surviving into the seventh, eighth, and ninth decades of life, but also stimulate inquiries regarding the hypothesis that those surviving beyond seventy-five years may exhibit special characteristics distinguishing them from nonsurvivors.

These statistics also indicate a major source of impetus for the present and growing interest in old age in the United States and in other societies. Clearly, we are a graying society, and we want to know why and how this is so, what it means to us now, how it will affect our society and our world tomorrow, and what we should be doing about it.

One recurring question associated with this age trend is: How do we define old? Nearly everyone acknowledges some difficulty with that question. Bernard Baruch, industrialist, philosopher, and advisor to presidents, when asked in his eighties whom he would call old, is said to have remarked, "Anyone who is fifteen years older than I am." Undoubtedly, definitions of "old" are influenced by the age of the person responding. Age-grading (and hence definitions of "old") has largely been determined by society's attitudes and expectations.

TABLE 1–1. Percentage of Increase for Different Cohorts, 1970–1980

Age Group	Increase
Under 45	11.5
45–64	15.9
65+	21.1
65–74	13.0
75+	37.1

Source: Weg (1983).

TABLE 1–2. Age Groups in the United States, 1970–2000

	Number (in thousands)				Percent distribution				Percent change		
Age	1970	1975	1985	2000	1970	1975	1985	2000	1970–1975	1975–1985	1985–2000
All ages	203,235	213,137	232,880	260,378	100.0%	100.0%	100.0%	100.0%	4.9	9.3	11.8
Under 18	69,689	66,294	62,293	68,977	34.3	31.1	26.7	26.5	−4.9	−6.0	10.7
18–64	113,574	124,444	143,283	159,579	55.9	58.4	61.6	61.3	9.6	15.1	11.4
65 & over	19,972	22,400	27,305	31,822	9.8	10.5	11.7	12.2	12.2	21.9	16.5
65–74	12,443	13,874	16,545	17,436	6.1	6.5	7.1	6.7	11.5	19.3	5.4
75–84	6,122	6,650	8,172	10,630	3.0	3.1	3.5	4.1	8.6	22.9	30.1
85+	1,408	1,877	2,588	3,756	0.7	0.9	1.1	1.4	33.3	37.9	45.1

Sources: 1970 and 1975—U.S. Bureau of the Census, *Current Population Reports,* ser. P-25, no. 614, tables 2 and 4; 1985 and 2000—U.S. Bureau of the Census, *Current Population Reports,* ser. P-25, no. 704, table 8.

In this century in the United States, at least, the onset of old age has typically been associated with the index of chronological age adopted by the Social Security system in the 1930s, namely, age sixty-five and beyond. Although a recent Harris poll suggests some consensus on the mid-sixties as the point of entry into old age (Harris, 1981; see Table 1–3), the degree to which this is in fact relevant or even appropriate continues to be questioned from time to time by the public, by public policy makers, and by gerontologists.

Divisions of the Lifespan

In an earlier era the lifespan was segmented by common usage into three relatively simple, straightforward categories: childhood, adulthood, and old age. Detailed studies of the early third of the lifespan have produced fine-tuned descriptions of age-graded developmental and maturational sequences, which in turn have generated a number of age-specific categorizations. All too familiar are references to such life cycle stages as the **neonate,**[1] young child, preadolescent, adolescent, postadolescent, young adult, early middle-ager, and late middle-ager. Each category invokes particular connotations regarding age-specific **behavioral correlates.**[2] In parallel fashion, the recent tendency has been to differentiate age categories within the general period of old age by reference to the "young-old" (approximately sixty-five to seventy-five years of age) and the "old-old" (seventy-five and older). One reason given for this differentiation is that studies comparing the old-old to the young-old suggest that certain characteristics may significantly distinguish long-livers from younger age cohorts.

Whether this sort of age category differentiation has any utility is not certain. Age-specific categories can be related to well-investigated and well-described behavioral correlates. On the basis of such evidence, predictive accuracy relative to physical and psychological outcomes can be expected to

[1] *neonate:* newborn infant
[2] *behavioral correlates:* behaviors which are related to (but not necessarily determined by) certain factors (e.g., age, sex, race)

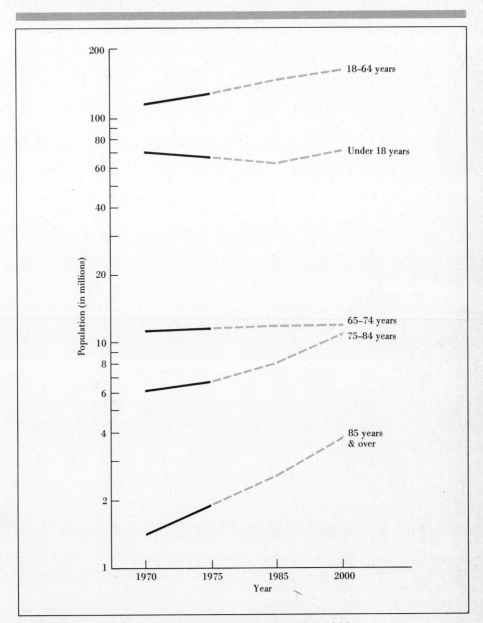

FIGURE 1–1   Age Groups in the United States, 1970–2000

Source: Redick, R. W. & Taube, C. A. Demography and mental health care of the aged. In J. E. Birren and R. B. Sloane (Eds.), Handbook of mental health and aging. Englewood Cliffs, N.J.: Prentice-Hall, Inc. p. 58.

increase. On the other hand, however, age-grading of behavior can also raise unrealistic and inappropriate expectations (Sontag, 1972).

Sontag argues in eloquent fashion that in less complex (usually agrarian) societies where social roles are clearly defined and accepted, chronological age differentiations rarely receive great attention. In more complex,

TABLE 1-3. The Age at Which the Average Man and Woman Become Old[1]

| | The Average Man | | | | | | The Average Woman | | | | | |
| | 1981 | | | 1974 | | | 1981 | | | 1974 | | |
Age of Respondents	Total	18–64	65 and over	Total	18–64	65 and over	Total	18–64	65 and over	Total	18–64	65 and over
	%	%	%	%	%	%	%	%	%	%	%	%
Under 40 Years	1	2	*	1	1	*	2	3	*	1	1	1
40–49 Years	4	4	1	4	5	2	5	6	2	5	5	3
50–59 Years	13	15	4	11	11	8	14	16	7	11	11	8
60–64 Years	19	20	12	12	12	11	19	21	12	10	11	8
65–69 Years	17	17	18	11	10	11	16	16	15	8	8	8
70–74 Years	18	19	16	10	10	8	14	14	14	9	10	7
75–79 Years	6	5	9	3	3	3	6	5	10	3	3	4
80 Years and over	5	5	6	1	1	4	5	5	8	2	1	2
Never	1	1	2	2	2	3	2	2	3	2	2	5
It Depends	10	9	20	22	23	23	10	9	19	23	24	23
When He/She Stops Working	1	*	1	4	4	4	*	*	1	2	2	2
When His/Her Health Fails	3	2	5	11	11	13	2	1	5	13	12	16
When She Can't Have Babies Anymore; Menopause	x	x	x	x	x	x	*	*	*	2	2	1
Other	*	*	*	3	3	2	—	12	—	3	3	2
Not Sure	2	2	4	5	4	8	2	2	5	6	5	10

Chronological Concept of Old Age (All Numerical Responses)	83	86	66	53	53	46	81	85	68	49	50	41
Nonchronological Criteria for Old Age (All Non-Age Responses)	15	13	28	42	43	45	14	13	28	45	45	49
Median Chronological Age		**66 Years**			**63 Years**			**65 Years**			**62 Years**	

Source: Harris & Associates (1981).

[1]This table is based on the responses to the following questions:

Q: I'd like to start by asking you at what age do you think the average man becomes old? Just think about men, not women.

Q: At what age do you think the average woman becomes old?

*Less than 0.5%.

x = Not asked.

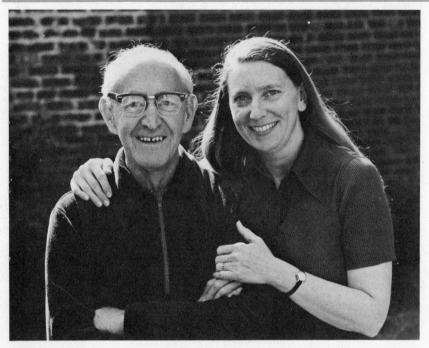

An older person's self-esteem is enhanced when emotional interdependence between generations is acknowledged and cultivated.

highly industrialized, high-technology societies (and especially in urban centers), where social roles are more indeterminate and are in the process of change, differentiation and identification by age appear to be necessary, and much more common. One interpretation of these observations may be formulated in terms of the sense of self-identity. When one's social and work roles are clear-cut, consistent, and continuing, then chronological age adds little if anything to the full dimensions of self-identity for individuals well integrated into the fabric of their society. Conversely, where social roles are unclear, fluid, or otherwise ill-defined, then age-specific determinations serve as a major and necessary index or anchor of self-identity. On this basis, we may then hypothesize that presently surviving centenarians often have difficulty determining their own age not so much because of poor memory or record keeping, but rather because within the social context of their adult development chronological age as such was simply not important to them.

Life Stages Approach

At one conceptual level, life has been characterized as a series of developmental stages; old age has been characterized as the final stage in a series of developmental stages. Organizing life experience into a series of sequential stages has considerable appeal both to the general public and to behavioral scientists. "Oh, they are just going through a stage" is a familiar remark in reference to children and adolescents; now it is sometimes made about middle-aged and elderly persons as well. Sociologists and social psychologists in particular have found the stage approach to lifespan development a convenient and congenial **paradigm**[1] (Clark & Anderson, 1967; Havighurst, 1973; Kohlberg, 1973; Kuhlen, 1968; Newman & Newman, 1975; Williamson, Munley, & Evans, 1980).

Stages are usually described in terms of age-specific periods of life, to which are assigned moral, social, or psychological "tasks" or dilemmas that must either be accomplished or resolved before one moves on to the next developmental stage. Especially to be noted in the stage approach is the fact that invariably stages and tasks are linked to particular periods of chronological age.

A good example is the work of Charlotte Buhler and several of her students (1935), who developed a life stages schema using biographical and autobiographical materials gathered during the 1930s in Vienna. Her major interest was in relating the course of life to biological development (not unlike the interests of Freud, reflected in his own early work on developmental stages). Buhler and her associates developed the following sequence of developmental stages, based on the life stories of some four hundred people:

Age Stage (approximate)	Developmental Theme or Task
0–15 years	Early growth in the home; prior to self-determination
15–25 years	Unfolding of sexual capabilities; testing of self-determination of life goals
25–45 years	Stable growth; crystallization of self–determined life goals
45–65 years	Phasing out of reproductive capacity; self-review and assessment of life goals
65 and beyond	Biological decline; continuation of life-satisfying activities or return to need-satisfying orientations of childhood

Although Buhler's perspective places a useful emphasis on the individual process of goal-setting for living, it fails to emphasize the full human potential for expansion of skills and psychological growth in the later years. Buhler's description reflects a view of the life cycle limited to maturation, growth, and development in the early third of life, a plateau effect in midlife, and contraction and decline in the later life cycle. The implication of this conventional and widely accepted point of view is the *inevitability, irreversibility,* and *universality* of decrement and decline across time, assumptions which should not be accepted without question. Rather, they warrant careful

[1]*paradigm:* abstract model, framework, or representation

examination and thought. For this reason, a critical discussion of this issue, the first of a number offered in the chapters which follow, is presented.

CRITICAL DISCUSSION ▬▬▬▬
Is Aging the Enemy?

The irreversible decremental model of aging has become the most pervasive view of old age not only among the lay public but among many professionals as well. This perspective implicitly assumes that decrement, decline, and loss are an inevitable accompaniment to old age, and that deteriorative features of later life occur as a matter of course, and virtually without exception. Instances where this is not the case are taken to be dramatic exceptions that simply prove the rule. If the assumption about decrement and deterioration as intrinsic is held to be valid, then it follows that, because aging is irreversible, decline is irreversible.

There appears to be little reason to argue whether decrement and deterioration do in fact occur, especially with respect to physiological factors. They do. What has not been demonstrated is that such outcomes are, in *all* instances and under *every* condition, an inherent, innate characteristic of the biological nature of the human organism.

Further, the generalization from physiological decrement to psychological and social decline with the passage of time is an even more questionable assumption. Too many of the conclusions about functional decline are based on inappropriate and sometimes invalid measures and on equivocal findings that lend themselves to bias. In addition, even now too little is known about intervening factors that can affect the behavior of the old. Many of the deficits reported in the biology and psychology of aging lean heavily upon statistical correlations, but a major tenet of scientific methodology warns that correlation is not to be confused with causation.

The irreversible decremental model of aging is vulnerable to serious criticism because it offers essentially a negative, even hopeless, picture of the aging process. Within this framework, there is little if any incentive to maintain the elderly as an integral part of society's mainstream. If decrement, decline, and deterioration are in fact inherent in the aging process itself, one cannot account for the great amount of variability (positive and negative) evident in the lives of so many elderly persons. Too many exceptions to the rule raise the possibility that we have come to accept an invalid rule. In assessing the irreversible decremental model, what is required is more careful, well-controlled observation, and research conducted with valid measures and more appropriate research strategies.

Another developmental theorist, Erik Erikson (1963), formulated his well-known scheme of life stages from his clinical impressions, and on the basis of Freudian and Jungian psychology. Erikson's contribution consists of his set of descriptions of "eight ages" of human life, a series of crucial turning points from birth to death. Each stage represents a "crisis," or developmental task which must be mastered before the individual moves on to the next sequential stage of life. Success or failure in the later developmental tasks depends, according to this view, upon having come to grips with and having mastered the earlier crises.

Stage	Task
1. Oral/sensory	Trust vs. basic mistrust: testing of relationships, development of confidence
2. Muscular/anal	Autonomy vs. shame and doubt: learning to hold on and to let go
3. Locomotor/genital	Initiative vs. guilt: developing assertiveness, rivalry, morality
4. Latency	Industry vs. inferiority: developing task orientation, personal competence
5. Puberty/adolescence	Identity vs. role confusion: to find one's role in life as a sexual, productive, responsible adult with consistent attitudes about self
6. Young adulthood	Generativity vs. stagnation: expansion of ego interests, assuming adult responsibilities
7. Adulthood	Intimacy vs. isolation: flowering of "genitality," mutuality with others
8. Maturity/old age	Integrity vs. despair: emotional integration, making sense of one's life

The major emphasis in this schema is on the childhood stages of life, with relatively little attention given to the later years. Once again, the relatively scant attention paid to the later years of life in Erikson's approach implies that old age offers little significant data for fruitful study, and that the later years are merely the tag ends of life, hold little promise beyond a kind of tying up of the already completed package, simply foreshadow death, and have little of the substantiveness of the earlier years.

Weaknesses of the Life Stages Approach

The life stages approach to human development has generally enjoyed wide appeal because of its conceptual orderliness, its relative simplicity, and its **face validity**.[1] This approach, however, is not without its weaknesses. Stages of development often do not occur in the proscribed, expected sequence, and in certain instances the theorized developmental tasks may become associated with a time frame other than that anticipated (Sheehy, 1977). In fact, one may not complete or resolve an earlier developmental task—in effect, skip a stage—and go back to the unresolved or uncompleted task later in life. In other words, the developmental growth process is not as uniform and well-ordered as life stage theorists would have it.

[1]*face validity:* apparent effectiveness or utility as commonly judged

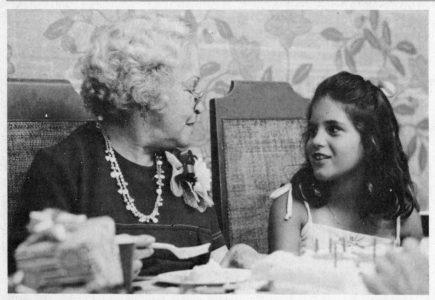

As more people live longer, society's younger members are discovering that their elders have much value to offer.

Nor can the criticism of the life stage approach by developmental psychologists be overlooked. From their perspective, the stage approach, insofar as it is linked to time sequences, attributes certain behaviors to an age or stage and thus bestows a magical quality to each birthday.

> Time as a gross indicator of physiological maturation, or of cumulative interactions with the environment, or both, does nothing to advance a functional analysis of behavior and development. . . . [In this sense,] time is not a variable but a dimension for recording events. . . . the field does not any longer need the grand theoretical designs proposed by Piaget, Freud, Erikson, Gesell, and Werner [Bijou, 1968, pp. 422–423].

Another weakness of the life stage approach to human development is that it places undue emphasis upon internal psychological and cognitive events linked to biological maturation and change, and fails to take into account the enormous impact of the external environment (including social and physical environmental components) upon human behavior. This flaw appears to be a fatal one, especially with respect to observations of growth and development in the later years. Just how and to what extent external environmental variables influence the aging process is not clearly identified.

It is largely within the past decade that the interrelationships between individuals and their environments have been brought into sharper focus by a considerable amount of attention to and research on what have been called "person-environment transactional variables." This perspective, adopted throughout this textbook, holds that internal psychological factors and events are necessary considerations in accounting for behaviors of the aged, but are by no means sufficient. Life is not merely a stage upon which human behavior takes place, with the external environment serving as a kind of indeterminate background or "scenery" which can be moved about or modified without unduly affecting the "actors." Just as various kinds of environmental variables may profoundly affect the behavior of an individual, so may that person's behavior have a marked impact upon the external environment; with respect to this, the elderly are no exception (Aloia, 1973; Lawton, 1974; Schooler, 1969; Schwartz, 1974; Schwartz & Proppe, 1969; Seligman, 1973). To reiterate, this view assumes that one cannot truly understand the older person's perspective or behavior independent of their environmental context. This issue will be discussed in some detail in ensuing chapters.

Age Changes versus Age Differences

The familiar phrase "generation gap" directs attention to an important caution that must be observed in evaluating the array of findings and conclusions from research on aging. Extreme care must be taken to distinguish *age changes* (reflecting growth, development, and maturation) from *age differences* (reflecting cohort- or generation-specific variability).

Most of the research that has been done in the field of aging is cross-sectional research. In a cross-sectional study, the investigator identifies and selects samples of individuals representative of two or more distinct age groups (e.g., a sample of individuals aged twenty to thirty, fifty to sixty, and eighty to ninety years old). Each group is measured with respect to a selected variable or series of variables of interest to the investigator, such as life satisfaction, response time on a specific task, and attitudes toward retirement. The measured differences, if any, between groups (assuming that the tests and procedures are reliable and valid) suggest generational rather than developmental values, and are thus described in terms of age differences.

For example, an eighty-one-year-old man who is tested today was born sometime shortly following the turn of the century. His life experiences include growing up before the advent of television and jet air travel, in a largely rural area within the context of the extended family, with fewer opportunities and less inducement for education beyond the eighth grade, and living through a severe economic depression and two world wars. This man belongs to a cohort (generation) significantly different experientially from the member of the research project who was born thirty years later. Differences measured in that way, therefore, may be attributable as much to different life experiences and a different sociocultural and historical environment as to the mere passage of time (chronological age).

To examine age changes, longitudinal research strategies are most commonly employed. Following an individual or a group of individuals across a number of years and periodically measuring selected variables of interest may reflect differences in behavior over various periods of time. Assuming

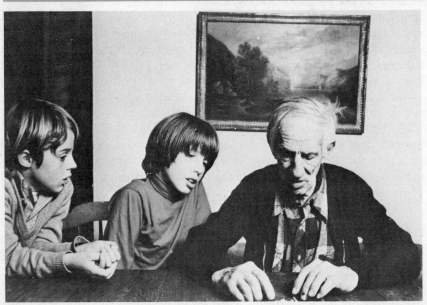

Children need grandparents as much as grandparents need children, who discover their family "roots" in the reminiscing stories of their grandparents.

that all other variables have been controlled, the investigator concludes that these differences are best described as age changes, because they occur within individuals over time and thus are characteristic of personal growth and development.

Although there may be general agreement that the longitudinal strategy of investigation offers distinct advantages over cross-sectional research methods in the study of aging, there are positive and negative features of both approaches that cannot be overlooked. A number of these advantages and disadvantages are listed in Table 1–4. A more recent technique that has been developed attempts to trade on the advantages while avoiding the pitfalls of cross-sectional and longitudinal research strategies (Baltes, 1968; Schaie & Strother, 1968). This technique, the cross-sequential method of aging research, is discussed in terms of its major features and other pertinent considerations in Appendix A.

Framework for the Study of Aging

It must be apparent from the preceding account of the history and development of gerontology that the pioneers who contributed our first major insights into the aging process came from a great variety of intellectual fields.

TABLE 1–4. Major Advantages and Disadvantages of Traditional
Developmental Research Designs

Design	Advantages	Disadvantages
Cross-sectional	Quick data collection	Different environmental exposure at various ages
		Difficulty to obtain equally representative samples in all age groups
Longitudinal	Individual trends can be investigated	Time-consuming
		Expensive
	Increased statistical power	Methods may become obsolete
		Participants may not be representative of population
		Selective attrition may bias results
		Increased age associated with increased test experience
		Increased age associated with more recent environmental exposure

Source: T. A. Salthouse. *Adult cognition: An experimental psychology of human aging.* New York: Springer-Verlag, 1982, p. 23.

From its inception, gerontology has had a *multidisciplinary* focus. Physiology, psychology, sociology, and environmental studies, among others, have contributed unique findings from their respective domains. No single disciplinary approach is sufficient to explain or describe fully the aging process, however; for this reason, gerontology is also characterized as *interdisciplinary*. It is only when we can interface and interrelate the contributions from each area of study that we can begin to formulate truly realistic, holistic explanations of what happens daily to the individual older person. In this book we will look at the contributions of each discipline and then synthesize their complementary findings and component parts into a comprehensible, meaningful, holistic view of the aging process.

Summary

Gerontology is defined as the study of the aging process. Its primary objective is to produce new knowledge and information and to deepen our understanding of this multidimensional, complex process. Some of the issues to which scientists studying aging and providers of direct services to the old must address themselves grow out of theoretical considerations. Many other issues derive from the everyday experiences of older persons. In any case, the study of aging has a strong tradition of pragmatism which leads new knowledge toward practical applications in the service of older persons.

Interest in longevity dates back to early recorded history. Magical and superstitious notions about longevity were typical of prescientific approaches to aging, and a residue of such thinking remains embedded in many popular concepts of aging even today. With the dramatic increase in the number and proportion of persons surviving into later life, however, we are presented with a striking and challenging new phenomenon as the subject of scientific investigation and research.

Despite the growing number of scientific studies of aging within the past century, a single, succinct definition of aging has yet to be formulated. One conceptual framework with wide appeal describes old age as the last of a series of sequential life stages. These developmental stages appear to offer a relatively simple and orderly way to organize and describe maturation and growth throughout the life cycle. This approach is exemplified by the schemas developed by Charlotte Buhler and Erik Erikson, among others. Nonetheless, the notion of life stages is vulnerable to criticism, due to certain conceptual weaknesses stemming from this perspective. A major weakness is the fact that the potential for continued growth and development in the later years appears to be either ignored or severely limited.

The focus within recent years on the person-environment transactional perspective offers a much more positive and optimistic view of aging than does the more conventional and pervasive view of irreversible decrement as characteristic of the later years. The major emphasis of the person-environment transactional theorists is on the interaction between the aged and the environments in which they live. One cannot fully understand the behaviors or perspectives of older people unless one takes into account the sociocultural, historical, and physical environmental framework of their lives.

A critically important caution for all who study, plan for, or serve the elderly is the necessity of making a clear distinction between age changes and age differences. Confounding these two factors remains the chief hazard in the interpretation of research data, regardless of the type of design employed.

Most important of all in the study of aging is to recognize the multidimensional nature of this complex process. Because of its nature, an interdisciplinary, multidisciplinary approach is required to provide the integrated, holistic view of aging that will enable us to put together the many complementary and often seemingly disparate chunks of information about the aging process. This book follows the interdisciplinary path in hopes of achieving a comprehensive and comprehensible grasp of the complexities inherent in the study of aging.

References

Aloia, A. J. Relationships between perceived privacy options, self-esteem, and internal control among aged people. Doctoral dissertation, California School of Professional Psychology, 1973.

Baltes, P. Longitudinal and cross-sectional sequences in the study of age and generational effects. *Human Development,* 1968, **11**(3).

Bijou, S. Ages, stages, and the naturalization of human development. *American Psychologist,* 1968, **23**(6), 419–427.

Birren, J. E., & Clayton, V. History of gerontology. In D. Woodruff & J. E. Birren (Eds.), *Aging: Scientific perspectives and social issues.* New York: Van Nostrand, 1975. Pp. 15–27.

Buhler, C. The curve of life as studied in biographies. *Journal of Applied Psychology,* 1935, **19**.

Butler, R. Successful aging and the role of the life review. *Journal of the American Geriatrics Society,* 1974, **22**, 529–535.

Clark, M., & Anderson, B. *Culture and aging.* Springfield, Ill.: Charles C. Thomas, 1967.

Copley, F. *On old age.* Ann Arbor: University of Michigan Press, 1967.

Erikson, E. *Childhood and society.* (2nd ed.) New York: Norton, 1963.

Freeman, J. T. Medical perspectives in aging (12–19th century). *Gerontologist,* 1965, 5 (1, pt. II), 1–24.

Harris, L., & Associates. *Aging in the eighties: America in transition.* Washington, D.C.: National Council on the Aging, 1981.

Havighurst, R. J. History of developmental psychology: Socialization and personality development through the lifespan. In P. B. Baltes & K. W. Schaie (Eds.), *Life-span developmental psychology: Personality and socialization.* New York: Academic Press, 1973.

Hendricks, J., & Hendricks, C. D. *Aging in mass society.* Cambridge, Mass.: Winthrop, 1977.

Kohlberg, L. Continuities in childhood and adult moral development revisited. In P. B. Baltes & K. W. Schaie (Eds.), *Life-span developmental psychology: Personality and socialization.* New York: Academic Press, 1973.

Kuhlen, R. G. Developmental changes in motivation during the adult years. In B. Neugarten (Ed.), *Middle age and aging.* Chicago: University of Chicago Press, 1968.

Lauer, R., & Goldfield, M. Creative writing in group therapy. *Psychotherapy: Theory, Research and Practice,* 1970, 7(4), 248–251.

Lawton, M. P. Coping behavior and the environment of older people. In A. Schwartz & I. Mensh (Eds.), *Professional obligations and approaches to the aged.* Springfield, Ill.: Charles C. Thomas, 1974.

Lickorish, J. The therapeutic use of literature. *Psychotherapy: Theory, Research, and Practice,* 1975, **12**(1), 105–109.

Newman, B., & Newman, P. *Development through life.* Homewood, Ill.: Dorsey Press, 1975.

Reedy, M. N., & Birren, J. E. *Life review through guided autobiography.* Poster presented at the Annual Meeting of the American Psychological Association, Montreal, Canada, Sept. 3, 1980.

Schaie, K. W., & Strother, C. R. A cross-sequential study of age changes in cognitive behavior. *Psychological Bulletin,* 1968, **70**.

Schooler, K. The relationship between social interaction and morale of the elderly as a function of environmental characteristics. *Gerontologist,* 1969, 9(1).

Schwartz, A. A transactional view of the aging process. In A. Schwartz & I. Mensh (Eds.), *Professional obligations and approaches to the aged.* Springfield, Ill.: Charles C. Thomas, 1974.

Schwartz, A., & Proppe, H. *Perception of privacy among institutionalized aged.* Proceedings of the 77th Annual Convention of the American Psychological Association, Washington, D.C., 1969.

Seligman, M. Fall into helplessness. *Psychology Today,* June 1973.

Sheehy, G. *Passages.* New York: Bantam, 1977.

Sontag, S. The double standard of aging. *Saturday Review,* Sept. 23, 1972, 29–38.

Weg, R. B. The old: Who, what, where, how? (Mimeographed report.) Andrus Gerontology Center, University of Southern California, Los Angeles, 1977.

Williamson, J. B., Munley, A., & Evans, L. *Aging and society.* New York: Holt, Rinehart & Winston, 1980.

For Further Reading

Beauvoir, S. de. *The coming of age.* New York: Putnam, 1973.

Binstock, R., & Shanas, E. (Eds.). *Handbook of aging and the social sciences.* New York: Van Nostrand Reinhold, 1976.

Birren, J. E. (Ed.). *Handbook of aging and the individual.* Chicago: University of Chicago Press, 1959.

Butler, R. *Why survive? Being old in America.* New York: Harper & Row, 1975.

Kalish, R. *Late adulthood: Perspectives on human development.* Monterey, Cal.: Brooks/Cole, 1975.

Kimmel, D. *Adulthood and aging.* New York: Wiley, 1974.

Puner, M. *To the good long life: What we know about growing old.* New York: Universe Books, 1974.

Ryder, N. B. The cohort as a concept in the study of social change. *American Sociological Review,* 1965, **30**.

Sarton, M. *As we are now.* New York: Norton, 1973.

Scott-Maxwell, F. *The measure of my days.* New York: Knopf, 1968.

Physiological Aspects of Aging

Chapter 2

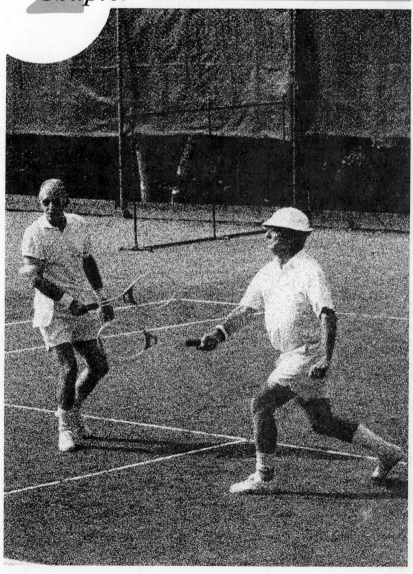

When I was forty, my doctor advised me that a man in his forties shouldn't play tennis. I heeded this advice carefully and could hardly wait until I reached fifty to start again.

Justice Hugo Black

Biological, genetic, and physical factors represent an initial basic set of facts upon which to build strong scientific studies of the aging process, as already indicated in the first chapter of this text. Although physical and health factors alone do not in any sense constitute sufficient explanations of aging, they are unquestionably important constituent elements of the whole picture. Gerontology, therefore, will continue to pay considerable attention to these variables.

As a guiding principle in gerontology, the notion that "aging is an infinitely eliminable variable" (Birren, 1959) takes precedence. Many outcomes and events are initially attributed to age until a different cause is identified, whereupon age is eliminated as the causal agent. And so the process is repeated with each new discovery: age per se accounts for increasingly less variability in behavior.

A number of biomedical researchers have formulated theories of aging based upon physiological and genetic data. The student of gerontology must have at least a nodding acquaintance with these biomedical theories because they are important contributors to our understanding of the complex patterns of aging. At the same time, caution must be exercised in evaluating these theories because of the temptation to be seduced into biological reductionism—the tendency to pare down the complex events that make up the total experience of human aging to the level of mere biological processes. When that occurs, the significance of other important and influential factors is lost. In our efforts to understand the total process in aging, reduction of the human organism and its experience to biology alone would be just as misleading as dissecting a flower, placing its parts side by side, and then examining the several parts in an effort to discover the "nature" or the beauty of the flower.

The following paragraphs present a sample of biomedical formulations which may be explored in greater detail through the references and suggested readings at the end of this chapter.

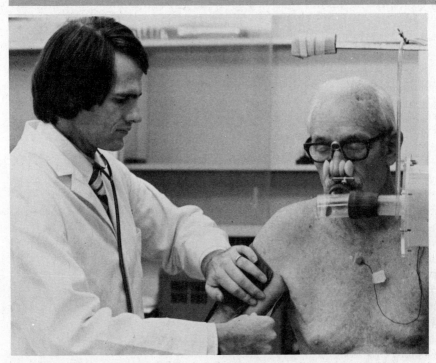

Investigations into various aspects of the physiology of aging have become very complex and sophisticated. Such research has contributed to the growing identification of gerontology with basic science.

Biomedical Theories of Aging

There are numerous theories of aging (Comfort, 1964, has listed at least twenty), but many of them remain untested and are not generalizable across organisms. Biological theories fall into two major categories: *genetic,* referring to the way that information is transferred from DNA molecules in biochemically determined patterns and sequences, and *physiological,* referring to the interactions among cells, tissues, and organ systems (Shock, 1977). In any case, some kind of genetic program apparently exists which sets the upper limits of the lifespan for any given species. What that limit may be for humans is not at all clear, because other factors may intrude and attenuate life expectancy before the potential for the full lifespan is realized.

Reservoir Theory

One such theory of aging (now considered outdated and of relatively little explanatory value) might be labeled the reservoir theory (Curtis, 1966).

It derives from the notion that each individual begins life with a specific, limited amount of energy or vitality, and that the more rapidly this energy is expended, the faster the reservoir becomes depleted or drained. An interesting parallel to this concept is the formerly common belief that too much or too vigorous sexual activity on the part of men during their early years would use up their potential for sexual vigor, "drain the reservoir," and leave them depleted in their later years. Another version of this is the notion of exhaustion of energy over time, analogous to the winding down of a watch spring.

Wear-and-Tear Theory

A separate theory of aging which bears some resemblance to the reservoir theory and still apparently enjoys some credence is the wear-and-tear theory (Shock, 1977). This theory views the human body as if it were a machine, and suggests that just as a machine's parts may wear out and contribute to its ultimate breakdown and malfunction, so it is with the parts of the human body. As with so many arguments from analogy, however, this theory is flawed by its inability to account for the many exceptions to the rule it proposes. Many of the body's organ systems, unlike mechanical systems, are capable of repairing themselves and can thereby compensate for specific tissue damage, loss, or dysfunction. Furthermore, this repair system in humans is not only more sophisticated but also appears to be more effective and efficient than that of lower organisms (Sinex, 1977).

Free Radical Theory

Another theory holds that the accumulations of chemical (cellular) waste products within the body may account for the deteriorative aspects of the aging process. A good example of this type of formulation is the free radical theory of aging suggested by Harman (1956, 1969). According to this particular version of the contributions of cellular waste to the aging process, the normal life of a cell includes its potential destruction through the oxidation of its surrounding membrane(s) and, subsequently, its internal structures. Cell destruction is hastened by the presence of "free radicals," or potentially chemically active molecules which combine readily with various substances in the cellular environment. Cell membranes are especially susceptible to oxidation and thus to production of free radicals because they contain a relatively high concentration of unsaturated fat molecules, which are very reactive in the presence of oxygen. When oxidation occurs at the membrane level, cellular functioning is significantly disrupted. The waste products that result from the combination of oxidized unsaturated fat molecules with other substances may themselves be free radicals, capable of promoting further free radical damage through a chain reaction (autoxidation), or may revert to less active, relatively stable substances collectively known as lipofuscin (age pigment). The process of oxidation and age-pigment formation (and thus, presumably, the process of aging itself) may be retarded by a decrease in unsaturated fat intake in the diet and/or by an increase in the consumption of antioxidant substances, such as vitamins C and E and the mineral selenium, according to this theory. In addition, a drug by the name of centrophenoxine (used to improve memory functioning in older adults in recent experiments) has been reported to limit the production of lipofuscin as well as remove existing stores of this age pigment in neural cells of sub-human organisms (Schneider & Nandy, 1977; Spoerri & Glees, 1975).

Gains in longevity due to these dietary and drug-based modifications, however, appear to be negligible in healthy organisms and only somewhat more effective in organisms whose lifespans have been seriously affected by major dietary insufficiency and other debilitating conditions. In other words, the normal lifespan is apparently seldom extended to a significant degree if these proscriptions are followed by a relatively healthy organism. Interestingly, free radical reactions are also implicated in certain disease mechanisms and processes which become increasingly more manifest in the later years. Due to a variety of methodological problems involved in the control and measurement of specific free radical reactions, however, this theory has yet to be widely accepted as a valid explanation of the aging process.

Stress Theory

Another theory of aging which seems to integrate various aspects of the reservoir, wear-and-tear, and cellular waste accumulation formulations is Selye's theory of the impact of stress on the individual across the lifespan. Stress, according to Selye (1976), is "the state manifested by a specific syndrome which consists of all the nonspecifically-induced changes within a biologic system" (p. 64). Furthermore, it is "the common denominator of all adaptive reactions in the body" (p. 64). Stress is understood as the state one is in, rather than the agent that produces that state. Stress-producing stimuli may be physical, psychological, or social, and may originate from within the individual or from an outside source.

The "specific syndrome" which occurs in response to a stress-inducing stimulus is described by Selye as the general adaptation syndrome, or GAS, and includes (1) an *alarm reaction,* during which "the direct effect of the stressor upon the body" (p. 56) is initially registered and the body's available adaptive resources are mobilized into action; (2) a *stage of resistance,* characterized by "internal responses which stimulate tissue defense or help to destroy damaging substances," (p. 56) and in which the body begins to adapt by reaching a new level of homeostasis or balance in its continuing response to the stressful agent(s); and finally, (3) a *stage of exhaustion,* during which "internal responses which cause tissue surrender by inhibiting unnecessary or excessive defense" occur (p. 56).

Selye contends that every individual is born with a reserve of adaptation energy, the quantity of which is biogenetically determined. This energy actually exists at two levels, one superficial (which can be depleted through participation in stressful activities but can subsequently be replaced), and one at a deeper level (which serves to empower the body to respond in general and from which reserves are drawn to replenish the superficial store). The stress theory thus parallels the reservoir theory in that it suggests that there are limits to the individual's total energy reserves, which can be expended slowly by avoiding stressful situations or rapidly by engaging in and seeking out stressful situations. Aging occurs as these reservoirs become more and more depleted over time, and can vary in rate as a function of exposure and ability to adapt to stress.

The stress theory bears resemblance to the wear-and-tear theory of aging as well. As Selye explains it, stress has differential effects on the various parts of the body such that some "wear out" sooner than others. He comments:

> We invariably die because one vital part has worn out too early in proportion to the rest of the body. Life, the biologic chain that holds our parts together, is only as strong as its weakest vital link. . . . there is always one part which wears out first and wrecks the whole human machinery, merely because the other parts cannot function without it. . . . The lesson seems to be that, as far as man can regulate his life by voluntary actions, he should seek to equalize stress throughout his being, by . . . the frequent shifting-over of work from one part to the other [pp. 432–433].

Thus, for Selye, normal or optimal aging entails the distribution of stress in relatively equal amounts over the body; death occurs when the cumulative effects of stress on one part of the body complete the entire GAS sequence and the adaptive energies of the body become totally exhausted.

Finally, the stress theory may be thought of as a "waste product" theory. Selye further observes that any stress which requires adaptation on the part of the organism leaves a "residuum" of impairment from which the organism never recovers completely. In a sense, the depletion of the reservoir of adaptive energy and the accumulation of residuum stores over time may be viewed as complementary events; with increasing stores of residuum as a function of responses to stress over a lifetime, adaptive energy is reduced. When residuum stores are distributed relatively equally throughout the body, the decline in adaptive energy which results is referred to as aging; when residuum effects are relatively concentrated in one location in the body, the decline in adaptive energy which results predisposes the organism to disease or death.

Although many people view stress as a negative response and stressful events as negative stimuli, it must be pointed out that "nonspecifically-induced changes within a biologic system" may also result from positive challenges to the system. Indeed, a life without such challenges would be exceedingly dull. The key to successful adaptation in the face of stress, whether interpreted positively or negatively by the organism responding to a stressful event, is the ability to balance stress responses characteristic of the GAS sequence throughout the body.

Suggested Theoretical Criteria

An important biologically based formulation which seems to be applicable to aging has been offered by Strehler (1977). He proposes that the criteria which any age-associated change should meet before being considered a part of any basic age process include the following four concepts: (1) universality, (2) intrinsicality, (3) progressiveness, and (4) deleteriousness. The first, universality, refers to phenomena associated with aging that occur in all older members of the species. Intrinsicality assures that aging is distinguished from the operation of age-correlated factors outside the organism. Because aging is usually considered to be a process rather than a sudden event, progressiveness is included in the list of criteria. For example, a stroke or a tumor may be associated with age, but neither of these can be considered part of the aging process. Some age-correlated changes which meet the first three criteria may be excluded because they represent later-life adaptive responses which may actually result in an improvement in the individual's capacity to survive. These age-correlated changes should not be confused with aging itself. Only those changes which are deleterious to the organism and reduce its chances of survival, and which also fit the other criteria mentioned above, should be considered part of the aging process.

Case Illustrations

It is perhaps instructive in this context to look at some samples of real-life situations. The following brief descriptive summaries have been extracted from detailed case studies originally conducted by a senior counselor in gerontology. Names, dates, and places have been changed, of course, but the essential facts and circumstances are true.

CASE ILLUSTRATION
Optimistic at Eighty-nine

Mr. M. L. Z. is an eighty-nine-year-old white male of Eastern European origin. He lives in a midsized nursing home in the Middle West. Many of his daily activities revolve around his circulating among the facility's residents, chatting, playing cards, reading to them, and "fetching things." Most important, Mr. Z. carries his old battered violin about with him and at the drop of a hat will play a tune or break into song in a surprisingly strong, clear, melodic voice. He claims to be able to sing songs in any one of seven languages, and with the least encouragement will try out several for anyone who will listen.

Mr. Z. is small (5'3"), frail-looking, and completely bald. He has facial scars and wears extremely thick-lensed glasses. He seems to be known and well-liked by practically all residents and staff of the facility in which he resides, and by many visitors there as well.

He recalls a colorful history. He "escaped" his homeland at the tender age of fifteen and a half to avoid compulsory military service, and fled to Russia. There he was inducted into the army, and was subsequently sent off to duty in Siberia, where he lived for about six years. After another tour of duty in a border patrol he deserted, made his way across Europe, and eventually came to the United States. Here he took odd jobs, educated himself, and in time "got into show business": he became a vaudeville prompter. In time his contacts in entertainment took him around the world. Yet time took its toll.

He tells of marrying a woman with whom he lived for "almost forty years." They had no children and she died some fifteen years ago. Following her death, he began to experience a series of physical difficulties. An operation for cataracts left him with the need for very thick glasses. At one time he had a toupee made, which he has not worn for some time. One leg was amputated because of a diabetic condition and he now wears a prosthetic leg. In addition, he wears a hearing aid, false teeth, and, for the last year, a heart pacer. Several years ago he experienced what he calls a "small stroke," which left him "mixed up" for a few days. But he "worked this out," he reports, by "walking a lot," an activity in which he engages frequently.

Mr. Z. says he has never smoked and drinks only on "occasions" or holidays, and then only to a limited degree. He scorns food fads, and eats "mostly" fresh fruits and "lots of vegetables"; he loves fish and drinks a lot of tea.

Despite all his troubles, Mr. Z. maintains what is apparently a cheerful, optimistic view of life and circumstances, while he pursues his "hobby" of energetically helping his fellow residents keep their spirits up and their interests high.

He is very highly regarded and seen as filling a very important role in his nursing home as a story-teller and entertainer.

CASE ILLUSTRATION
"A Lady Who Gives No Trouble"

Mrs. R. P. is an eighty-one-year-old woman who came to America when she was an adolescent. She is quite tall and very thin, has a beautiful shock of white hair, and speaks hesitatingly, with a marked accent.

She resides in a large nursing home located in a large metropolitan area on the West Coast. Her living arrangements do not contribute much to her happiness; she doesn't "have many friends and there isn't much to do." But she says she has "become accustomed to it." She has been widowed for about five years, and has two children: a married daughter who lives sixty miles away and a son who lives on the East Coast. Visits from her children are few.

Mrs. R. P. wears glasses for a severe visual deficit and has chronic diabetes which for some years has been controlled by diet. Other than some mention of mild arthritis in her hands, she seems to have no further complaints about her health. Her general mood appears to be one of sadness, helplessness, and resignation. She had been a wife, homemaker, and mother. Now she expresses feelings of uselessness tinged with boredom. She is perceived by the staff of the facility in which she lives as "a very quiet, pleasant lady who gives no trouble."

Given the theories of aging indicated earlier, what would gerontologists say about Mr. Z. and Mrs. R. P.? What kinds of questions are asked about older persons like these? Perhaps the following will provide some clues:

1. Should such older persons be characterized as chronically ill, or are they simply persons with disabilities (chronic ailments)?

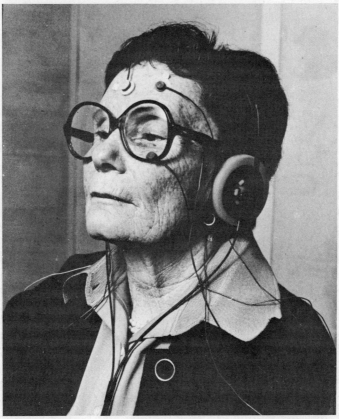

Psychophysiological testing has enabled researchers to uncover many important clues as to the nature of physical and health factors in later life.

2. What do physical changes mean to the older person?
3. How do physiological changes affect behavior?
4. From a physical point of view, are Mr. Z. and Mrs. R. P. typical of the elderly in our society?
5. What are the physical changes commonly experienced by the aged?
6. Is decline in physical health an inevitable accompaniment of old age?
7. Do all older people put physical health at the top of their list of concerns?

Physical Change and Loss

The most obvious fact about aging, one on which all gerontologists can agree, is the element of change. Many, if not most, changes associated with aging may be placed in the matrix of loss. Indeed, the characteristic most commonly used to describe aging is multiple loss. At the same time, geron-tologists emphasize that loss itself is neither a function of nor intrinsic to the aging process, but rather is *associated with* the aging process.

Physical and health factors represent a major category of change and loss variables. These factors influence the course of aging itself in individual cases and also exert substantial impact upon how **senescence**[1] is personally experienced. There is good reason, then, why health factors have captured much of the attention of gerontological researchers. Outcomes from such research provide much raw material for those who develop public policy and those who initiate programmatic planning and provide direct services to the elderly.

A life changes schedule developed by Holmes and Rahe (1967) has demonstrated respectably high predictive validity for incidences of change-related illness. In other words, recent life situation changes, while differing in degree of impact upon individuals, increase the probability of dysfunction and physical illness. In their studies, Holmes and Rahe and associates have rank-ordered recent life events (those occurring within the preceding six or twelve months) and assigned a number value to each one according to its relative degree of emotional impact. On the basis of scores derived from the use of such a scale, the incidence of illness can be predicted. Table 2–1 shows a compressed version of the recent life changes schedule. A further discussion and application of this schedule will be elaborated in the next chapter.

Chronic and Acute Conditions

Surveys of health status among elderly persons repeatedly have shown increases in illness and illness-related incapacities to be associated with the passage of time. Much of this is linked to chronic conditions, in contrast to acute episodes: diminution of cardiovascular and pulmonary competence,

[1]*senescence:* the normal aging process

TABLE 2-1. Social Readjustment Rating Scale

Rank	Life Event	Mean Value
1	Death of spouse	100
2	Divorce	73
3	Marital separation	65
4	Jail term	63
5	Death of close family member	63
6	Personal injury or illness	53
7	Marriage	50
8	Fired at work	47
9	Marital reconciliation	45
10	Retirement	45
11	Change in health of family member	44
12	Pregnancy	40
13	Sex difficulties	39
14	Gain of new family member	39
15	Business readjustment	39
16	Change in financial state	38
17	Death of close friend	37
18	Change to different line of work	36
19	Change in number of arguments with spouse	35
20	Mortgage over $10,000	31
21	Foreclosure of mortgage or loan	30
22	Change in responsibilities at work	29
23	Son or daughter leaving home	29
24	Trouble with in-laws	29
25	Outstanding personal achievement	28
26	Wife begin or stop work	26
27	Begin or end school	26
28	Change in living conditions	25
29	Revision of personal habits	24
30	Trouble with boss	23
31	Change in work hours or conditions	20
32	Change in residence	20
33	Change in schools	20
34	Change in recreation	19
35	Change in church activities	19
36	Change in social activities	18
37	Mortgage or loan less than $10,000	17
38	Change in sleeping habits	16
39	Change in number of family get-togethers	15
40	Change in eating habits	15
41	Vacation	13
42	Christmas	12
43	Minor violations of the law	11

Source: Holmes & Rahe (1967).

changes in connective tissues (especially collagen), decline in the acuity of various senses, chronic arthritis and diabetes, loss of teeth, and the like. The corollary also obtains; that is, younger persons are more subject to acute episodes of illness or disease than older persons, and, obviously, less subject to chronic conditions.

From Table 2-2 we can see a clear trend of diminution of acute condi-

TABLE 2–2. Number of Acute Conditions Per 100 Persons Per Year, by Age, Sex, and Condition: July 1969–June 1970

Sex and Condition Group	All Ages	Under 6 Years	6–16 Years	17–44 Years	45 Years & Over
Male					
All acute conditions	196.9	352.1	261.6	176.0	106.4
Infective and parasitic diseases	24.6	53.5	40.3	17.0	9.1
Respiratory conditions	107.1	205.7	134.6	97.3	56.7
Upper respiratory conditions	61.4	140.7	79.5	48.5	30.2
Influenza	39.1	44.3	48.0	44.4	23.2
Other respiratory conditions	6.7	20.7	7.2	4.4	3.3
Digestive system conditions	10.2	10.9	15.2	9.9	6.3
Injuries	33.5	35.7	45.7	35.0	20.7
All other acute conditions	21.5	46.3	25.8	16.9	13.6
Female					
All acute conditions	212.2	340.8	264.5	208.6	138.0
Infective and parasitic diseases	24.3	57.5	34.8	22.0	9.0
Respiratory conditions	118.5	193.3	155.2	111.9	76.3
Upper respiratory conditions	69.9	135.5	105.2	57.6	38.5
Influenza	43.0	43.3	45.1	49.5	33.8
Other respiratory conditions	5.5	14.5	4.9	4.8	3.9
Digestive system conditions	11.8	14.9	16.0	11.9	7.7
Injuries	22.3	21.4	25.6	22.5	20.0
All other acute conditions	35.3	53.8	32.8	40.4	25.0

Source: National Center for Health Statistics (1972).

Note: Excluded from these statistics are those conditions that do not involve restricted activity or medical attention.

tions with advancing years and a greater incidence of the same in the younger years. Also of interest is the relatively larger number of illnesses reported for females in contrast to males for all conditions. The occurrence of acute conditions reported is similar for both sexes with respect to infectious and digestive diseases—conditions which are very likely to demand the attention of a physician and, perhaps, hospitalization. In the case of the last category, "all other conditions," however, the occurrence for females is greater across age groups than for males. This may give additional confirmation to the common observation that women are more likely to seek medical attention than men, especially when the option of doing so is not highly motivated by a state of emergency.

Illness and Functional Capacity

The finding that older people are more likely to exhibit ailments of a chronic nature, are more likely to report a higher incidence and greater prevalance of "permanent" disabilities, and are more likely to complain of multiple disabilities is generally supported in the literature (Shanas, 1974; Shanas & Maddox, 1976).

High blood pressure, heart ailments, rheumatism, diabetes, and arthritis show up as the most common chronic disabilities affecting individuals from midlife and beyond. Although they can also limit activities, such disabilities as asthma and hay fever are less common chronic conditions in later life.

Nevertheless, in spite of pervasive attitudes that still equate old age with sickness and incapacity, gerontologists recognize that by far the largest proportion of the elderly retain at least adequate levels of health and, from a physical point of view, remain remarkably functional. According to a U.S. Vital and Health Statistics Survey, although some 37 percent of persons aged sixty-five years and older experience some kind of limiting chronic disability, more than 62 percent of all older people are able to carry on most of the activities of daily living. Only 16.4 percent, according to the same survey, are judged unable to carry on primary activities of daily life. Obviously this is in sharp contrast to the popular view of old people as generally "sick and disabled."

The extent to which disease and varying degrees of disabling conditions set limits on activities, especially activities of daily living (ADL) can be seen in Figure 2–1.

The fine line between a person with a disability and a disabled person becomes particularly important for planners and rehabilitation specialists

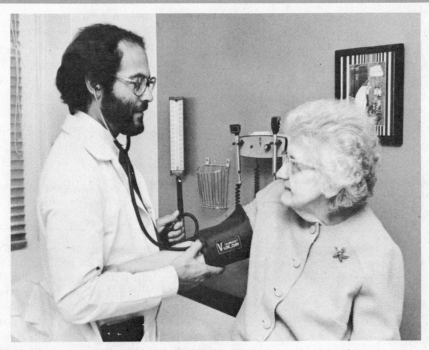

Health is a major concern but not necessarily the highest priority of the aged. One high priority is to train health professionals so as to minimize age stereotypes and generate multi-disciplinary strategies and positive attitudes.

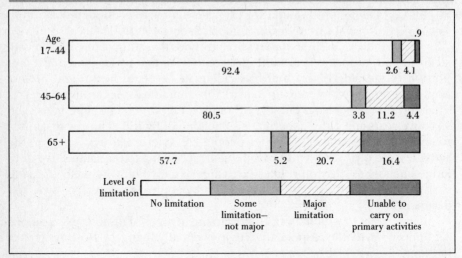

FIGURE 2–1.   Percentage of Adults with Various Degrees of Limited Activity, 1970

Source: Limitation of Activity Due to Chronic Conditions, United States, 1970, Vital and Health Statistics, ser. 10, no. 80. Washington, D.C.: Government Printing Office, April 1973. Table, p. 5.

(Wright, 1958). It will also make a great difference in general expectations of later life and perceptions of the capabilities and potentials of the aged. The fundamental issue has to do with how we choose to define sickness, ill health, and chronic illness. Definitions are affected by global societal expectations, and by the disciplinary biases of health professionals (nurses, physicians, clinical psychologists, psychiatrists, etc.). Moreover, individual characterizations of personal state of health may differ significantly from one person to the next.

CRITICAL DISCUSSION

To Be or Not To Be!

The World Health Organization (WHO) and organizations like the American Medical Association (AMA) correctly insist that health is more than simply the absence of disease. Yet most definitions of health, including those of WHO and the AMA, are deficient on at least two counts (Carlson, 1975). First, health is too often measured against some objective and extrinsic standard (e.g., absence of pathology, freedom from overt disability). Second, health is erroneously conceived of as a static state of an organism, rather than as a dynamic conflux of conditions.

Health is not merely the absence of disease; in fact, it often cohabits with disease (Carlson, 1975). A woman who develops chronic diabetes or arthritis or a heart murmur or defective vision may be said to be, therefore, not sick, but merely a different person than she was before; that is, she is now a person with certain constraints on her activities. Within those limitations such a person can be as healthy as anyone else. This is precisely the point made by Beatrice Wright (1958) more than two decades ago: being a person with a disability is not the same as being disabled. Ray Charles, the blind singer-pianist, is a person with a disability. He is hardly a disabled person, even though blindness places some constraints upon his behavior and necessitates some assistance. Nevertheless, sightlessness is not a relevant factor in his functioning as a musician. Apropos of this, studies indicate (Maddox, 1964) that older persons tend to assess their personal state of health in terms of subjective, functional grounds (e.g., ability to "get around") than in terms of more objective criteria (e.g., physician's diagnostic evaluation).

Following Carlson's formulations, then, any redefinition of health must include at least four major elements. The first is an environment which is supportive and harmonious. The rationale for this has been discussed elsewhere (Schwartz, 1974). The second element is readily obtained resources to assist the individual in becoming or staying healthy. This simply recognizes the fact that some contingencies lie beyond the individual's immediate control. The third element is self-esteem, which includes the need for someone who cares, someone to care about. The fourth element is the individual's own participation in and responsibility for health. That is, health is likely to elude those who maintain a strictly passive, disinterested role with respect to health.

It is precisely these issues and these values that have raised serious questions about the caretaking of institutionalized elderly and the criteria established to monitor and evaluate nursing homes. Of concern are the appropriateness of caretaking patterns and the enormous sums of money spent inappropriately in Medicare and Medicaid programs (Tiberi, Schwartz, & Albert, 1977), problems that will be discussed more fully in a later chapter.

What all this implies with respect to a great many aged people, then, is that although many may suffer from one or more chronic conditions, they are not ill, nor are they sick in the conventional sense of the term, that is, having an acute transient illness or disease amenable to therapeutic intervention leading toward cure. On the contrary, such elderly individuals should more appropriately be considered persons with one or more disabilities. These disabilities will certainly place some constraints on behavior or limit activity, but neither case requires the assumption of an "illness" role, or justifies treating such persons as if they were "sick," any more than one would be justified in treating a deaf person as "sick."

While considering issues of sickness and health in later life it is interesting to note how older people rank-order health with respect to other important life priorities. The 1981 Harris poll (see Table 2–3) indicates the

TABLE 2–3. "Very Serious" Problems: Personal Experience of the Elderly Vs. Public Expectations

Rank as Actual Very Serious Problem for 65 and Over		1981			1974		
		Personal Experience "Very Serious" Problems Felt Personally by Public 65 and Over	Public Expectation "Very Serious" Problems Attributed to Most People Over 65		Personal Experience "Very Serious" Problems Felt Personally by Public 65 and Over	Public Expectation "Very Serious" Problems Attributed to Most People Over 65	
			By Public 18–64	By Public 65 and Over		By Public 18–64	By Public 65 and Over
#		%	%	%	%	%	%
4	Not having enough money to live on	17	68	50	15	63	59
3	Poor health	21	47	40	21	50	53
6	Loneliness	13	65	45	12	61	56
10	Poor housing	5	43	30	4	35	34
2	Fear of crime	25	74	58	23	50	51
8	Not enough education	6	21	17	8	19	25
8	Not enough job opportunities	6	51	24	5	47	32
7	Not enough medical care	9	45	34	10	45	36
1	High cost of energy, such as heating oil, gas, and electricity	42	81	72	x	x	x
5	Getting transportation to stores, to doctors, to places of recreation, and so forth	14	58	43	x	x	x

Source: L. Harris & Associates. *Aging in the '80s: America in transition.* Washington, D.C.: The National Council on the Aging, 1981.

x = Not asked

degree of disparity between older persons' priorities and the expectations or opinions of the rest of the population. Most younger people assume that health issues are by far the greatest preoccupation of old folks. This poll indicates that a mere 21 percent of the older people included in the sample considered this to be so. While this does not mean that health is not a concern for most older people, it does indicate rather convincingly that health issues are not necessarily a top priority for the elderly in general. Health may indeed be important, but other concerns are even more so, and take precedence over health in the vast majority of instances.

Observable Indications of Age

Many kinds of age-related changes, such as those in health, may be assessed and described at the **molar**[1] as well as at the molecular level. Most true biological age changes are not readily visible, but occur as complex, internal events well-hidden within the organism. Other classes of age changes are clearly apparent and in many instances can appropriately be called "cosmetic" changes. We will examine in this section some molar indications of aging to which society often responds (at least initially) by making assumptions about other molecular changes presumed to occur at the same time in aging individuals.

Usually the most obvious indicators of age are changes in physical appearance. Hair tends to thin out and to gray or whiten. The skin begins to wrinkle. With age the ears become longer, the earlobes thicken, and the nose becomes somewhat broader. Skin discolorations ("liver spots") appear, most frequently on the backs of the hands. Imbalance in the hormone chain tends to produce a "neutering" effect; that is, a slight increase in body and facial hair growth appears in women, a slight decrease of these characteristics in men. Pitch and tone of voice are usually less stable, although this kind of change is more commonly associated with lung capacity and efficiency, breath control, voice production, and hearing level than it is with physical changes in the vocal apparatus. Along with these changes, reductions in muscle size and tone and a characteristic sagging of muscles are observed in older individuals who fail to attend to continuing and appropriate body maintenance. Where some loss of weight has also occurred the skull may appear slightly larger than before.

CRITICAL DISCUSSION ▬▬▬▬
Lines as Signs and Bad Images

Lines are unmistakable, observable signs that older individuals have left their youth well behind them. Unfortunately, in our society at least these very signs generate negative attitudes and produce some less-than-

[1] *molar:* pertaining to the whole as opposed to its detailed parts

desirable effects. In nonindustrial societies, most people are not certain exactly how old they are. When the span of human life is divided into long periods of stable responsibility and clearly marked social and vocational roles, the exact number of years one has lived seems to be a rather trivial matter. In more highly industrialized, complex technological societies, where, by contrast, roles are less stable and less clearly marked and fixed, people seem haunted by the numbers game of chronological age. When the scorecard of birthdays is tallied up, for most purposes anything above a low total is considered bad news. Youth becomes the metaphor for vitality, vigor, productivity, and assertiveness, old age the metaphor for depletion, illness, incompetence, and passivity (Sontag, 1972). And now especially, when more people than ever are living longer, what amounts to the latter half (or more) of everyone's life is shadowed by the poignant apprehension of irretrievable loss, decay, and devaluation of one's worth as a human being.

In just this way, negative expectations, myths, and stereotypes of old age and old people are nourished and continue to grow. This can most easily be seen in much of the humor about the elderly. Examine a sample of birthday cards addressed to middle-aged celebrants and you will discover numerous snide, pejorative references to aging. Many of the roles assigned to TV actors portraying the old depict them in unrealistic ways: either as benignly witless or as doddering, mean, forgetful incompetents. Cases in point are the cruel caricatures that have been presented with some frequency on Johnny Carson's and (previously) Carol Burnett's comedy programs, both of which have been severely criticized for this very reason.

Negative attitudes toward the old are not always blatant, nor are they limited to the general public. The AARP/NRTA[1] News Bulletin of October 1981 reported a survey conducted by a University of Miami professor of nursing which indicated widespread prejudice on the part of nurses against older patients. The survey, which sampled 581 Florida R.N.s working in hospitals, nursing homes, and home health agencies, suggested that those who care for the elderly with the greatest frequency hold the least favorable attitudes toward them. Some participants in the survey, in fact, reported such acute feelings of dislike or fear of aged persons that they were described as having "gerontophobia" (exaggerated fear of aging). The reluctance of many mental health professionals to become significantly involved in providing direct services to the old, as well as the persistent practice of using the term "dementia" and referring to certain behaviors of elderly persons as "demented," with all the term's negative connotations, when alternative descriptions are readily available, likewise raises the question of subtle but very real negative attitudes on the part of such professional helpers.

The prestige of youth afflicts almost everyone in our society. In spite of the fact that men are just as prone to periodic bouts of the "blues" about growing old as women, Susan Sontag has made an insightful case for what she calls "the double standard of aging" (1972). Her thesis is based upon these observable "cosmetic" signs of age. Society

[1]AARP/NRTA: American Association of Retired Persons/National Retired Teachers Association

is much more permissive about aging in men, she argues. That is, men are "allowed" to age without penalty in several ways that women are not.

> This society offers even fewer rewards for aging to women than it does to men. Being physically attractive counts much more in a woman's life than in a man's, but beauty, identified as it is for women with youthfulness, does not stand up well to age.

> Perhaps all of this helps account for a society which "combats" age and the appearance thereof with creams, dyes, lotions, and face lifts, as well as with denials of age through euphemisms and pejorative humor. It is hard to avoid concluding that information and knowledge about aging and the technology of services to the elderly have advanced farther and more rapidly than have personal attitudes toward aging and the aged.

Height and Weight Changes

Human anatomical changes with age have produced considerable data, which must be accepted with reservations, however, because of the preponderance of cross-sectional analyses. The comparative aspects of changing height over time among different groups show rather small increases from age twenty to forty but a decline in stature generally beginning in about the fortieth year and tending to be progressive in succeeding decades. These changes parallel the activities and functioning of bone tissues throughout the lifespan as they **absorb**[1] and **resorb**[2] relatively greater or lesser amounts of crystalline material from or into the fluid environment surrounding the bones. During the earliest phase, more material is absorbed into the skeleton than resorbed from it, leading to a net gain in bone tissue. At maturity, absorption and resorption reach equilibrium, and bone tissue mass remains relatively constant. Past maturity, particularly beyond the age of forty years, less crystalline material is absorbed into the skeleton, more is resorbed back into the surrounding fluid environment, and the thinner, less dense, more porous bones which characterize osteoporosis result. Vertebral compression fractures which commonly accompany osteoporosis in the later years may account for the loss of height which begins in the fourth decade. Lifetime loss of height is estimated at approximately 4.9 cm in females and 2.9 cm in males (Rossman, 1977); while observable to some degree, these decreases nonetheless are rather small.

Studies of weight related to age in industrialized societies also support the well-known notion of increasing weight in the middle years with a subsequent decrease in old age. The incidence of obesity is more prevalent in higher than in lower income groups.

[1] *absorb:* collect and store deposits of materials in a more concentrated form
[2] *resorb:* break down and disintegrate deposits of materials from a more concentrated to a more dispersed and less concentrated form

In the 1965 Health Examination Survey (cited by Rossman, 1977), males achieved maximum average weight between thirty-four and fifty-four years of age, with a decline in weight through age seventy-nine. Weight changes for women were different. For women, weight levels continued to climb for two decades longer, and the decline into old age was proportionately less.

Changes in Vision

Gerontological researchers refer to two dimensions of vision: visual perception and visual communication. Visual perception refers to those processes within the individual that are necessary to sense, interpret, and respond to visual information. Visual communication refers to those physical and psychosocial processes involved in transferring visual information between individuals, and within groups (Fozard et al., 1977).

As age increases, so does the likelihood of visual impairment. The visual capability of three out of five persons over age seventy-five is likely to be affected to some degree, more often in females than in males. The National Center of Health Statistics reports that by age sixty-five about half the population has 20/70 visual acuity or worse. This is about five times the number of those with 20/70 vision at age forty-five.

A study by the National Society for the Prevention of Blindness (1966) revealed that the incidence of legal blindness (defined as an acuity of 20/200 or worse) increases from about 250 to 500 to 1,450 persons out of every 100,000, in age groups ranging from forty to sixty-four, sixty-five to sixty-nine, and sixty-nine years and older, respectively.

Such surveys highlight the visual problems of aging but do not tell much about the causes or the practical significance of such problems. They also demonstrate that losses of visual acuity and the occurrence of blindness are by no means universal phenomena of aging. The same holds for other sense modality changes in aging.

Many of the practical problems of vision encountered by the elderly are related to glare and poor visibility. Such circumstances can only exaggerate any visual losses that come from structural changes in the seeing apparatus.

The lens increases in thickness to the point that by age eighty it is 50 percent larger than it was at age twenty. At the same time the size of the pupil decreases, reducing the amount of light reaching the retina. This, along with the diminished ability of the eye to adjust to changing amounts of light, can seriously interfere with visual perception. Cataracts (clouding of the lens) and glaucoma (excessively high intraocular pressure) can also increase the hazard to vision in older persons (Fozard et al., 1977).

Another observable effect associated with aging is the restriction in the use of one's eyes—for example, restriction in the range of upward gaze in older individuals (Snyder, Pyrek, & Smith, 1976). There are no limitations in the lower range of gaze, but studies do show a rising incidence of constriction of upward gaze for monocular vision from ages five to ninety-four years. The practical significance of this for an older individual's perception of signs, landmarks, storage space, safety hazards, and the like, all of which are often placed high in the angle of regard, is obvious.

Changes in Hearing

Hearing loss can usually begin in the early twenties and *may* increase, especially in the upper tonal registers, as age increases. As with vision, hearing deficits are not universally an age-related phenomenon (Corso, 1977). However, unilateral and bilateral hearing impairments and deafness do occur with some frequency. Approximately 13 percent of individuals aged sixty-five and older show advanced signs of **presbycusis**,[1] and approximately 30 percent of the older population shows some signs of hearing loss.

The auditory system consists of the ear and its associated neural pathways, which are organized into subsystems running parallel to each other. With advanced age, deterioration may occur in the neural structures at any level, as well as in the peripheral components directly involved in sound transmission. Presbycusis represents neural loss, whereas **otosclerosis**[2] adds a component of conductive hearing loss. Surgery for the latter condition may be quite beneficial but will not completely restore hearing in most cases.

Because hearing plays such a major role in communication and interpersonal relations, any impairment frequently produces negative consequences for both the psychological and social adjustment of elderly persons (Corso, 1977). Commonly, the frequency and intensity of social contacts become the earliest casualties. While blindness has more easily recognized "signals" (dark glasses, white canes, Seeing Eye dogs), a mild to moderate hearing impairment is not readily apparent to others. No response at all on the part of hard-of-hearing elderly, or an inappropriate response because a few words have been missed here and there in a conversation, can easily be misconstrued by others as "confusion," "senility," or even antisocial behavior, rather than simply as a hearing deficit. The self-consciousness and embarrassment which often accompany the experience of such a deficit may induce an individual to avoid social situations and contacts, which in turn leads to greater social isolation.

Not least among the difficulties and obstacles that hard-of-hearing or deaf elderly face are household and safety hazards. Appliances that feature auditory signals (bell timers, buzzers, telephones) are obviously inappropriate and generally useless. For the hearing person, water basins, toilets, garbage disposals, motorized heating units, and the like are ordinarily judged to be functioning adequately from the sound of their operation. These common auditory cues are missed by those with severe hearing loss. Warnings or

---

[1]*presbycusis:* difficulty in hearing (i.e., detecting and discriminating) high-frequency sounds in the later years of life due to loss of neural function

[2]*otosclerosis:* difficulty in detecting and discriminating sounds due to the progressive hardening and increasing loss of mobility of the bones of the inner ear; represents a loss of bone conductivity

threats to safety which are inherent in traffic sounds, auto horns, and smoke-sensor units are missed, creating special penalties and hazards for the hard-of-hearing. Obviously, these are important factors to which service providers must sensitively attend.

A related form of loss is **aphasia**.[1] When external auditory signals fail to reach the brain centers because of neural or conductance loss, the resulting state is referred to as "receptive" aphasia. When auditory stimuli are processed properly but not effectively translated by the individual into appropriate responses, this is referred to as an "expressive" aphasia.

Although this kind of event is associated with brain damage, experience has shown that a knowledgeable therapist or helper can, with persistence and skill, successfully retrain the sufferer to regain much, and in many instances all, of his or her previous ability to perform.

Changes in Smell and Taste

The gustatory and olfactory modalities are closely dependent upon each other and will therefore be treated together in the following discussion.

It has been conventional to measure these sense modalities in much the same manner as vision and hearing are measured, namely, via **psychophysical**[2] investigations of increased or decreased units of difference in acuity. The appropriateness of such methodology has been questioned. Taste and smell appear to be poorest in discriminating differences in concentrations of a single substance and best in discriminating distinctions between qualitatively different substances (Engen, 1977).

When an aged resident in a nursing home complains that the food is not palatable, or when an elderly mother is very reluctant to bake her "famous" cookies because "they don't taste good anymore," these persons may be speaking the literal truth. The number of taste buds may decrease as much as 75 to 80 percent by the time we reach the age of eighty-five, but data on this remain inconclusive. Some studies have shown a decline in taste sensitivity during the sixth decade of life, while other studies have suggested a decreased ability among older persons to detect sweet substances. Consistent evidence also indicates a diminishing ability with advanced age to discriminate between sweet, bitter, sour, and salty tastes, although there is less reduction in sensitivity to sour. Sex and state of health appear to be important factors in determining differential taste sensitivity in the later years. Old men showed a deficiency in detecting salty-tasting substances, but old women did not, for example (Bourliére, Cendron, & Rapaport, 1958; Cooper, Bilash, & Zubek, 1959). Yet other studies have found no significant age decline in taste sensitivity to salty, bitter, sour, or sweet stimuli (Cohen & Gitman, 1958). When taste *preference* is measured (sweet seems almost universally liked

[1] *aphasia:* inability to process and produce speech properly or normally, either due to sensory (incoming) or motor (outgoing) neural loss or disability
[2] *psychophysics:* study of behavior that attempts to relate physical stimuli and sensation

and bitter, disliked) individual differences in long-standing habits and specific momentary needs also play an important part.

Findings on the sense of smell suggest that odor preference may be largely a result of cultural influences. There is some lessening of smell sensitivity with age, but the evidence once again is inconclusive; that is, the sense of smell does appear to remain stable in older persons.

In spite of the difficulties in measuring these sense modalities and the lack of conclusive findings as to the cause of change, gerontologists recognize that many older persons do not taste food exactly as they did years ago. Many older persons, too, may not recognize and respond as quickly to noxious odors that can warn of potential hazards to safety and well-being (e.g., toxic fumes or poisonous substances). In practical terms, an older person with a failing appetite may not necessarily be "cranky" but rather may be reporting the fact that food really doesn't taste the same. What food providers need to consider, therefore, is not blander food but instead tastier, spicier food, depending, of course, upon individual life-style and preference.

In a clinical context, evaluation of taste and smell responses must take into account a number of possible contributing elements, including (but not limited to) individual preference, familiarity with the substance, state of health, emotional stress or dysfunction (such as grief or depression), and the possibility that expressed distaste or loss of appetite may be symbolic or symptomatic of other life dissatisfactions. Lack of dentition or ill-fitting dentures which make biting or chewing painful, a decline in ability to salivate, and shrinking gums can also contribute to eating problems and diminished satisfaction.

Touch and Temperature

Changes in sensitivity to touch and temperature should not be thought of as a function of aging per se. These changes can be understood and accounted for within the context of the whole anatomical and physiological picture. Further, it is a mistake to assume that such deficiencies are going to occur universally in the aged.

Sensitivity to all stimuli applied to the feet starts to decrease at an earlier age than that applied to the forearm. In 5 to 10 percent of elderly tested there is some decline in sensitivity to vibration, temperature, pain, and light touch in the upper extremities. This occurs in more than 40 percent of individuals when sensitivity in their lower extremities is tested. Loss of sensitivity to light touch occurs in only 25 percent of elderly persons. Nor is it unusual to find some loss of sensitivity in one mode (such as **kinesthesia**[1]) but little or no loss in others (Kenshalo, 1977).

The criteria for thermal comfort do not appear to change with advancing years. But the capability of the body's temperature-regulating system to cope

---

[1] *kinesthesia:* "motion sensitivity," the sense of one's physical self (body) mediated through end-organ receptors in muscles, tendons, and joints

with temperature changes does seem to diminish. Thus an elderly woman who complains of a chilly room and insists on a shawl when younger people in the room are quite comfortable may not necessarily be acting unreasonable. By the same token, an elderly man awakening in the middle of the night may be responding to too many blankets or an overheated room. A rise in body temperature of as little as one degree can be enough to waken a light sleeper.

Convincing evidence of change in cutaneous pain sensitivity with advanced age is still lacking; findings relevant to this issue are mixed. What complicates such research is the well-accepted fact that pain is more than a sensory phenomenon. Clinicians especially are familiar with the cognitive (intellectual/symbolic) and affective (emotional) aspects of personality that can influence and affect individual reactions and responses to various kinds and intensities of pain stimuli.

Such factors, if they are to be correctly assessed, must be teased out and identified in the clinical setting, whether it be medical or psychosocial. Studies have shown, for example, that highly anxious patients report pain at lower stimulus intensities than do nonanxious patients (Kenshalo, 1977). Also, particular instructions to experimental participants can make both age and sex differences disappear and reappear. Participants not informed that an experiment involves the experience of pain report higher pain thresholds than those so informed.

With respect to the sense modalities in general, then, deficiencies and impairments can and do occur with increasing age. But these are not universal phenomena, nor do they occur consistently in a given individual. They affect a relatively modest proportion of the elderly and are reflected in marked individual differences as well as in differential sense thresholds among older individuals.

Changes in Sexual Response

That older persons are capable of continuing normal and rewarding sexual experiences in later life (an issue to be discussed further in a later chapter) does not mean that no changes occur. Patterns of sexual response in old age might be characterized by the phrase "a long time coming." That is to say, older persons respond to affectional and sexual stimulation (kissing, hugging, caressing) quite readily but usually require further stimulation of this kind over a more extended period of time before full sexual arousal is achieved.

Changes attendant to later life usually are not serious, but older persons need to be aware of them and to know how to cope with them in order to increase sexual fulfillment. An adequate description of physical changes associated with age is contained in the discussion of "Geriatric Sexual Response" in the book *Human Sexual Response* (Masters & Johnson, 1966). The findings of Masters and Johnson are summarized here.

For females, it is noted that:

1. The vagina loses length, width, and vaginal-wall thickness and a "significant degree of involuntary ability to expand under sexual tension." But the loss is less for those females who have a consistent sexual relationship during the middle and early later years.

2. Lubrication due to sexual stimulation is delayed in comparison to younger women, but for most women can be produced in one to three minutes.

3. Orgasms follow the general process as in the younger years, but their duration is shorter.

4. The intensity of reaction is diminished. But "the aging human female is fully capable of sexual performance at orgasmic response levels."

5. If there are conditions such as vaginal burning, pelvic distress, and painful uterine contractions associated with orgasms, these can be corrected by adequate endocrine replacement.

6. Women who have regular sexual expression once or twice a week maintain sexual capacity.

For males, it is noted that:

1. The older the male, the more time it takes for full penile erection.

2. The erection may be maintained in older men "for extended periods of time."

3. Once an erection is lost in older men, it will not return as soon as would be the case for younger men.

4. The number of expulsive contractions during orgasm are fewer for the older male.

5. In general the male (as well as the female) loses some physiological efficiency as he ages.

6. The more consistent the male's sexual history during middle and early old age, the greater his chances for a healthy sexuality in his later years.

7. Most males over the age of fifty who have "secondarily acquired impotency" can be restored to potency. Impotency in the older male is accounted for by boredom with a dull and repetitive sexual regime; such great concentration on economic and occupational goals that no energy or time is left for sexual enjoyment; overindulgence in alcohol or food; physical or mental losses of either the individual or the partner; or fear of sexual failure.

Physiological Adaptation: Successes and Failures

A major hypothesis regarding physical and health factors in aging questions the effectiveness (or failure) with advanced age of a variety of control mechanisms that are known to regulate the interaction of different organ systems and tissues (Birren & Renner, 1977). Primary control mechanisms operate through either the endocrine system or the nervous system in conjunction with the vascular system. The corticosteroids, for instance, can have various physiological effects. They influence electrolytic and water balance, and moderate metabolism and the functional capacities of the cardiovascular system, kidneys, skeletal muscles, and central nervous system. They also influence the capacity of the body to cope with change and stress. In contrast, one might examine the breakdown of causes of death in the United States. Table 2–4 very clearly shows how diseases of the heart and circulatory system have become the major cause of death from middle through old age in our country. No doubt that is why such diseases, associated with the circulatory system and exacerbated by stress factors, have come to be labeled "diseases of the industrialized West."

This phenomenon draws attention to the central role of psychosocial factors in the total picture of physical well-being of the population from the middle through the later years of life. Thinking of the older person as a social being, then, let us look at some subsystems from the physiological point of view and try to imagine how the physical and psychosocial dimensions interrelate, especially in old age.

Physiologically, the human body is an intricate mechanicochemical system which controls a constant flow of energy in the form of incoming nutrients, water, and gases and outgoing waste products, water, heat, and gases. Such a paradigm, suggested by Abbey (1975), provides a useful framework for the study of physical factors in aging.

Consider, for example, the shape of a fairly typical elderly person. Arms

TABLE 2–4. Death Rates per 100,000 Population in the United States During 1973

Cause of Death	Age								
	1–14	15–24	25–34	35–44	45–54	55–64	65–74	75–84	85 and Over
Major cardiovascular diseases	1.6	4.0	14.3	73.3	268.1	762.6	1,914.5	5,229.4	12,914.7
Malignant neoplasms, including neoplasms of lymphatic and hematopoietic tissues	5.6	7.2	15.4	54.9	181.4	428.6	778.2	1,208.1	1,457.7
Influenza and pneumonia	2.2	2.0	3.7	7.6	14.6	31.0	79.9	228.3	875.5
Diabetes mellitus	0.1	0.4	1.7	4.4	11.4	33.1	82.0	171.1	227.0
Bronchitis, emphysema, and asthma	0.1	0.2	0.5	1.9	8.3	32.2	79.8	134.2	123.9
Accidents	24.1	71.0	51.6	45.3	49.2	52.2	75.2	157.0	404.9

Source: U.S. Public Health Service (1974).

and legs are relatively thin while the trunk, particularly around the abdomen, is fat. In the context of heat control or conservation, the spindly arms and legs, with marked decrease in blood circulation, act to prevent heat loss, while the fatty tissue around the belly tends to conserve heat in the area of the major organs, where it is most needed.

The body gets rid of excess heat arising from cellular activity by sweating, and through dilation of blood vessels in the extremities. The elderly person with a less functional heart and vasculature (circulatory system) thus does not tolerate extremes of heat and cold well. An elevated temperature is ordinarily more serious in an elderly person because in addition to reduced energy reserves, vascular adaptation is much more limited. If the arteries are **atherosclerotic**,[1] the capillary beds of the lungs are decreased, and thickened **alveoli**[2] all work to limit gaseous exchange (the normal process of breathing). The overall cardiopulmonary system can be said to be less adaptive and, possibly because of less sensitivity to adaptation "signals," cannot adjust properly to the increased demands in rate and volume.

Cardiovascular System

The heart becomes the central actor in this physical health drama. With advancing years the heart muscle typically shows a decrease in size and strength. It does not fill as well or squeeze as tightly, factors possibly related to the body's decreased ability to convert nutrients to mechanical energy as efficiently as it did when it was younger. By age sixty-five cardiac output decreases approximately 30 to 40 percent. Cardiac rate remains stable, but under conditions of exertion the heart rate takes longer to increase and the rate is not as fast as it formerly was.

Prolongation of the period of contraction occurs and aortic elasticity diminishes considerably in the later years. With exercise, an increase in cardiac output can result in a rise in arterial blood pressure. This makes the blood-pumping mechanism less efficient and less able to adapt to stressful, demanding situations.

The circulatory problems of aging are well known. Perhaps less well known (and associated with the familiar "midnight jitters") is that insomnia is often related to diminished cerebral blood flow, which can accompany reduced mental or emotional stimulation. In such instances a sedative can actually be dangerous. Much better would be something warm and sweet to drink (like hot chocolate) and someone to talk to for awhile. In addition, a gentle backrub or some mild exercise can also help circulation and reduce emotional stress.

---

[1] *atherosclerotic:* lined with fatty deposits which constrict the flow of blood
[2] *alveoli:* tiny thin-walled chambers surrounded by very small blood vessels (capillaries); the basic site of gas exchange

Respiratory System

The fact that all metabolic activities form acid end products focuses attention on the two major systems for acid-base control, the lungs and the kidneys. The lungs are a passive system, in that they are limited to gaseous exchange and cannot make electrolyte corrections, are unable selectively to conserve or excrete, and are totally dependent for effective functioning upon an intact rib cage and musculature (and are thus affected by posture). It is the nervous system that controls the respiratory muscles and causes breathing. The lungs themselves do not act as primary sensors for gaseous concentration, respiratory rate, or depth. If respiratory difficulties persist over a protracted period of time, the respiratory centers in the brain "reset" to cause breathing only at a higher concentration of acid and carbon dioxide in the blood. This will, of course, decrease the rate of respiration and materially lessen the amount of oxygen taken in. A backup receptor system then becomes the sole cause of breathing, and unfortunately does so only when the oxygen concentration in the blood drops to about 60 percent of the normal level. The individual thus breathes only when the amount of available oxygen is low.

This phenomenon can become a special problem in hospitals or nursing homes, or even in affluent private homes where bottled oxygen may be available. In such a circumstance, an elderly individual given nasal oxygen without careful observation can drift off to sleep, stop breathing, and die of acidosis. A very simple test of function is to request the elderly person to blow out a match held six inches from the mouth with the mouth wide open. If this cannot be managed one may conclude that respiratory function is compromised and that the individual needs close observation and help. In that event there is also a high probability that the individual will not be able to cough adequately, either.

The other system involved in acid-base management is the kidneys. Kidney function decreases in efficiency almost 50 percent, with a steady decline in ability to concentrate urine, between twenty and ninety years of age. Problems with dehydration as well as the possibility of bladder problems become potential threats to the physical well-being of elderly persons.

Stress and Perception of Health

Within the large body of research on the effects of stress in general, there is a growing emphasis on those elements of stress in the environment that generate a specific impact on the aging process. Convincing evidence demonstrates not only the psychological and emotional trauma but also the noxious physical consequences of environmental stress (Kiritz & Moos, 1974). Studies indicate a closer linkage of physical and health factors in the overall well-being of the elderly to environmental determinants than to any other single disease-inducing variable. These issues will be discussed in more detail in Chapter 10.

Health profiles of the aged are, typically, developed on the basis of the number or frequency of disease syndromes, pathological entities, and disabilities or "impairments." Gerontologists have begun to emphasize that in any such health evaluation what must also be taken into account is the equally important fact that disabilities vary greatly in intensity and effect upon each individual. Disabilities also vary with respect to duration. Disabling conditions of mild intensity and brief duration may have little effect upon the older person. Other disabling conditions of high intensity and greater chronicity are presumed to have much greater impact. Also to be considered are variations of these factors.

CRITICAL DISCUSSION

"Step on a Crack, Break Your Mother's Back"

Osteoporosis, described previously in this text, is a normal, progressive process through which the mature individual's bones become thinner, less dense, and more porous over time. Because this process is slow and continuous, it is difficult to detect accurately at the molecular level until significant quantities of bone tissue have been lost. The most obvious molar manifestations of osteoporosis are broken bones, most commonly involving the wrist, vertebrae, and hip. These fractures result in varying degrees of pain and may further interfere with normal functioning, depending on the location of the fracture. Wrist fractures are the least serious, requiring only minor modification of function; vertebral fractures, as noted before, may result in an apparent shortening of stature which is often associated with the aging process. Hip fractures, however, are the most serious, due to their immobilizing effect on the individual. Indeed, Gordon (1971) has observed that fewer than two-thirds of older individuals with hip fractures survive for a full year following the incidence of the fracture. This type of fracture occurs three times as often in women as in men (Zisserman, 1973) and, according to Heaney (1971), "is perhaps the most sinister manifestation of osteoporosis. . . . Some degree of deterioration in total life adjustment is a nearly inevitable consequence of those who survive" (p. 59).

An interesting fact about osteoporosis is that lighter-skinned individuals are more likely to sustain fractures than darker-pigmented people; in addition, women are generally at greater risk of suffering broken bones than men. Women begin to report a greater incidence of fractures between the ages of fifty and sixty, while men report a similar increase between the ages of sixty and seventy. (Darker-skinned individuals of both sexes appear to be affected a few years later than their lighter-skinned counterparts.) Although a relatively straightforward explanation exists to account for these sex and racial differences, for many years it was largely ignored in favor of a seriously biased interpretation—the "crack" that "broke mother's back." According to Albright, Smith, and Richardson (1941), the greater risk of fracture in older women in general was caused by the "pathological" state associated with the menopause. Because no premenopausal women ever suffered from clinical symptoms of osteoporosis, and those who did were all postmenopausal, Albright et al. mistakenly concluded that the loss of the female sex hormone estrogen at the menopause must be causally related to what they described as pathologically accelerated bone loss in women (associated with the earlier onset of clinical manifestations of bone loss in women as compared to men). Despite the lack of evidence to support the hypothetical connection between estrogen insufficiency and accelerated osteoporosis, estrogen therapy was (and in some cases, still is) prescribed for postmenopausal women who suffered bone fractures in an attempt to retard the process of bone resorption. As might be expected, this form of therapy was largely ineffective in reducing bone loss, and moreover became associated with an increased risk of cancer of the uterine lining (endometrium) in those women who underwent such therapy. When estrogen therapy was shown to be relatively ineffective in combating osteoporosis, other forms of therapy for older women were developed—again, with little success and, in many cases, unpleasant side effects for the women being treated for a "disease" (accelerated or secondary osteoporosis) which in fact does not exist. Interesting to observe, too, is that the erroneous hypothesis proposing estrogen deficiency as the cause of this "disease" could not account for the racial differences in the onset of clinical symptoms. Why should darker-skinned women (and, for that matter, men) be more resistant to broken bones than their lighter-skinned counterparts, if the event of the menopause were indeed the causal agent in bone deterioration?

As it turns out, there is no apparent connection between estrogen loss and osteoporosis, other than time. The factor which determines risk of fracture with normal bone loss in aging is the amount of bone tissue present in the individual at maturity. In general, men have larger skeletal structures than women at maturity, and darker-skinned people similarly have larger amounts of bone tissue than lighter-skinned people at maturity, all of which accounts for the sex and racial differences in incidence of fracture with age. It has been estimated that an individual can expect to lose an average of 15.6 gm of bone tissue annually past the age of forty years, regardless of sex or race (Trotter & Hixon, 1974). Although this amount is constant in absolute terms, relatively speaking it represents a greater proportion of bone loss in women than in men and in lighter-skinned than in darker-skinned people. Women generally lose about 1 percent of their bone tissue each year at age forty and beyond, while men generally lose slightly less than half this proportion of bone tissue over the same period of time (Garn, 1975; Newton-John & Morgan, 1970). Thus a woman of fifty-five to sixty years of age will likely have lost about 15 to 20 percent of her bone tissue, and would be roughly comparable in terms of bone loss to a man aged sixty-five to seventy.

So we can see that a "pathological" agent in the relatively more serious bone loss of women over time is unnecessary to explain normal osteoporosis. Because bone mass at maturity is the predisposing factor in determining risk of fracture in later life, the best way to reduce the risk is to increase bone density prior to maturity through proper nutrition. This suggestion obviously is of little help to those who at present are mature or aging adults, but may be useful in allowing the next generations to become "fracture-free" aged.

A counterpart or discontinuity hypothesis, proposed by Birren (1976), states that it is only when a physiological function becomes "abnormal" that the physical function affects behavior variables. Physical factors within a normal range not affecting the behavior of young persons may affect the behavior of older persons when the physical function reaches an abnormal level of intensity or duration. Such a notion is not inconsistent with the findings that most elderly tend to underestimate the "seriousness" of certain health factors in overall subjective judgment.

As was pointed out earlier, perceptions and assessments of personal health status may vary greatly from one aged individual to another. Even more curious is the fact that many older persons may rate their health as "good" or "pretty good," in spite of a number of decrements and deficiencies disclosed by medical examinations. Why this discrepancy between subjective assessment and objective evaluation?

Selye's stress theory, as we have noted, incorporates the notion of a residuum of impairment from which the individual (or organism) does not fully recover following an episode of stress. Taking this hypothesis to its logical conclusion, we may postulate that the perceived level of health after each episode of illness or stress gradually reduces the health "threshold" over time. At any given point a range of variability in the perception of health by any individual exists. The range of variability is influenced concurrently by personal expectations and biases, by objective measures and assessments, and by comparisons of personal health and well-being with the health status of others (such as age peers).

The schema displayed in Figure 2–2 offers a heuristic model of changing perceptions of health and well-being from earlier through later life.

The range of variability in perception of health status or well-being increases through the lifespan (or until the "terminal drop") and is hypothesized to influence subjective responses to health status following each health decrement event (E_1, E_2, E_3, . . . E_n).

For example, individual X, after experiencing a series of health decrement episodes of greater or lesser severity, may perceive her health status (or well-being) to be poor or precarious at the minimum. Individual Y, by contrast, after experiencing even greater traumatic events, may report a subjective perception of "average," "fair," or even "good," in spite of a negative objective evaluation (cf. Lazarus, 1982; Maddox, 1964). These individuals thus present quite different behavioral pictures as a function of differing subjective evaluations of health or well-being. Individual X says "my health is

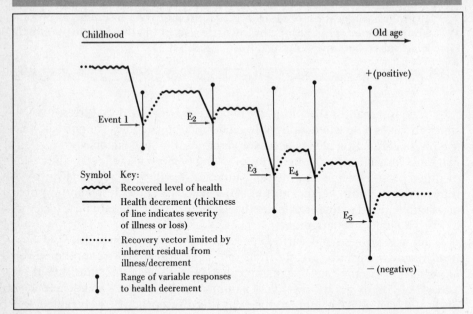

FIGURE 2–2. Schematic Model of Subjective Perception of Health Status across the Lifespan
Source: Arthur Schwartz.

poor," and assumes an invalid or quasi-invalid role; individual Y says "my health is good," and remains busy and active. Figure 2–2 depicts the increasing ambiguity of normative health and well-being referents with advancing age, and the increased variability of perceptions and subjective definitions of health and well-being as a function of greater and more frequent comparisons with the judgments of peers, richness of experience, and objective measures.

Drugs and the Aged: Use, Abuse, Misuse

A potentially major contributing factor to physiological disruption and behavior dysfunction in older persons is the misuse and abuse of drugs, a phenomenon which is increasing at an alarming rate among the aged in our drug-oriented society. One significant observation is that aged persons as a group consume a disproportionate share of drugs, both prescription and over-the-counter substances (Lee, 1978).

In part, the extent of the problem can be visualized from data reported by a British consultant geriatrician, along with his descriptive comments:

—37% of all women aged 75 and over receive psychotropic drugs;
—75% of the whole population aged 75 and over receive drugs of some kind;

two-thirds receive one to three drugs, and one-third four to six drugs simultaneously;

—25% of all adults are taking medicines first prescribed more than one year previously;

—75% of prescriptions are repeat prescriptions;

—50% of patient's bottles seen in a geriatric outpatient clinic have no dosage directions (personal observation);

—80% of patients admitted to geriatric wards are receiving drugs; for most of these patients, and for patients seen in geriatric outpatient clinics, it is impossible to be certain what the drugs are; and

—10% of admissions to geriatric wards are due to iatrogenic disease caused by drugs.

In the past, placebos, or the bona-fide medicines of the day, were often unpleasant, but they seldom had the powerful physiological actions of today's drugs, nor were they so freely available. Today the elderly are the main victims of modern drugs and the system by which they are administered. The reasons for this are: (1) multiple pathology of the elderly, (2) polypharmacy, (3) increased sensitivity of the elderly to drugs and side effects, (4) doctors' lack of training in geriatric prescribing, (5) unsuitable drug packaging and instructions, (6) poor supervision of elderly patients, and (7) dual prescribing systems in hospitals and in general practice, which prevent doctors from being fully responsible for their own prescribing [Bliss, 1981].

An investigation of drug use by older persons in the United States was undertaken by faculty researchers at the University of Southern California School of Pharmacy (Cheung & Kayne, 1975), who studied the use of drugs within randomly selected long-term-care facilities in Los Angeles County. The study revealed that on the average, 8.9 drugs were ingested daily by sample participants; the average medication error rate was reported to be 21.8 percent. Medication errors included administration of the wrong drug or an incorrect dosage; incorrect dosage intervals; missed dosage; and administration of a drug to the wrong person. The most frequent type of medication error reported was missed dosage (52 percent).

It is often difficult to differentiate the effects of "normal" aging from the effects of degenerative disease. Peter Lee has drawn attention to the inevitable overlap resulting from the increasing incidence of atherosclerosis, emphysema, diabetes, and hypertension with advancing age, which makes clear distinctions difficult to draw. Further complicating the issue is the fact that some drug effects and physiological changes are exaggerated by social and psychological factors, such as isolation, institutionalization, and loss of spouse, job, independence, and self-esteem (Lee, 1978).

Included in age-associated decrements of physical function are a number of tissue and organ system changes which are implicated in the older individual's differential response to drugs. Included among such organ, organ system, and tissue changes are decreases in brain weight, nerve conduction velocity, cardiac sufficiency (Harris, 1975), and renal (kidney), hepatic (liver), and lung efficiency (Lindeman, 1975; Shock, 1968). Changes in renal and hepatic efficiency with advanced years make the older person more prone to dire effects and adverse reactions (Eisdorfer & Stotsky, 1977).

These effects are magnified by those individuals who tend to be "physician shoppers," going from one physician to another and in the course of time accumulating a substantial stockpile of drugs prescribed for a variety of purposes. Outdated medications can be useless or worse, and exchange of drugs among friends can increase the potential hazards of toxicity through inappropriate use. Probably more important for the multiple-drug-taking older person are the potential hazardous interactions which may result from the combined use of such substances as ferrous salts, antacids, anticholinergic drugs, and various laxatives, which can modify the absorption of other drugs (Lee, 1978).

Increased sensitivity to drugs may require a lower dosage of psychoactive agents for elderly persons (over 50 percent less in many cases). For example, a dosage appropriate for a thirty-year-old can produce overwhelming or even lethal effects in the eighty-year-old. Also, the interaction of certain medications (e.g., **diuretics**,[1] corticosteroids, **barbiturates**,[2] and even multivitamin preparations containing vitamin K) can decrease drug sensitivity. Antidepressants, sedatives, and tranquilizers (such as Mellaril, Valium, and Librium) as well as **analgesics**[3] and **vasodilators**[4]—all frequently prescribed for older persons—are capable of generating toxic effects in certain elderly individuals which may be manifested in senile-like behavior (Eisdorfer & Faun, 1973).

To help avoid some of the hazards of drug therapy in the older patient, Peter Lee (1978) has proposed these guidelines:

1. Weigh the older patient for estimate of lean weight
2. Check blood pressure carefully
3. Look for organic causes of insomnia first
4. Reduce the dose of drugs excreted by the kidney
5. Reduce the dose of most CNS (central nervous system) drugs
6. Remember heart failure decreases hepatic blood flow and may prolong the half-life of drugs
7. Remember that the older person may make mistakes in taking medication, especially if the instructions are complicated
8. Reassess periodically the continued need for each drug.

In addition, Bliss (1981) adds:

All drugs should be stopped if they are not helping the patient, and most drugs, even those that are apparently being effective, should be tailed off and stopped from time to time to see if they are still necessary.

[1] *diuretics:* drugs which help to dilute and thus increase the volume of urine to be discharged
[2] *barbiturates:* drugs which calm and reduce activity
[3] *analgesics:* drugs which help reduce pain
[4] *vasodilators:* drugs which help to dilate or expand the blood vessels and improve circulation

Nutrition

An optimal state of physical and emotional well-being is highly dependent upon adequate dietary or nutritional regimens. The familiar saying "We are what we eat" may indeed have special significance for the elderly. Many different but related elements strongly influence customary dietary patterns among the elderly: social, motivational, financial, cultural, and physical factors, habit patterns, knowledge base, and the like. Adequate nutrition for an elderly person invariably becomes a problem when there is a breakdown in one or some combination of these elements.

One possible contributor to poor nutrition with advanced years is the incidence of periodontal disease, which increases with age to over 90 percent of individuals from sixty-five to seventy-five years old. Such difficulties include the failure to use dentures at all or the persistent use of ill-fitting dentures. Consequent pain or discomfort in biting down and chewing can tempt an elderly person to concentrate on nutritionally deficient junk foods, adopt a bread-soaked-in-milk diet, or engage in other nutrition-poor eating behavior.

Gastrointestinal changes with age can also spark dietary deficiencies and poor eating habits. For instance, delay in emptying of the esophagus which may lead to difficulty or pain in swallowing is not rare in later life. Digestive secretions diminish markedly beyond the age of sixty, although the quantity of enzymes necessary for carbohydrate and protein digestion appears to remain at a sufficient level.

The overall conclusion of nutritionists and dietary experts familiar with the eating habits of the aged is that where nutritional deficiencies are found among older persons, these deficiencies appear to be more closely linked to level of income, general health, feelings of well-being, and other factors than to old age itself. In point of fact, only a relatively small percentage of those in the later years are found to suffer from malnutrition to any significant extent (Barrows & Roeder, 1977). Nonetheless, Table 2–5 indicates the suggested daily amounts of selected nutrients for older people, with special attention to those nutrients which are most likely to be deficient with increasing age.

When cognitive dysfunctions (e.g., confusion, disorientation, and memory lapses) occur, or when intellectual functioning is impaired, these behaviors must be carefully examined to determine the extent to which the nutritional status of the aged individual may be implicated. Certain toxic states (which may also be caused by the interaction of certain drugs or by inappropriate drug dosages), inadequate supply of thiamine or nicotinic acid, avitaminosis, endocrine disorders, or anemia are all capable of producing the so-called signs of senility mentioned above. These are essentially transient conditions, and to the degree to which they are linked to eating habits can be practicably minimized or eliminated altogether by effective dietary

TABLE 2-5   Selected Recommended Daily Dietary Allowances

	Males	Females
Age	51+ yrs	51+ yrs
Weight	70 kg	55 kg
Height	178 cm	163 cm
Energy (kcal)	2,400 (51–75 yrs)	1,800 (51–75 yrs)
	2,050 (76+ yrs)	1,600 (76+ yrs)
Protein (g)	56	44
Vitamin A (μg RE)	1,000	800
Vitamin D (μg)	5	5
Vitamin E (mg α-$\gamma\epsilon$)	15	10
Vitamin C (mg)	60	60
Thiamin (mg)	1.2	1.0
Riboflavin (mg)	1.4	1.2
Niacin (mg Nϵ)	16	13
Vitamin B6 (mg)	2.2	2.0
Folacin (μg)	400	400
Vitamin B12 (μg)	3.0	3.0
Calcium (mg)	800	800
Phosphorus (mg)	800	800
Magnesium (mg)	350	300
Iron (mg)	10	10
Zinc (mg)	15	15
Iodine (μg)	150	150

Source: Recommended Dietary Allowances. (9th rev. ed.) Washington, D.C.: National Academy of Sciences, National Research Council, 1980.

modifications. The appropriate addition of vitamins and other nutritional supplements also helps. When these temporary conditions are removed, the related cognitive dysfunctions can be significantly improved or eliminated as well. Clearly, factors associated with poor dietary patterns (solitary eating, lack of money, lifestyle habits, and so on) need to be assessed and taken into account in any appropriate intervention or service-delivery strategy.

Exercise

Along with nutrition, exercise plays a large role as one of the important elements in prevention of deterioration and maintenance of physical as well as psychological well-being in the later years (De Vries, 1975). The amount and kinds of exercise in which older persons participate serve not only as antidotes to certain kinds of physical change and stress and the subjective experience of pain, but also have a direct (and often immediate) effect upon states of emotional stress, boredom, general morale, and outlook.

With aging, muscle cells decrease in number. Also the transmission rate of impulses through nervous tissue decreases approximately 15 percent in

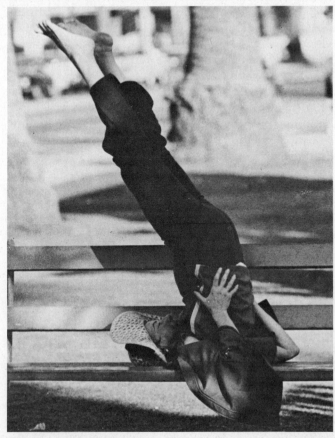

Appropriate exercise enables people to maintain their zest and a high level of well-being as they grow older.

motor nerves and 30 percent in sensory neurons between twenty and ninety years of age. In addition, there is loss to some degree of vibratory sensation and a lessening of tendon reflex responses. Regularly performed exercise can increase the capacity for ventilation, the amount of oxygen used, cardiac output, and blood flow, and not only slow the rate of muscle loss but cause the functioning cells to grow and react faster. As long as nerve tissue is intact, impairment of functioning in aging muscles can be actively, and often successfully, combated.

An important bonus to be obtained from regular, appropriate exercise in later life is its tranquilizing effect. Exercise has a significantly greater calming effect (with no undesirable side effects) than does meprobamate, one of the most frequently prescribed tranquilizing drugs (De Vries & Adams, 1972). This should not be overlooked when a tranquilizing effect is desired. A fifteen-minute walk at a moderate rate, for example, may be sufficient to provide a tranquilizing effect for at least one hour afterward, according to De Vries.

Exercise appropriate for elderly persons has been found to decrease arterial blood pressure. A clear-cut case can also be made for the importance of habitual, lifelong, rigorous physical activity as a preventive measure against obesity and its attendant ills.

De Vries (1971) also points out that only if exercise in later life is appropriate and carefully moderated will its benefits be maximized and its potential hazards minimized. Unless the intensity of exercise is vigorous enough to raise the heart rate more than 40 percent above the resting rate it is unlikely to produce significant benefits to the cardiorespiratory system, even though lower-intensity exercise may benefit other muscles as well as joints. De Vries and other physiologists point out that appropriate exercise means avoiding or minimizing high activation of small muscle masses and static (isometric) contractions. Much more desirable exercise regimens for the elderly emphasize the rhythmic activity of large muscle masses. Activities such as walking, dancing, jogging, bicycle riding, running, and swimming are best suited for this purpose.

Summary

A common denominator in the rapidly expanding gerontological literature is the notion of multiple loss. Physical and health factors, because they represent a major category of change and loss and also provide a large base for planners and practitioners, have received much attention from researchers.

Chronic conditions are more frequent in an older population than are acute physical ailments. Yet most elderly are able to function quite adequately. Chronic disabilities may limit activities but need not identify such persons as sick.

Cosmetic signs of aging are highly visible and may elicit negative attitudes, especially toward women. Other losses associated with aging, such as the changes in the sense modalities, may penalize older persons in more subtle ways. These physiological changes interact in various ways to affect the health as well as the mental competence and emotional well-being of older individuals. Because of the great variability in perception and assessment of subjective health and well-being among older people, a heuristic model is offered as a hypothetical construct to account for a self-rating of "good health" by elderly persons with evident health deficiencies. At the same time, it is to be noted that many decrements to physical health and well-being are reversible and preventable. The major maintenance and prevention strategies in this regard have to do with nutrition and exercise.

References

Abbey, J. Physiology of the aged. Mimeograph of lecture delivered at Andrus Gerontology Center, University of Southern California, Los Angeles, 1975.

Albright, F., Smith, P., & Richardson, A. Postmenopausal osteoporosis: Its clinical features. *Journal of the American Medical Association,* 1941, **116**, 2465–2474.

Barrows, C., & Roeder, L. Nutrition. In C. Finch & L. Hayflick (Eds.), *Handbook of the biology of aging.* New York: Van Nostrand Reinhold, 1977. Pp. 561–577.

Birren, J. *Handbook of aging and the individual.* Chicago: University of Chicago Press, 1959.

Birren, J. Psycho-physiological relations. In J. Birren, R. Butler, S. Greenhouse, L. Sokoloff, & M. Yarrow (Eds.); *Human aging I: A biological and behavioral study.* USDHEW, Public Health Service, National Institute on Aging. DHEW Publication No. (ADM)77-122, 1971, reprinted 1976.

Birren, J., & Renner, J. Research on the psychology of aging: Principles and experimentation. In J. Birren & K. W. Schaie (Eds.), *Handbook of the psychology of aging.* New York: Van Nostrand Reinhold, 1977. Pp. 3–38.

Bliss, M. R. Prescribing for the elderly. *British Medical Journal,* 1981, **283** (July 19, 1981), 203–206.

Bourliére, F., Cendron, H., & Rapaport, A. Modification avec l'age de seuils gustatifs de perception et de reconnaissance aux saveurs salée et sucrée chez l'homme. *Gerontologia,* 1958, **2**, 104–111.

Carlson, R. *The end of medicine.* New York: Wiley, 1975.

Cheung, A., & Kayne, R. An application of clinical pharmacy in extended care facilities. In R. Davis (Ed.), *Drugs and the elderly.* Los Angeles: University of Southern California, Andrus Gerontology Center, 1975.

Cohen, T., & Gitman, L. Studies in the gastrointestinal tract in the aged. *Journal of Gerontology,* 1958, **13**, 441 (abstract).

Comfort, A. *Aging: The biology of senescence.* New York: Holt, Rinehart & Winston, 1964.

Cooper, R. M., Bilash, I., & Zubek, J. P. The effect of age on taste sensitivity. *Journal of Gerontology,* 1959, **14**, 56–58.

Corso, J. Auditory perception and communication. In J. Birren & K. W. Schaie (Eds.), *Handbook of the psychology of aging.* New York: Van Nostrand Reinhold, 1977. Pp. 535–550.

Curtis, H. *Biological mechanisms of aging.* Springfield, Ill.: Charles C. Thomas, 1966.

De Vries, H. Exercise intensity threshold for improvement of cardiovascular-respiratory function in older men. *Geriatrics,* 1971, **26**(4), 94–101.

De Vries, H. The physiology of exercise and aging. In D. Woodruff & J. Birren (Eds.), *Aging: Scientific perspectives and social issues.* New York: Van Nostrand, 1975. Pp. 257–276.

De Vries, H., and Adams, G. Electromyographic comparison of single doses of exercise and meprobamate as to effects on muscular relaxation. *American Journal of Physical Medicine,* 1972, **51**, 130–141.

Eisdorfer, C., & Faun, W. (Eds.) *Psychopharmacology and aging.* New York: Plenum Press, 1973.

Eisdorfer, C., & Stotsky, B. Intervention, treatment, and rehabilitation of psychiatric disorders. In J. Birren & K. W. Schaie (Eds.), *Handbook of the psychology of aging.* New York: Van Nostrand Reinhold, 1977. Pp. 724–774.

Engen, T. Taste and smell. In J. Birren & K. W. Schaie (Eds.), *Handbook of the psychology of aging.* New York: Van Nostrand Reinhold, 1977. Pp. 554–559.

Fozard, J., Wolf, E., Bell, B., McFarland, R., & Podolsky, S. Visual perception and communication. In J. Birren & K. W. Schaie (Eds.), *Handbook of the psychology of aging.* New York: Van Nostrand Reinhold, 1977. Pp. 497–528.

Garn, S. Bone loss and aging. In R. Goldman & M. Rockstein (Eds.), *The physiology and pathology of human aging.* New York: Academic Press, 1975. Pp. 39–57.

Gordon, P. The probability of death following a fracture of the hip. *Journal of the Canadian Medical Association,* 1971, **105**, 47–51.

Harman, D. Aging: A theory based on free radical and radiation chemistry. *Journal of Gerontology,* 1956, **11**, 298–300.

Harman, D. Prolongation of life: Role of free radical reactions in aging. *Journal of the American Geriatric Association,* 1969, **17**(8), 721–735.

Harris, R. Cardiac changes with age. In R. Goldman & M. Rockstein (Eds.), *The physiology and pathology of human aging.* New York: Academic Press, 1975.

Heaney, R. Menopausal effects on calcium homeostasis and skeletal metabolism. In K. Ryan & D. Gibson (Eds.), *Menopause and aging.* Summary report and selected papers from a Research Conference on Menopause and Aging, Hot Springs, Arkansas, May 23–26, 1971. Bethesda, Md.: USDHEW, 1971. Pp. 59–67.

Holmes, R., & Rahe, R. The social readjustment rating scale. *Journal of Psychosomatic Research,* 1967, **11**, 219–225.

Kenshalo, D. Age changes in touch, vibration, temperature, kinesthesis, and pain sensitivity. In J. Birren & K. W. Schaie (Eds.), *Handbook of the psychology of aging.* New York: Van Nostrand Reinhold, 1977. Pp. 562–575.

Kiritz, S., & Moos, R. Physiological effects of the social environment. In P. Insel & R. Moos (Eds.), *Health and the social environment.* Lexington, Mass.: D. C. Heath, 1974. Pp. 13–35.

Lazarus, R. S. Stress and coping as factors in health and illness. In J. Cohen, J. W. Cullen, & L. R. Martin (Eds.), *Psychosocial aspects of cancer.* New York: Raven Press, 1982.

Lee, P. V. Drug therapy in the elderly: The clinical pharmacology of aging. *Alcoholism: clinical and experimental research,* 1978, **2**(1), 39–42.

Lindeman, R. Age changes in renal function. In R. Goldman & M. Rockstein (Eds.), *The physiology and pathology of human aging.* New York: Academic Press, 1975.

Maddox, G. Self-assessment of health status: A longitudinal study of selected elderly subjects. *Journal of Chronic Diseases,* 1964, **17**, 449–460.

Masters, W., & Johnson, V. *Human sexual response.* Boston: Little, Brown, 1966.

National Center for Health Statistics. *Acute Conditions: Incidence and Associated Disability, United States, July, 1969–June, 1970.* Vital and Health Statistics, ser. 10, no. 77. Washington, D.C.: Government Printing Office, 1972.

National Society for the Prevention of Blindness. *Estimate of statistics on blindness and vision problems.* New York: Author, 1966.

Newton-John, H. F., & Morgan, D. B. The loss of bone with age, osteoporosis, and fractures. *Clinical Orthopaedics and Related Research,* 1970, **71**, 229–252.

Rossman, I. Anatomic and body composition changes with aging. In C. Finch & L. Hayflick (Eds.), *Handbook of the biology of aging.* New York: Van Nostrand Reinhold, 1977. Pp. 189–216.

Schneider, F. H., & Nandy, K. Effects of centrophenoxine on lipofuscin formation in neuroblastoma cells in culture. *Journal of Gerontology,* 1977, **32**(2), 132–139.

Schwartz, A. A transactional view of the aging process. In A. Schwartz and I. Mensh (Eds.), *Professional obligations and approaches to the aged.* Springfield, Ill.: Charles C. Thomas, 1974.

Selye, H. *The stress of life.* New York: McGraw-Hill, 1976.

Shanas, E. Health status of older people, cross-national implications. *American Journal of Public Health,* 1974, **64**, 261–264.

Shanas, E., & Maddox, G. Aging, health, and the organization of health resources. In R. Binstock & E. Shanas (Eds.), *Handbook of aging and the social sciences.* New York: Van Nostrand Reinhold, 1976. Pp. 592–618.

Shock, N. The physiology of aging. In J. Powers (Ed.), *Surgery of the aged and debilitated patient.* Philadelphia: Saunders, 1968.

Shock, N. Biological theories of aging. In J. Birren & K. W. Schaie (Eds.), *Handbook of the psychology of aging.* New York: Van Nostrand Reinhold, 1977. Pp. 103–115.

Sinex, F. M. The molecular genetics of aging. In C. Finch & L. Hayflick (Eds.), *Handbook of the biology of aging.* New York: Van Nostrand Reinhold, 1977. Pp. 37–58.

Snyder, L., Pyrek, J., & Smith, K. Vision and mental function of the elderly. *Gerontologist,* 1976, **16**(6), 491–495.

Sontag, S. The double standard of aging. *Saturday Review,* Sept. 23, 1972, 29–38.

Spoerri, P., & Glees, P. The mode of lipofuscin removal from hypothalamic neurons. *Experimental Gerontology,* 1975, **10**, 225–228.

Strehler, B. *Time, cells, and aging.* (2nd ed.) New York: Academic Press, 1977.

Tiberi, D., Schwartz, A., & Albert, W. Envy vs. greed: proposed modifications of Medicare policy. *Long Term Care and Health Services Administration Quarterly,* 1977, **1**(3), 275–292.

Trotter, M., & Hixon, B. B. Sequential changes in weight, density, and percentage ash weight of human skeletons from an early fetal period through old age. *Anatomical Record,* 1974, **179**, 1–18.

U.S. Public Health Service. National Center for Health Statistics. *Vital Statistics of the United States: 1970. Vol II: Mortality.* Washington, D.C.: Government Printing Office, 1974.

Wright, B. *Physical disability: A psychological approach.* New York: Harper & Row, 1958.

Zisserman, L. Fractures of the aged, with special reference to the femur. *Journal of the American Geriatric Society,* 1973, **21**, 193–199.

For Further Reading

Cohen, J., Cullen, J. W., & Martin, L. R. (Eds.) *Psychosocial aspects of cancer.* New York: Raven Press, 1982.

Dietz, A. A. (Ed.) *Aging—its chemistry.* Proceedings of the third Arnold O. Beckman Conference in Clinical Chemistry. Washington, D.C.: American Association for Clinical Chemistry, 1979.

Loeb, M., & Howell, S. (Eds.) Nutrition and aging: A monograph for practitioners. *Gerontologist,* 1969, **9** (3, part II).

Masoro, E. J. Physiologic changes with aging. In M. Winick (Ed.), *Nutrition and aging.* New York: John Wiley & Sons, 1976.

Rahe, R. Life change and subsequent illness. In E. Gunderson & R. Rahe (Eds.), *Life stress and illness.* Springfield, Ill.: Charles C. Thomas, 1974.

Winick, M. (Ed.) *Nutrition and aging.* Vol. 4, Current Concepts in Nutrition. New York: John Wiley & Sons, 1976.

Wolf, S., & Goodell, H. *Behavioral science in clinical medicine.* Springfield, Ill.: Charles C. Thomas, 1976.

Wu, R. *Behavior and illness.* Englewood Cliffs, N.J.: Prentice-Hall, 1973.

Psychological Aspects of Behavior in Later Life

Chapter 3

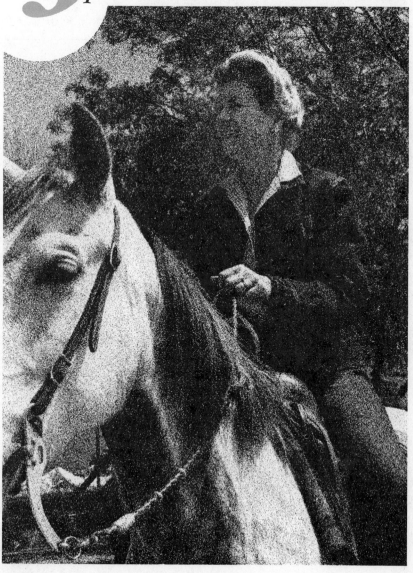

> Enjoy your achievements as well as your plans. . . . Be yourself . . . take
> kindly the counsel of the years, gracefully surrendering the things of
> youth. . . . Beyond a wholesome discipline, be gentle with
> yourself. . . . You are a child of the universe no less than the trees and
> the stars; you have a right to be here.
> *Allegedly found in Old St. Paul's Church, Baltimore, Maryland, dated 1672*

Gerontologists are as much interested in generating knowledge about behavior in later life as psychologists are in discovering general laws of human behavior at every age. More than this, students of human behavior continually try to identify the specific "laws" or principles that will account for unique individual behavior styles. For the gerontologist, the degree of success in accomplishing this determines the extent to which behavioral responses in late maturity can be not only more fully understood but also anticipated or predicted. The present state of the art is such that gerontology can claim only a limited understanding of the dynamics of behavior in old age. While most research findings are not at all conclusive, and much of our knowledge is at best an approximation of the "whole truth," still we are faced with an embarrassment of riches with respect to information about many psychological aspects of aging. Much of this information will require further testing and integration into the larger body of knowledge before it will be relevant to theory building and before it can be applied without restriction.

An important theme throughout this book is the uniqueness of the individual experience of aging. This theme assumes the psychological uniqueness of perception as the older person attempts to cope with events in later life. The following brief essay, reprinted in its entirety from *The New York Times* (1977), is one woman's portrayal of the intense feelings associated with a particular crisis in the later years. This essay presents an individual perspective with which many older persons may identify.

CASE ILLUSTRATION

How Old is Old?

I have recently been retired. I use the passive voice deliberately. This retirement was no act of mine; it was forced upon me by a computer that simply threw up a name to be discarded. It was no act of an admin-

70

istrator who rationally considered the worker and her work. The worker with an excellent record of attendance, responsibility and reliability, whose vigor and willingness were in no way diminished, had to be dismissed. The years of experience were less than nothing.

For some time I had been uneasy, aware that however fit I might be, students, growing up in a society in which the emphasis is on the youth, would think of me as diseased. After all, old age is a disease in America. The aged person becomes a leper, to be put away in an institution, or, if lucky, and affluent, in an expensive colony, separated from the rest of mankind.

I found myself beginning to feel apologetic for my continuing tenure. I felt that I should do as everyone said, go away and make room for a younger person, someone with little or no experience, whose chief asset would be youth, and therefore with more right to the position.

Accordingly, when that dire notice arrived, my reaction was to disappear quietly, to let no one know that I had been struck down with that dread "disease." I was no longer an active, intelligent human being, but a supernumerary to be put out of the way. I wanted no testimonials to my condition. I was ashamed.

Walking about my own neighborhood in the light of day, I would not reveal the truth to inquiries about my idleness. I was on leave, I was writing a book, I was on sabbatical. I could not confess that I was now a relic. I edged away from organizations for the retired, shunning my own kind. I refused to take advantage of the privileges for "senior citizens," continuing to pay full fares, full charges.

But some things are unavoidable, and the whole apparatus of Social Security hit me: papers to be filled out, official ukases to be interpreted, the mimeographed word to be construed, the muddy language of the computer to be painfully transmitted to the understanding, figures to be added up again and again.

Just now, when this great change in my life is taking place, and I need a structured routine, the structure is cut down under my slipping feet. I get up in the morning, just as early, or even earlier, for now I cannot sleep, then go through the household chores, and have nothing further to do.

There is not the stimulation of a shared experience with colleagues, the preoccupation with the work. There is only the lonely house and the lonelier walk. Entertainment soon palls; the freedom of one's own time, the time that stretches endlessly, is not used. But there is also the prickling awareness that that very time is limited, that it must be used at once, or it will be gone. And then one thinks, "What the hell, let it go, it doesn't matter."

Everything seems to be coming to an end anyhow. With the cut in income there is also a cut in benefits, to which I am no longer entitled. So I begin to worry about money: Should I spend it all now—there's so little future left; or should I watch every penny, I may get sick and need private nurses; there will be no one to take care of me when I'm destitute. Should I move, can I afford it, is it worth the effort?

Then there is the question of relationships with former colleagues. I have the time, but they're working, taking on new loads; they're occupied. I must proceed carefully so as not to intrude into their precious time, careful not to injure the fragile bond, careful not to become an annoyance.

Some of these colleagues have expressed envy of my freedom. I used to bewail the fact that I had not enough free time; there were so many things I wanted to do. Now I have all that time, but not the will to do anything. I used to bake bread on those Sundays when I had five sets of papers to mark. I managed to find the time and the energy. Fatigue? It was well-earned fatigue, I had a right to pamper myself. Now I have no right, I have not earned it, I cannot go on that long trip.

The doctor tells me I am "in very good shape." My mind is teeming with ideas, but no one wants them. I don't want to fill in the time before I die. I want to use the time. I need to work, not make-work, not a hobby, not volunteer work. I need a job. I want my old job back. I was good at it.

To be considered unfit for the very job for which I was trained, in which I have many years of experience, is the cruelest kind of rejection.

Then I am truly unfit, no good at anything. There is no longer any incentive to work; there is only the overwhelming fear of further rejection. Nothing else matters, nothing else affords any kind of compensation.

We do not know many details of this anonymous writer's life and circumstances. Still, this brief autobiographical essay suggests some of the questions with which the psychology of aging is concerned:

1. How do we identify the "continuities" and the "discontinuities" between behavior in old age and in the middle years?
2. In what ways is old age "connected" to earlier life experience?
3. Do cognitive processes (e.g., perception, learning, memory, decision making, etc.) change significantly with advancing age? If so, what is the nature of such change and how does it affect functional competence in the elderly?
4. Are cognitive factors in aging more or less important than motivational or personality factors?
5. Are changes in some levels of functional competence to be construed as "senility?"
6. Does personality change over the lifespan?
7. How do we define "mental health" for the elderly population?
8. Is "senility" (often referred to as "senile dementia") a useful label, and is this an inevitable result of growing older?
9. Are there basic criteria for intervention in old age, or are we to believe that *any* kind of helping is "good?"

Theoretical Perspectives

The development of a comprehensive theory to explain and predict normative psychological processes in later life has posed a formidable challenge to gerontologists in their attempts to organize and integrate current knowledge and information about constancy and change across the lifespan. Detailed studies of older persons, more and more of whom are surviving well into their seventh, eighth, and ninth decades and beyond, confirm that while there exist common patterns of adaptation to the tasks and demands of the later years, individual differences in cognitive styles and strategies, responses to motivational variables, and personality structures which occur in the context of diverse physical and social environments appear to be even more the rule than the exception. Clearly, more than one theory is required to describe and define the behavior of the elderly under such diverse circumstances.

Just as theories of child behavior have evolved to explain the development of cognitive processes and intelligence, affect and motivation, and personality and social behavior, so it is that theories which address the psychol-

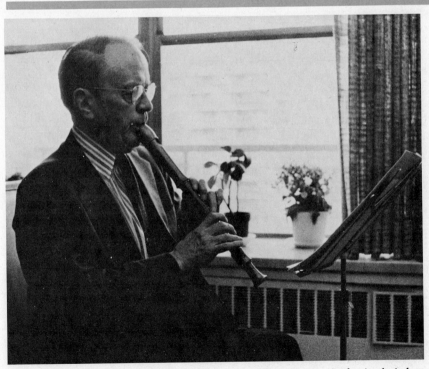

Many older persons are able to function very well, even creatively, in their later years. Many factors in the early and middle years contribute to psychological well-being in old age.

ogy of aging are focused on specific behavioral domains. Indeed, some gerontologists have argued for the extension of theories of child and adolescent behavior (e.g., psychoanalytic theory, Piagetian cognitive theory) through adulthood to provide lifespan continuity to our understanding of human life, rather than the formulation of age-specific theories to account for smaller chunks of the psychological puzzle at various stages of life. Regardless of the extent to which theories of psychological functioning in the later years can be incorporated into a lifespan framework, however, they must be able to accommodate qualitative as well as quantitative change in behavior in the sociocultural and physical environment in which it occurs. The nature-nurture dilemma which pervades the study of psychological processes at any age is best resolved through reference to the person-environment transactional perspective, which maintains that the behavior of any given individual at any point in the lifespan cannot occur independently of social and physical environmental variables. It further provides a functional interface between individual characteristics and patterns of behavior and their environmental contexts (see Chapter 10 for further discussion).

Cognitive Processes

Cognitive processes are described as hypothetical mental events through which individuals indirectly come to know about themselves and their environment. These processes are assumed to operate on cognitive "structures" (i.e., organizational hierarchies, schemas, strategies, or frameworks; cf. Scott, Osgood, & Peterson, 1979) which organize, categorize, and impart meaning to objects and events that are analyzed and synthesized in the individual's cognitive "space" (Saltz, 1973). Evidence for the existence of cognitive processes and structures and of cognitive space is often inferred from the performance of individuals and groups on various tasks administered largely in laboratory settings. Of interest to gerontologists and geropsychologists is the extent to which cognitive processes and structures vary over the course of the lifespan within and between individuals as functions of history and life experience or of maturation and development. Reference to these hypothetical constructs provides a basis for the study of intellective functioning in the later years.

The development of cognitive processes and intelligence in childhood and early adolescence was studied by Piaget and his colleagues over a highly productive fifty-year period of investigation that continues even today. Among the products of these inquiries into the nature of intelligence and its **ontogeny**[1] in the young was the formulation of a stage theory of cognitive development. This theory assumed that intellectual growth is qualitative in

[1] *ontogeny:* development of an individual organism or being

nature and requires the active participation of the child or adolescent in assimilating and accommodating new information into his or her cognitive structures or schemas. According to Piaget, four periods of cognitive development progress in a fixed sequence from birth.

The final period of development, *formal operations,* was assumed to extend throughout the adult years without further qualitative differentiation. Yet it seems reasonable that cognitive processes and structures which mediate behavior in the middle and later years should differ in at least some ways from those which are operational in adolescence and young adulthood, as a function of depth and breadth of experience gained through the years. To this end, Riegel (1975) has proposed an additional developmental stage, that of *dialectical operation,* to account for adult intellective behavior in the face of the situational diversity, ambiguity, and contradiction with which adults are confronted in their daily lives. Labouvie-Vief (1980) has observed that

> the [adult] individual does not function at *one* stage only, but is characterized
> by a degree of multilevel operation in which the highest level of competence
> is achieved only under optimal circumstances. . . . the task of adulthood
> becomes instead to attempt to utilize best one's knowledge towards the
> management of concrete life situations [p. 152–153].

In the same vein, Schaie (1979) has drawn finer distinctions in the sequence of adult cognitive development, while collapsing Piaget's periods of childhood and adolescent development into a single stage. Following this initial *acquisitive* stage, in which cognitive tools and skills are acquired for application in later life periods, is the stage of *achievement.* This second stage, which characterizes young adulthood, is the first major interface between the acquisition of cognitive skills and their application to practical situations as a function of environmental demands. Middle age is differentiated into two parallel stages, one in which greater integration and sophistication in coping with social and environmental challenges and tasks is developed (*responsible* stage), and another, more specialized *(executive)* stage entailing the use of specific, technical strategies and skills in the solution of complex problems which may be superimposed upon the general responsibilities of the middle adult years. Finally, in old age (*reintegration* stage), the information, experiences, and strategies of earlier years are reorganized and resynthesized on the basis of personally salient and efficient characteristics and features. This reorganization process, which reflects the unique impact of the individual on the environment and vice versa, implies an idiosyncratic schema which may contribute to increasing individual differences in performance throughout the later years. Although this schema requires greater elaboration, testing, and evaluation, it provides a useful model for the study of life-span development which is consistent with the person-environmental transactional approach to aging adopted throughout this book.

Information Processing

The study of cognitive processes is a complex, multifaceted approach to the analysis of human behavior at any point in the lifespan. Because of the many different ways information about the individual and his or her environment may be obtained and interpreted, psychologists and gerontologists alike have found it convenient for purposes of investigation to focus upon more limited domains of cognitive processing. These subprocesses generally include (but are not necessarily limited to) attention, sensation, perception, imagery, thinking (e.g., abstract reasoning, **hypothetico-deductive**[1] thought), language acquisition and use (reading, writing, linguistic creativity, oral expression), learning (rote learning, spatial learning, cognitive learning, verbal learning, concept formation and acquisition, motor skills acquisition), memory (encoding, decoding, storage, recall, recognition, retrieval, forgetting), decision making, and problem solving. Our knowledge of cognitive processing in the later years of life has grown rapidly—although in a somewhat piecemeal fashion—over the past few decades as a result of intensive efforts to understand the nature of these more limited functional domains across the lifespan.

With the advent of highly sophisticated computer technology in recent years, one convenient (albeit mechanistic) approach to the systematic organization of information about cognitive processes has been that of information processing (IP), which "can be viewed as a continuous flow of input from receptors at the periphery to the brain" (Hoyer & Plude, 1980, p. 227). The IP approach describes how "sensory input is transformed, reduced, elaborated, stored, recovered, and used even when [cognitive processes] operate in the absence of relevant stimulation" (Neisser, 1966, p. 4).

Well-received by the majority of psychologists and gerontologists alike since the 1950s, IP has proved highly useful as a conceptual frame of reference for the study of cognition, although a number of critical questions about the validity of this approach have been raised (see the following Critical Discussion for details).

While some variation among specific models of information processing does exist, the three-stage model described by Craik (1977) is generally representative of the state of the art. In the first stage of processing, effective sensory inputs are **transduced**[2] by their respective sense organ systems. The resulting copies of sensory experience or *icons* are held in their respective sensory registers for a very brief period of time (generally no more than two seconds). During this period, information may be lost or otherwise obscured by previous or subsequent inputs to the system. If the individual attends to the information in his or her sensory registers, however, it will be further

---

[1] *hypothetico-deductive:* logical system of reality testing through which certain outcomes are expected to follow certain antecedent conditions

[2] *transduction:* process of energy transformation from physical or chemical energy to a nervous impulse

processed in the second stage, referred to as *short-term* or *primary memory.* If information in the form of memory traces is rehearsed sufficiently, it will proceed into the *long-term* or *secondary store.* As information moves from one stage to the next, relevant features may be selected and irrelevant features dropped in keeping with the processing demands and capacities of each stage. While the first two stages are limited in terms of processing time and maximum information capacity, the final stage is capable of storing an infinite amount of information over an indefinite or infinite period of time, providing the information has been well rehearsed and properly encoded.

Now that a brief overview of the IP model has been presented, we will turn our attention to a sample of the aforementioned cognitive subprocesses in order to discover the relationship of this **heuristic**[1] tool to the ways in which the elderly gain knowledge of themselves and their environment.

CRITICAL DISCUSSION
"Now You See It, Now You Don't"

The study of cognitive processes and structures developed as the result of growing dissatisfaction with the behavioristic tradition in psychology, which dominated research and training in the field during the first part of this century. Many psychologists felt that behaviorism's mechanistic stimulus-response (S-R) paradigm ignored or overlooked important organismic variables that contributed significantly to the behavior of organisms, particularly human ones. As the "black box" of organismic variables was slowly opened, initially by Tolman and his colleagues in the 1930s and 1940s, an increasing number of psychologists began to realize the apparent value of casting these variables in a revised stimulus-organism-response (S-O-R) framework.

Today, with the support of the information processing model, cognitive psychology has become a functionally autonomous field of investigation. Entire scholarly journals are devoted to the publication of hundreds of articles describing various aspects of cognitive functioning throughout the lifespan as they relate to the modern technology of the computer. Yet some serious questions have been raised as to the utility and validity of invoking a computer-based model to explain human behavior.

Perhaps the most obvious criticism is that human beings are active perceivers, learners, "rememberers and forgetters," decision makers and problem solvers, while computers must be programmed with certain instructions which subsequently dictate their passive responses. Humans move around their environments; computers are relatively stationary. Humans experience feelings and emotions; computers cannot. Humans make mistakes; computers themselves do not (unless programmed incorrectly by a human, or short-circuited by variations in

---

[1]*heuristic:* helpful in its application in a problem-solving context, but of no intrinsic value beyond that context

human-engineered electrical flow; cf. Estes, 1980). To suggest that humans, too, are "programmed" to respond in certain ways implies that there are miniaturized versions of computer programmers residing somewhere in our bodies (in our brains, perhaps?) who provide us with a service similar to that which humans provide to computers. In other words, "all forms of cognitive processing imply cognition so as to account for cognition" (Gibson, 1979, p. 253), clearly a circular and indefensible position. Neisser has argued for the study of cognitive processes simply "because they are there" (1966, p. 5), but a number of psychologists have challenged even the claim that these processes exist at all.

Aside from these pitfalls in arguing the case for cognitive information processing in humans by analogy to computers, there are other issues that must be addressed with respect to the ways through which humans come to know about themselves and their environments. One is the nature of cognitive processes themselves, and another is how they are studied and analyzed.

As mentioned previously, cognitive processes are hypothetical mental events that are assumed to mediate incoming information and subsequent behavior. Thus, humans come to know about themselves and their environments only indirectly; information is, in a sense, "screened" to provide a subjective picture of reality. Gibson (1966, 1979), among others, has argued that the vast array of hypothetical mental events and structures posited by cognitive theorists are in fact unnecessary to our understanding of behavior. According to his "ecological approach," information about ourselves and our environments is obtained by means of active "information pick-up," through which we directly sample the "affordances" of the environment, i.e., the structural and transformational invariants of the environment, "what it *offers* . . . , what it *provides* or *furnishes,* either for good or for ill" (1979, p. 127). "An affordance points both ways, to the environment and to the observer" (p. 129); "information to specify the utilities of the environment is accompanied by information to specify the observer himself" (p. 141). This process of information pick-up is direct, requiring no mediating processes, structures, or space, and provides a subjective view of reality based upon where we are relative to environmental affordances. Gibson's approach appears to have much utility as well as validity for explaining the ways we gain information about ourselves and our surroundings, and provides a serious challenge to cognitive theorists' attempts to explain such behavior.

Finally, it must be pointed out that cognitive processes and structures, as hypothetical constructs, are neither tangible nor measurable entities. Their existence is **inferred**[1] solely on the basis of performance (response) variables, which are typically investigated under controlled laboratory conditions. The extent to which performance under such relatively sterile and impoverished conditions represents performance in the rich context of everyday life is an unresolved, highly controversial issue (cf. Bugelski, 1981). The generalizability of research findings so

---

[1] *inferred:* assumed to be

obtained is limited, as is their ability to account for behavior at any given point in the lifespan.

This is particularly true of research involving elderly participants who are recruited to serve in studies of cognitive (or other) behavior. A number of studies suggest that elderly individuals whose abilities or intelligence are measured in terms of performance on cognitive (or other) tasks may respond more cautiously than younger adults (Botwinick, 1978). In other words, the performance of the elderly on such tasks may not be truly representative of their abilities due to the effects of response bias, which can differentially mask their responses. Not all older people exhibit cautiousness in their response to such tasks, but it is not always possible to determine the existence of cautiousness and its effects on behavior independent of general task performance—a situation which can impair significantly the validity of research findings.

Related to this is the problem of interpreting the results of cross-sectional studies. Even if older persons are in fact more cautious in their responses to certain kinds of tasks than younger persons, this observation can be taken to mean that cautious behavior increases with increasing age (age change), or that generational differences exist in cautiousness (age difference), or both. Nothing more specific can be determined from the cross-sectional studies which report this phenomenon. It is possible that differences in performance (whether involving cautiousness or not) as well as changes in performance through the lifespan may be the result of inappropriate testing procedures and instruments. For example, many tests of intelligence employed to study cognitive behavior in elderly persons were devised for use with younger adult populations, and may be quite inadequate for properly testing older individuals. It goes without saying that the results of such studies are of questionable utility and validity in describing the ways in which older people come to know about themselves and their environments. Psychologists and gerontologists alike, regardless of their age or their cohort membership, would be well advised to exercise caution in interpreting research on cognitive behavior in the elderly.

Sensation and Perception

Sensation and perception represent the first molar dimensions of the information processing sequence. In general, studies of sensory and perceptual processes in the aged have focused upon changes in the efficiency of these aspects of the processing system in the presence of limited or impoverished information that is often presented in time intervals of very brief duration. Age differences that have resulted in these contexts suggest that the processing systems of older adults are generally less efficient than those of younger adults, and that timing and duration of stimuli to be processed are crucial variables in determining relative efficiency.

These findings have been reported in the study of a variety of sensory-perceptual phenomena. It appears that decreasing efficiency may be related to physiological changes in receptor organs and systems as well as changes in the efficiency and number of functional neurons, the effects of which are cumulative over the course of the lifespan and more notable with advancing age. Detailed descriptions of these physiological changes in the visual, auditory, gustatory (taste), olfactory (smell), haptic (touch), thermal (temperature), and somatic systems are provided in Chapter 2. However, other variables may be implicated in reports of declining efficiency.

A small sample of the tasks in which performance decrements in sensory-perceptual processing have been documented in the elderly will be presented to illustrate typical research efforts in this field. This sample is strongly biased toward the modalities of vision and audition, and thus is not entirely representative of the full range of sensory-perceptual processes.

The absolute threshold is an index of perceptual sensitivity, defined operationally as the lowest level of stimulus energy which can accurately be detected on 50 percent of the occasions in which this level of energy is presented to an observer. Absolute thresholds can be determined for any modality. Many studies designed to determine the level of the absolute threshold for vision and audition as well as the other modalities indicate, in general, that with increasing age, stimulus energy levels must be increased in order to be perceived—in other words, the absolute threshold rises as a function of age (cf. Birren, Bick, & Fox, 1948; Luria, 1960; and Robertson & Yudkin, 1944, on perception of light following periods of dark adaptation; Corso, 1963a, 1963b, for perception of pure tones; and Feldman & Reger, 1967; Farrimond, 1961, for perception of speech).

Other studies, however, call into question the notion that thresholds are valid indices of sensory-perceptual ability and efficiency. Because it is a unitary index, the threshold cannot provide information about the relative influences of perceptual ability and response strategies or bias. As Szafran (1968) has observed, certain response strategies based on cumulative experience may play an important role in an individual's reactions to the presentation of stimuli, particularly in those instances where stimulus energy levels are difficult to perceive (as is the case with absolute thresholds). More recent studies employing signal detection methods (Tanner & Swets, 1954) provide additional evidence for this point.

The advantage of signal detection methods is that they provide independent indices of response bias and sensory-perceptual sensitivity or discriminability. In studies of auditory sensitivity, Craik (1966) and Rees and Botwinick (1971) reported no age differences in ability to perceive pure tones, but discovered significant age differences in response bias: older persons apparently adopted a more "cautious" criterion in their decisions to respond. Indeed, although Rees and Botwinick found that the auditory thresholds of their participants rose with advancing age, the index of sensory/perceptual sensitivity remained relatively constant across the age groups tested. Quite obviously, the contributing factor to age differences in thresholds was response bias and not ability. In a study of visual illusion perception using signal detection methods, Snyder (1979) also found no age differences in sensory-perceptual ability, in contrast to a number of earlier studies reporting age differences in thresholds relative to this phenomenon (e.g., Comalli, 1965; Gajo, 1966; Wapner, Werner, & Comalli, 1960). These studies suggest that perception is by no means a "pure" process, but is affected by (and, in turn, affects) other cognitive processes.

Other tasks in which age differences in sensation/perception appear to exist are those that investigate critical flicker frequency (e.g., Weale, 1965), figural aftereffects (e.g., Eisdorfer & Axelrod, 1964), visual masking (Kline & Birren, 1975; Kline & Szafran, 1975; Till, 1978; Walsh, 1976; Walsh, Till, & Williams, 1978), and many more. These findings must be evaluated and interpreted, however, in light of several critical observations:

1. Sensory/perceptual studies are designed, for the most part, as cross-sectional investigations reflecting age differences rather than age changes. To interpret these studies, incorrectly, as indicative of declining efficiency (change) overlooks generational or cohort differences which may, in fact, be largely responsible for the statistical trends obtained.

2. Because sensation and perception are hypothetical constructs, they cannot be directly measured, but instead are assessed indirectly through task performance. It may be that any observed decline in processing efficiency in the later years is the result of extraneous task- or performance-related factors which mask the true ability and capacity of the elderly to function, in comparison to their younger counterparts.

3. In most instances, the purported decline in processing efficiency in older adults is observed in the context of laboratory experiments rather than under "real life" conditions. The control of variables made possible in a laboratory setting raises the important question of whether such measures are valid indicators of the ways in which older persons (or persons of any age, for that matter) truly function. The paucity of information presented to experimental participants, and the extreme time constraints they are under, have little resemblance to the rich array of information normally present over longer periods of time in an individual's typical daily environment. If laboratory studies are not valid indicators of sensory-perceptual functioning, then differences in performance which have characterized the literature in this area of study may be **statistical artifacts**[1] in many (if not most) cases—at least insofar as these differences are construed to be caused by age. A "decline in sensory/perceptual efficiency" reported for laboratory-tested older persons does not necessarily mean that an elderly individual's functional capacity and competence outside the laboratory are on the wane.

4. Various investigators account for reported decrements in sensory and perceptual processing by pointing to physiological changes in receptor organ sensitivity or the reduced efficiency or number of neurons (nerve cells) which occurs with age. Again, while there may be some relationship between physiological (molecular) change and behavioral (molar) variables, the

---

[1] *statistical artifacts:* methodologically-produced errors which may distort experimental results

human organism is highly adaptable; biology seems somewhat less important with age, while psychosocial and environmental factors play an increasingly important role in determining functional capacity and efficiency. It is quite possible, therefore, that while physiological factors are correlated with sensory/perceptual functioning, they do not necessarily determine processing efficiency in the elderly (cf. Corso, 1977).

5. Individual differences in responding to sensory/perceptual tasks are increasingly common with advancing age. Many older persons perform significantly better on such tasks than younger persons. Inappropriate sampling techniques can lead to the selection of less-than-representative samples of older people, which may bias group results. In any case, it is important to keep in mind that generalizations about the capacity and competence of the entire population of older persons based on evidence obtained from a small sample of aged individuals are not necessarily warranted.

Learning and Memory

The old adage "You can't teach an old dog new tricks" dies hard. In spite of the fact that little experimental evidence of learning in old dogs has been reported, recent research suggests what experience confirms: the old adage is outdated when referring to learning in elderly humans (Arenberg & Robertson-Tchabo, 1977).

This is not to suggest that we cannot distinguish the performance of younger from older learners. In most instances, comparisons of learning performance among different age groups favor young adults. But considerable progress has been made in indentifying conditions that impair or improve the learning performance of older individuals.

Although virtually all research strategies approach learning and memory as separate functions, the investigation of one is inevitably complicated by factors implicating the presence of the other. In other words, one cannot assess the efficiency of memory (recall, recognition, and retrieval versus forgetting) processes without considering whether initial learning has taken place. Nor can one test the effectiveness of a learning procedure independent of memory processes.

Few studies have employed the longitudinal approach to study learning and memory in older adults, a method more appropriate to determining developmental change over time. One such study, reported by Gilbert (1973), tested people in their twenties and thirties on a verbal learning task and then retested them on the same task thirty-five to forty years later. In the study of verbal learning, this test-retest method has been commonly used to study the efficiency of learning and recalling words presented in discrete pairs (paired-associated learning) or in sequence (serial list learning) under highly controlled conditions.

Research in this area has shown a decline in performance among older participants. One question that researchers raise is whether retesting the same individuals at a later time introduces a "retesting bias" that improves performance. Although early reports of learning and retention scores show a decline with age, vocabulary scores remain high. Therefore, Arenberg's caution regarding such studies must be heeded: it is necessary to control for retest effects and to control for effects of noncomparability of testing materials when studying aging in this context (Arenberg & Robertson-Tchabo, 1977).

Of special importance in interpreting age differences is the distinction made between learning and memory on the one hand and performance on the other. Learning and memory, as mentioned earlier, are hypothetical constructs; learning represents the more global acquisition of general information, knowledge, and rules, memory the retention of specific events occurring at a given time and place. They cannot be measured directly, but rather are inferred from performance on various tasks. For example, an older man

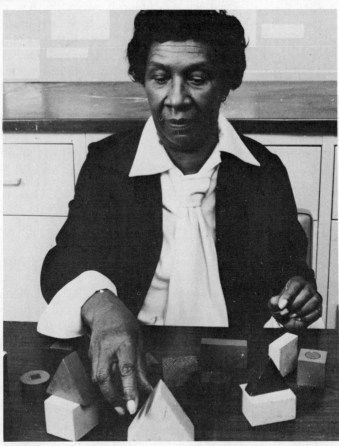

Psychological and intelligence tests must be used with great caution with the elderly so that they are not penalized or stigmatized by inappropriate or invalid test procedures.

may have memorized an item from a list as part of an experimental test of learning and memory, and yet fail to remember it in his response under certain conditions. Although he may have learned the item, his performance could at times suggest otherwise.

In addition to studies of verbal learning behavior in the elderly, several other kinds of learning have been investigated. Included among these are classical conditioning, psychomotor skills, and practical learning (Botwinick, 1978).

Classical Conditioning, Psychomotor Skills, and Practical Learning

In studies of classical conditioning, stimuli that reliably produce a reflexive response are paired with other (neutral) stimuli that normally do not elicit that response. Following repeated presentations of these paired stimuli to a research participant, an association between these stimuli develops so that when the formerly neutral stimulus is presented in the absence of the eliciting stimulus, a reflexive response occurs. Studies of classical conditioning in the elderly generally indicate that older persons are less resistant to learning under such conditions. In addition, once conditioning has occurred, older persons are less likely to continue responding to the formerly neutral stimulus when it is presented alone (i.e., older persons "extinguish" more rapidly) in comparison to younger persons (cf. Braun & Geiselhart, 1959; Kimble & Pennypacker, 1963).

Psychomotor skills provide the foundation for a wide range of behavior throughout the lifespan. Noble (1978) summarizes the results of several factor analytic studies designed to isolate the major components of psychomotor skills tasks. These include arm-hand steadiness, control precision, finger dexterity, manual dexterity, multilimb coordination, rate control, reaction time, response orientation, speed of arm movement, and wrist-finger speed. It is interesting to note that four of these factors are directly related to task pacing and speed, which appear to reliably distinguish the performance of older from younger subjects on a variety of tasks (e.g., Birren, Woods, & Williams, 1980; Cunningham, 1980; Stern, Oster, & Newport, 1980). Somewhat less distinguishable is the performance of older versus younger persons on untimed tasks which focus on mastery or power (Noble, 1978). The following observation has been made with respect to psychomotor performance and age:

> Sensory and perceptual abilities show an earlier and steeper impairment than do motor . . . abilities; complex tasks tend to produce greater differences among age groups than do simple tasks; [and] although general trends based on the averages of age groups are clear and replicable, there is considerable overlapping caused by individual differences [Noble, 1978, p. 318].

Studies of practical learning, while limited in number, tend to suggest that "all age groups can learn, and some methods of training are especially helpful to the older worker," when learning is assessed in occupational contexts (Botwinick, 1978, p. 305). One practical task that is largely dependent upon psychomotor skills learning and performance is driving an automobile. Figure 3–1 shows the number of licensed drivers among the elderly (based on 1974 data). While no information is provided on the ages of these individuals when they first learned to drive or the number of years they have been driving, this figure does suggest that a large proportion of older persons can perform the relatively complex functions involved in operating a motor vehicle at least well enough to obtain a license. No doubt familiarity and experience compensate for changes in reaction time and other factors that might otherwise interfere with successful performance of this practical task.

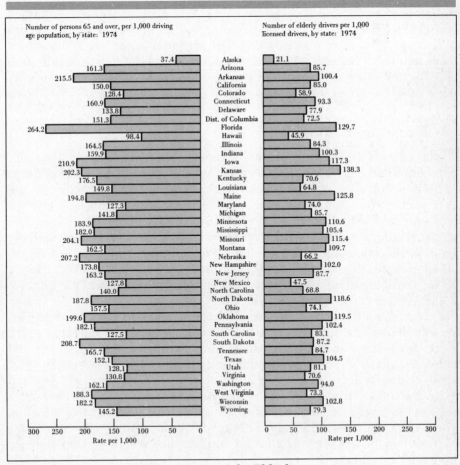

FIGURE 3–1.   Licensed Drivers among the Elderly

Note: Based on the 42 states reporting their number of licensed drivers in 1974.

Source: U.S. Department of Transportation, 1977.

Memory

Many findings and observations across a variety of learning tasks indicate that most age-associated memory deficiencies occur in recent short-term (primary) memory, while remote, long-term (secondary) memory tends to remain intact. We need to keep in mind that short-term memory, the initial stage of memory storage, is highly dependent upon the efficient operation of the sensory, perceptual, and learning components of information processing, and that it is also affected by many other social, psychological, and physical factors. The incredible number of variations in all these factors accounts for the wide range of differences that can be observed in older individuals' memory functions. Dealing with aged persons in a clinical context or any other one-to-one situation, therefore, demands individualized evaluation and instruction sensitive to these variations. A physician explaining a complicated therapeutic regimen to an elderly patient, a clinical geropsychologist or geropsychiatrist interviewing an aged client, a nurse seeking "informed consent" from an elderly patient, an instructor teaching a class that includes elderly students, a pharmacist filling a prescription for an aged customer, a bank teller or a Social Security clerk asking an elderly person to fill out a complicated form—in every case possible problems with primary memory must be taken into account.

Decision Making

Studies of the ways people of different ages react to different situations, coupled with the apparent need for more time on the part of older people to perform a variety of tasks, has been interpreted by some to mean that the elderly characteristically may be more reluctant to take a chance on giving a response about which they are uncertain. This means that for an elderly individual making a decision about whether to respond in a certain manner, the kinds of task materials presented, the nature and clarity of task instructions, and the degree of emotional support involved are important considerations; so are possible arousal or anxiety, the level of confidence, and the ultimate degree of success in task performance.

A commonly observed feature of response patterns among older persons in ability testing is the tendency to commit errors of omission much more frequently than errors of commission—in other words, not to respond rather than respond and risk committing an error (e.g., Botwinick, 1966, 1969; Eisdorfer, Alexrod, & Wilkie, 1963; Korchin & Basowitz, 1957; Wallach & Kogan, 1961). It is assumed that the difference in these two error rates reflects the level of confidence of older individuals in a demand situation. The reluctance to respond and the degree of "cautiousness" shown by older persons may in fact serve as a useful and adaptive self-protection strategy. Botwinick comments:

> It would seem that the elderly may be cautious when there is no reason to be otherwise. When, however, there is reason to take risks, they seem to be no

more cautious than anyone else. It may be wise to be risky only when there is a meaningful reason to do so [1978, p. 136].

Intelligence

The concept of intelligence has come to have an especially important status simply because intelligence tests have come to be so widely used as the basis for judgments and decisions affecting vocational and educational careers and perceived social status. Nevertheless, intelligence is an intangible construct. Psychologists have attempted to make it more tangible by defining certain ways of measuring it.

An extreme definition offered by Boring (1923) is that "intelligence is what intelligence tests measure." While this may be true from an operational perspective, the wide variety of intelligence tests devised over the past several decades would force us to conclude that there are as many definitions of intelligence as there are instruments to measure it. What, then, *is* intelligence, and what kinds of tests are most appropriate for its assessment? Does intelligence remain stable over the lifespan, or does it change as we grow older? What sampling techniques and research methods are best suited for evaluating intelligence in the later years? Inconsistencies in the answers to these and other related questions have been identified by Botwinick (1977) as some of the difficulties attendant to the study of intellectual functioning in the elderly.

Given the problems of validity associated with certain methods of research in gerontology, it is important first to distinguish between *age changes* and *age differences* with respect to intelligence in the elderly. Cross-sectional studies, for example, have typically shown a decline in intellectual ability beginning at midlife and extending throughout the later years. These findings contrast sharply, however, with data reported from longitudinal studies (Schaie & Strother, 1968).

As can be seen from Figure 3–2, follow-up studies undertaken in the early 1960s by Schaie and Strother in effect converted their earlier cross-sectional studies into a longitudinal paradigm. Schaie (1975) concluded that the relatively small declines in his longitudinal study reflected age differences between groups, rather than decremental age changes over the lifespan of the individual. That is, different generations appeared to perform at different levels of ability or proficiency. In addition, measures of performance gathered from an aging (longitudinal) sample also reflected instances within the sample where extraneous, intruding factors apparently interfered with the ability of individuals to respond.

Figure 3–2 depicts the results of a vocabulary recognition test as reported on appropriate age gradients within generations. Schaie draws attention to the fact that the peak functional age in the longitudinal sequence of this study is fifty-five, not thirty-five, as suggested by the cross-sectional data. Even at age seventy, according to these results, estimated performance is still at a higher level than it was at age twenty-five.

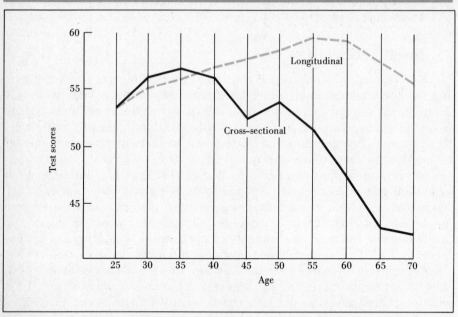

FIGURE 3–2. Comparible Cross-Sectional and Longitudinal Age Gradients for the Verbal Meaning Test

Source: Schaie, K. W., & Strother, C. R. A cross-sequential study of age changes in cognitive behavior. *Psychological Bulletin,* 1968, *70:* 671–680.

In another study of this phenomenon, when measures were taken over a fourteen-year period (from which three cross-sectional gradients were derived), the shape of the gradient (curve) of decline appeared identical for each age group (Schaie & Labouvie-Vief, 1974). That is, for each time period tested, later-born cohorts performed better than earlier-born ones. As a result, the age of peak performance keeps increasing over generations, a finding interpreted by Schaie to mean that "we are smarter than our parents were, and . . . our children, in turn, are likely to be smarter than we are" (1975, p. 119).

Generational differences arise from various sociohistorical changes which may contribute to the behavior (performance) measured on intelligence tests. These include the amount and complexity of general information disseminated in society; the speed of information dissemination (e.g., the differences between those who grew up before and after the invention and marketing of TV); the experience of living through a severe economic depression and a series of worldwide political conflicts; changes in formal educational attainment; changes in nutritional values and habits; and many other environmental variations that occur from one era to another and thus provide a different set of experiences from one generation to the next.

Specific situational factors may also contribute to age differences in performance. For example, it has been pointed out that because elderly persons are more likely to tire during extended periods of testing, fatigue may affect their performance. If this is the case, then any conclusions about age differences in intellectual capacity might be called into question on this count as well.

Furry and Baltes (1973) compared the performance of individuals in three age groups (eleven to fourteen, thirty to fifty, and fifty-one to eighty) on the Primary Mental Abilities (PMA) test. One procedure involved a twenty-minute pretest that was included to induce fatigue. Half the participants in each group were given this pretest, while the other half were not.

A statistically significant interaction between age and fatigue was found for three of the PMA subtests. On the Reasoning and Verbal Meaning subtests, the two younger groups were apparently unaffected by fatigue, in contrast to the adverse effects of fatigue on the performance of the oldest group. On the Word Fluency subtest, both adult groups were adversely affected by fatigue, but the adolescents were not; in fact, they actually performed better than when the pretest was omitted. The results of the two adult groups from the Reasoning subtest are shown in Figure 3–3, which clearly shows how a situationally induced factor like fatigue (F) can easily lower the performance of an older group.

Thus it is important to distinguish between performance-related versus

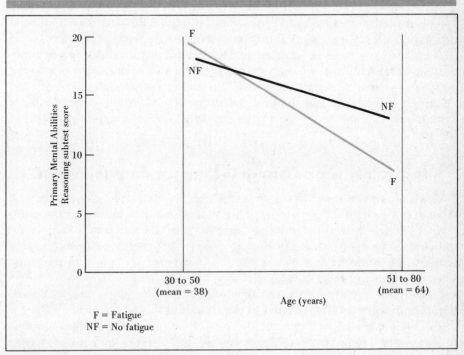

FIGURE 3–3. The Results of Two Adult Groups on the Primary Mental Abilities Subtest for Reasoning
Source: Furry & Baltes, 1973.

absolute capacity or ability factors in the accurate assessment of intelligence. Every effort should be made to control extraneous performance factors that may obscure the true ability of older persons, regardless of the research methods employed.

Performance factors as well as other extraneous variables appear to contribute to the minor changes observed in intellectual functioning in the context of longitudinal research studies as well. Again, while the nature of such change suggests a slight decline in cognitive ability, such decline is more likely due to methodological artifact than to aging per se. For example, increasing mortality rates with the increasing age of a study sample may mean that some individuals recruited for study participation may not survive to be tested again at a later date. This situation can result in a group which, at the end of a study, may be no longer representative of the sample originally selected for participation. Smaller group size may mean that individual differences in ability and other extraneous factors will be magnified in such a way as to distort the results of the entire group.

For example, Kleemeier (1962) and others have observed a phenomenon referred to as "terminal drop": impending death is often preceded by a relatively sharp decline in cognitive functioning. This phenomenon is not necessarily age-dependent, but seems to occur prior to the final collapse and demise of the individual at whatever age. A study of twins over a twelve-year period confirmed preliminary evidence of terminal drop (Jarvik & Falek, 1963). It may be that some longitudinal studies of intellectual functioning have included in their samples one or more individuals who have died relatively soon after being tested. If this has been the case we might expect group performance scores to be somewhat depressed due to the decline in functioning (terminal drop) reflected in the performance of participants who are rapidly approaching death. Thus it is altogether possible that, rather than declining in the later years, intellectual ability (considered independently of extraneous factors) may remain relatively stable throughout the adult lifespan.

Individual versus Group Differences in Intelligence

All of the studies touched on so far refer, of course, to group behavior. What about individual variations? Some elderly individuals may show intellectual decline, but so do some younger persons. By the same token, some individuals have shown a gain in performance between seventy and eighty years, while some have shown a decline between twenty and thirty years. What accounts for these variations?

We have already mentioned the rich complexity of events and conditions (both internal and external to the individual) that can either enhance or inhibit successful performance on tests of various kinds, including intelligence tests. Frequently the higher test scores of older persons who continue to be active in a richly stimulating environment confirm that the "use it or lose it" principle applies to intelligence.

A question that gerontological researchers ask in this connection is: how important, pragmatically speaking, are differences in intellectual performance between younger and older persons? Without question, behavioral scientists pay a great deal of attention to differences that are "statistically significant." All that really means is that the differences found are reliable; that is, they are quite likely to occur again if the same testing is repeated under the same conditions. It does not mean that the differences are necessarily large or important. In practical terms, some "statistically significant" differences turn out to be so small as to have no practical meaning for the activities of daily living (Schaie, 1975). Some differences do have practical consequences; other differences are inconsequential. The fact that an older person can recall four nonsense syllables fewer per three-minute interval than a younger person is likely to have little direct impact upon the life of anyone. In contrast, demonstrated age differences in spatial visualization may in fact require revisions in criteria for employment of older tool-and-die makers or airline pilots.

One conclusion to be drawn from the foregoing is that while differences in performance between successive generations have been observed and measured, the question of differences in capacity between later life and the earlier part of the lifespan requires much more careful study and astute interpretation before it is settled.

For example, differences in performance are often attributed to the slowing down associated with advancing age. That is the usual explanation for why elderly persons perform better on the Verbal Scale of the Wechsler Adult Intelligence Scale (WAIS) than the Performance Scale (the "classic aging pattern"). Most of the latter subtests are timed tests, and because they put a premium on speed of performance do not allow for individual self-pacing, and thus penalize the slower-performing older person. With regard to decrements in learning and memory efficiency associated with aging, even if it is true that older persons have more memory problems than do younger persons, no satisfactory answer as to why this is the case has yet been reported. Perhaps it is not only memory that changes with experience, as Estes (1980) has stated. Perhaps a first step toward that answer may be recognition that when we fail to recall a name or an event it is not that something is wrong with our memory but that something has changed in us (Bugelski, 1981). And to some extent, at least, the circumstances (environmental contingencies) that affect us all are different in terms both of objective contingencies and how they are subjectively perceived.

Motivation

The systematic identification and integration of motivational variables that determine or otherwise affect the behavior of the elderly are tasks of major importance to geropsychologists. Why is it that some older persons lead full, active, enriching, productive, and satisfying lives while others feel bored, tired, depressed, and useless, and withdraw from their social and physical environments?

Motivation has been viewed from various perspectives; yet it is, "at bottom, the control of action by subjective gains and losses" (Brown & Herrnstein, 1975, p. 112). The governing principle upon which action appears to be based is the *law of relative effect:* organisms generally behave in ways that are consistent with the relative quantity or quality of positive outcomes that result from their behavior.

While some psychologists have examined motivation in terms of physiologically based needs to which humans and other animals respond, others have recognized the equal—if not greater—role of cognitive, social, and environmental variables in the shaping of human action.

For the geropsychologist attempting to understand motivation as an intervening variable that may facilitate or impede behavior across the lifespan, the task is thus:

1. To identify gains and losses as sources of intrinsic versus extrinsic motivation.
2. To determine the relative importance of gains and losses to the elderly as a function of previous experience and current circumstance.
3. To determine the extent to which personal responsibility and attribution of control influence the functional integrity of older people.

Gains and losses are examined in greater detail in Chapter 9, but it is important at this point to distinguish the effects of these outcome variables on behavior. First, gains and losses can influence behavior *extrinsically*—that is, outcome variables that are separate from but dependent upon a person's responses can increase or decrease the possibility that the person will respond in a similar fashion in the future. For example, an elderly woman might walk a long way from her home to buy groceries at a distant market. If she arrives at the market and finds there all the items on her list (positive outcome or gain), it is likely that she will walk that distance again to shop there in the future. On the other hand, if she is unsuccessful in finding the groceries she wants, she may not choose to walk so far to that store at a later date (the negative outcome or loss results in a reduction in walking behavior, at least to the market). In this case, walking is a means to an end and is not necessarily perceived as rewarding in and of itself; its occurrence is controlled by other variables.

Some behavior, however, may be *intrinsically* motivated—that is, the behavior itself may be rewarding or punishing. This would be the case in our example if the elderly woman simply enjoys walking as a pleasant activity regardless of any extrinsic consequence that might follow from it. Intrinsically motivated behavior may also be said to be self-regulated, or under an internal locus of control of reinforcement, while extrinsically motivated behavior may be described as regulated by other persons or by the contingencies of the external environment, or under an external locus of control of reinforcement (De Charms, 1976; Rotter, 1966).

Some gains and losses that occur throughout the lifespan are not necessarily linked to specific or identifiable behavioral antecedents but may occur as the result of some fortuitous or unknown circumstance. Thus some gains and losses may at times occur independent of an individual's behavior. This point is relevant to our earlier question concerning the activity and productivity of some older people versus the passivity and feelings of uselessness characteristic of others in their later years. As we grow older we are more likely to experience multiple losses over which we have limited, if any, control. Examples might be the loss of sensory acuity (personal loss), a spouse or close companion (social loss), or of a job which includes the accompanying loss of income, social contacts, social status, and a familiar environment (social and environmental loss; see Chapter 9 for further examples). In the case of these and other time-related losses, in most cases the older individual cannot successfully exercise control over negative, punitive outcomes. In the case of mandatory retirement policies based solely on a person's chronological age, for instance, it is impossible to control the passage of time that leads to the loss of a job.

Each loss represents a decrease or limitation of personal freedom and autonomy, as the individual's functional capacity, social support network, physical environment, or all three are restricted in quality and scope. As these losses accrue in the later years, people who have come to expect that they themselves can do something about it (those with an internal locus of control) may be more motivated to change their situation by choosing alternative response strategies and patterns, by changing their social environment, or by changing their physical environment. Conversely, older people exposed to multiple loss who expect that there is nothing they can effectively do to change things (those with an external locus of control) will probably become less motivated and responsive and more passive as a result.

Interestingly, these observations are also consistent with Gibson's (1966, 1979) approach to ecological perception (see Critical Discussion earlier in this chapter), according to which people must actively engage in the process of "information pick-up" in order to perceive themselves and their environment accurately. To the extent that people or their environments are limited, information pickup will suffer and normal interactions with objects and events will be impaired. The noncontingent multiple losses that accumulate over time can restrict an individual's ability to engage in active information pick-up by restricting the individual's functional capacity through sensory, perceptual, cognitive, emotional, or psychomotor impairments; reducing the social network of family and friends, and increasing impersonal social controls over the range of the individual's behavior; and reducing environmental affordances through the restriction of appropriate environmental contingencies (Snyder, 1981).

Quite obviously, there is a wide range of individual differences in response to multiple loss among the elderly; the sense of being in control in the face of such loss may vary as a function of the type of loss experienced, the frequency of loss within a given period of time, the cumulative effects of various kinds of loss, and the nature of response to loss in the past, as well as many other factors.

Reactance, Adaptation, Competence, and Coping

One response to the loss of personal autonomy and freedom occasioned by the occurrence of loss is "psychological reactance" (Brehm, 1972)—an increase in motivation to regain personal freedom and control, resulting in renewed attempts to engage in the behavior that has been restricted. Perhaps the best examples of this are the activities undertaken by the Gray Panthers, a well-known advocacy and lobbying organization that has endeavored to restore personal control to the elderly and establish collective control by and for them in social, economic, and political affairs. In some cases, however, reactance may not be an appropriate response, particularly if it continually fails to result in positive outcomes (i.e., fails to restore a sense of internal locus of control).

Apparently the key to successful adaptation and coping is competence, "characterized by a flexible, adaptable, and personally rewarding response to environmental demands, whatever they may be" (Kuypers & Bengston, 1960). Indeed, McClelland (1973) has gone so far as to propose that we would do better to test for competency rather than for intelligence in the elderly, an argument further elaborated and documented in aging research by Fisher (1973). Competence is further defined as successful social-role performance; as the capacity to adapt to environmental change; and as personal feelings of mastery and internal control (Kuypers & Bengston, 1973). The sense of personal control plays a major role in determining older persons' responses to a wide range of stressful situations (Averill, 1973), and is strongly implicated as a contributor to life satisfaction in the elderly (Palmore & Luikart, 1972). According to Kobasa (1979), the sense of control is provided by:

1. Decisional control, or the option to choose from among several courses of action
2. Cognitive control, or the ability to interpret stressful life events in the framework of an ongoing life plan
3. Coping skills, or a greater repertoire of suitable responses to stress (Examples of coping skills include information seeking, direct action, inhibition of action, and intra-psychic coping; Lazarus & Launier, 1978.)

A "sense of commitment to various areas of life, such as work, social institutions, interpersonal relations, family, and self" (Kobasa, 1979), and a sense of humor, or the ability to gain a different and unusual perspective on even undesirable life experiences (Jewett, 1973), may further contribute to self-perceptions of control and to competent functioning. In addition, strong social support that "would allow elderly individuals to assume true competence in the sense of being their own locus of evaluation and control" (Kuypers & Bengston, 1973, p. 198) is an important factor in promoting adjustment in the elderly, and may involve at least five functions (Silver & Wortman, 1981):

1. The conveyance of positive feelings such as that one is cared for, loved, esteemed, and valued (cf., for example, Carl Rogers's concept of unconditional positive regard)
2. The validation of the stressed individual's feelings and thoughts as "normal"
3. The encouragement of an open expression of feelings and thoughts
4. The provision of material aid
5. The conveyance of information about belongingness to a mutually reciprocating social network.

Feedback provided in response to competent functioning of elderly persons such as successful performance of social roles and adaptation to

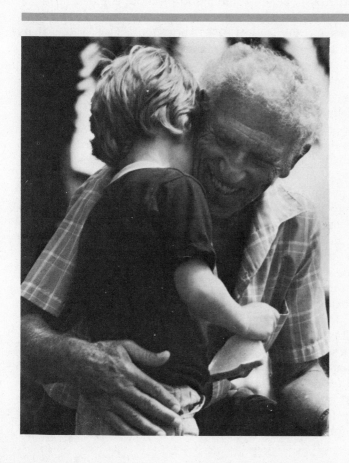

environmental change contributes not only to feelings of mastery and internal control, but also to feelings of personal worth, or self-esteem. And just as competent functioning promotes self-esteem, so self-esteem helps to maintain competent functioning (Schwartz, 1975).

Self-esteem is developed in the individual through those innumerable events, large and small, that provide emotional support and psychological reward. Such events can range from the cuddling and stroking the newborn infant receives to the public recognition represented by the award of certificates and other tokens of appreciation for the contributions of adult life. All these events mirror back to the individual an image of self that says, "You belong, you count, you are worthwhile, you are important." Accompanying these are the self-referent signals that denote mastery and control over oneself and the environment, one's personal space, that reassure the individual: "You are effective, you have an impact, you make a difference."

Threats to Competent Functioning and Self-Esteem

With the accumulation of multiple losses in the later years, the positive reflections that form the basis of self-esteem and promote competent functioning may become distorted, and in some cases reflections may convey negative messages. Kuypers and Bengston (1973) and Wigdor (1980) note that older persons seem to become more dependent upon external stimuli and "social labeling" for information about functional competence and self-worth. Yet our social value system offers little in the way of positive rewards and incentives for behavior which "is adaptive or appropriate to the changing life situations with advancing age" (Wigdor, 1980, p. 250). In large part, this is due to the lack of appropriate behavioral norms for the elderly. As a result, unfavorable comparisons may be made between older individuals and their middle-aged counterparts, for whom normative behavior is described in terms of achievement, competitiveness, and acquisition in the contexts of social and economic productivity. Without positive feedback to signify personal worth and effectiveness in the later years, behavioral options which serve to enhance self-esteem and functional competence become limited. In addition, exploratory as well as instrumental (goal-directed) activities may decline (Elias & Elias, 1977; Wigdor, 1980).

Older individuals who experience loss of internal control over behavioral options and outcomes may eventually learn to expect that they are incapable of producing positive results or change as the result of their behavior. If adaptive resources such as coping skills and social and environmental support are poorly developed, inappropriate, or unavailable, the older person may come to feel useless, worthless, and helpless.

One response that can further threaten the self-esteem and functional competence of the older individual experiencing "learned helplessness" is overzealous "helping" behavior on the part of other persons. Infantilization of the elderly is a trap into which unwitting professionals and family members too easily fall. It entails taking over the responsibilities of older persons,

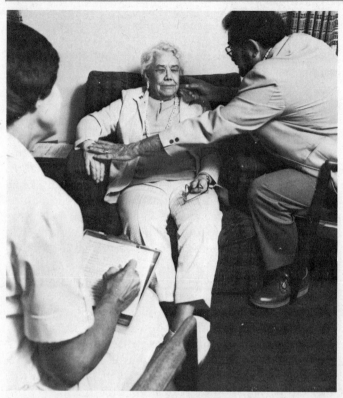

A gross screening technique for cognitive dysfunction, the Face-Hand Touch Test, is illustrated here. It must be used carefully, appropriately, and interpreted with extreme caution.

doing much more for older persons than they actually request or require. Although often performed in the interests of safety (as if all hazards in life could be eliminated), efficiency (as if dressing or performing other routine activities of daily life as quickly as possible were essential to life satisfaction), and cleanliness (as if spilling food from a tremulous hand were something to be avoided at all cost), this type of behavior is, nonetheless, destructive of the sense of competence and control. Getting things accomplished "in service to the elderly" in a brisk, efficient, neat manner—especially things that the elderly are capable of doing for themselves—infantilizes the old and erodes their sense of competence, self-worth, and self-esteem. It also devalues the ability of the elderly to function on their own. Social support providers, including family members and friends, must recognize the need to "deinvest their own power and control [in order to permit] self-determination by the elderly," and must find alternative means to provide "a source of exciting and relevant efforts to improve the condition of the elderly" (Kuypers & Bengston, 1973, pp. 199, 198).

Depression in the Old

The phenomenon of learned helplessness has been investigated by a number of researchers, most notably Seligman (1973, 1974, 1975), who has observed some striking similarities between learned helplessness and depression. Depression is one of the major and common manifestations of stress among older persons. It may vary in duration (from brief to extended episodes) as well as degree (from a mild state of pessimism to deep, pervasive black gloom or despair). In addition, a general withdrawal of interest may also be observed in an older person, and a slowing of activity, sometimes to the point of complete immobility in cases of pronounced depression. One common indicator of depression is the marked inclination to spend long periods of time dozing in a chair or asleep in bed (also associated with a high level of boredom). Typical physical signs of depression encountered in older persons include disturbances in appetite, weight loss, an unusual level of fatigue or feelings of malaise, and constipation (Pfeiffer, 1977). Also associated with depression is crying, although on occasion a person may report that he or she feels like crying but is unable to do so.

Seligman (1974) and others have observed that some older persons may die because they have come to feel useless, helpless, and depressed, and believe that they have no good reason to continue living. Frail elderly individuals are especially vulnerable to this feeling, often as the result of particularly inappropriate environmental contingencies (discussed in greater detail in Chapter 10). Again, the feeling of having control over oneself and one's environment appears to be of utmost importance in preventing the unnecessary dysfunction and perhaps untimely death of older people.

It is important to recognize that a depressed elderly person may deny feeling depressed while at the same time exhibiting physical signs and ailments that signal depression. This is the point at which the perceptive observer or interviewer will search for the relevant contributors to stress (including varying degrees of uncontrollable loss) in the depressed person's social and physical environment. An important, if not imperative, therapeutic role for professionals of all kinds working with old people is to go far beyond mere routine diagnostic procedures and to aim at mobilizing the elderly individual's strengths, coping skills, assets, and aspirations to facilitate competence, a sense of control, and self-esteem.

Personality

Psychologists define personality in terms of the probabilities of certain responses and the patterns of characteristic behaviors that flow from the way in which a given individual is dynamically organized. This is in contrast to common parlance, the pop definition of personality as "social impact"—that is, the effect or impact an individual has upon others in social situations ("warm," "outgoing," "lots of fun," "wet blanket," and so on).

The study of personality in aging follows from the premise that the behavior of the elderly is ordinarily not random but is consistent with certain general laws of behavior common to all humans (nomothetic laws), and consistent with specific laws unique to one given individual (idiographic laws). To answer properly the question "What personality changes are associated with chronological age in later life?" we must take into account not only the changes in behavior that do occur, but also what appears to be an underlying current of stability and consistency in personality across the lifespan.

Another dimension of the same issue has to do with the continuities versus discontinuities of personality and behavior. This dichotomy draws attention to the connectedness (or unconnectedness) of behavior at one time with behavior in an earlier period. But describing behavior in this way does not explain personality and behavior change.

Generally, the psychological literature describes age differences that may be observed on some measures of personality and not on others (Neugarten, 1977). This reminds us that personality, like intelligence, is a multifaceted hypothetical construct. Some excellent and intriguing work has been conducted on personality and behavioral changes with age that is relevant to the continuity versus discontinuity issue (Gutmann, 1977; Lowenthal, Thurner, Chiriboga, et al., 1975). According to these studies, men appear to progress from an active, instrumental, assertive pattern of behavior to a more passive, undemanding, dependent stance in later life. In contrast, women apparently move from a greater degree of helplessness and dependency to a more assertive, aggressive, independent, and energetic role in later life.

Such findings are often cited as evidence for intrinsic sex differences, even though the findings themselves may in fact be based upon inadequate or incomplete data. Differences in observed personality or behavior changes between men and women may reflect, not inborn qualities, but the differences in the ways men and women have been socialized into behavior consistent with their adult roles, including differing expectations and perceptions that men and women may have about themselves and their social roles (which may perhaps even be related to differential life expectancy in some ways).

If circumstances, environments, perception, and motivation remained unchanged—absolutely static—across the years, we might then be assured of perfect continuity in behavior and perfect consistency (stability) of personality from early life through the later years on any given repeated measure. But this is obviously not the case. Circumstances, environments, perception, and motivation (not to mention expectations) do change across the lifespan to varying degrees (Maehr & Kleiber, 1981). Elderly persons whose personalities remain relatively stable and whose coping strategies and perspectives remain relatively fixed tend to more frequently exhibit discontinuities in behavior when confronted with new and novel circumstances. These persons are often seen as more dissatisfied and less adaptive. By the same token, older persons whose personalities remain relatively stable but whose perspectives and coping strategies are flexible enough can maintain some continuities in the face of change and are usually viewed as more satisfied and adaptive. In other words, personality and behavior patterns that serve well at an earlier time of life may prove to be inappropriate or detrimental in later life. The reverse, of course, may also be true.

It is not inaccurate to say, then, that if a man or woman wishes to be a sweet, kindly, generous, active, and involved ninety-year-old, these qualities or traits need to be developed much earlier in life. At the same time, this observation does not preclude either the possibility or the need for continuing personal growth, development, and progress toward self-actualization throughout the second half of life.

Personality and Behavior Change with Age: Fact or Artifact?

Middle-aged sons and daughters sometimes notice what appear to be sudden, even dramatic changes in the behavior of their aging parents. An elderly mother, for instance, who was always seen by her children as a conscientious, even compulsively neat housekeeper is described as having "suddenly" lost all interest in keeping her house orderly and clean. She is observed to have become not only slovenly, but unwilling to invest time and energy in cooking. Not infrequently such changes are attributed to "senility" at worst, and "personality change" at best.

But a careful examination and fuller understanding of that woman's life patterns and motivations may reveal that she never liked either cooking or household chores. Now that her children are grown and away from home, and she is living alone with a husband whose appetite has diminished (or living by herself, or with a daughter who subtly discourages her attempts at housework), her earlier distaste for these chores surfaces. In effect, what has occurred is not a sudden change in personality; rather, underlying feelings of long standing are unmasked by changing life circumstances and motivations (Goldfarb, 1976).

A similar explanation can be advanced in the following case. An elderly woman was always known to her family as a quiet, compliant, self-effacing person in her younger and middle years. Now living alone with her retired husband, her children gone, she exhibits unusual behavior. "Suddenly" she has become loudly assertive, demanding, controlling. Again, a careful reading of her earlier history may reveal that she is a person who has consistently shown demanding, controlling characteristics over a period of many years. In the past, however, much of this behavior was displayed in the context of child-rearing, which took place in a home where her husband was a virtual stranger. Now he is constantly at home with her, and her controlling behavior is no longer siphoned off in child-rearing activities. What appears to be a sudden shift in personality is merely the redirecting of long-standing personality or behavior characteristics by dint of changed circumstances.

Mental Health

The phrase "mental health" is at best a very imprecise one. Because it is so widely used it is repeated here, but the authors much prefer the more descriptive and operational term "emotional well-being." Such terms as "mental health," "mental illness," "senility," "dementia," and "psychiatric impairment" tend to be used indiscriminately, and often have different connotations for different persons and disciplines.

Our concepts of aging and mental health are circumscribed by our limited knowledge of the aging process and by the medical biases implicit in the metaphorical term "mental health." Given the very real limitations on the systematic study and evaluation of lifespan mental and emotional well-being or distress, our concepts are "more often bound to metaphor than to data" (Birren & Renner, 1980; cf. Szasz, 1978).

Every attempt to articulate the positive and negative aspects of well-being in the later years of life confronts a complex and deeply embedded set of vague, ambiguous, and inconsistent values and criteria. These include imprecise terms and definitions, the use of metaphorical language (cf. Szasz, 1978), relativity of standards of judgment (Sarason & Sarason, 1980), concepts of dubious validity and utility, inappropriate methods of assessment and measurement, and much too frequently, the use, misuse, or abuse of inadequate or insufficient data (cf. Wang, 1977).

It should be apparent by now that a clear, comprehensive set of behavioral norms appropriate to the later years remains embarrassingly elusive. A related truism is that most norms assumed to be representative of later life tend to be negative norms; further, most behaviors of aged persons in our society tend to be judged against the standard of middle-aged norms (particularly those ascribed to white, middle-class males).

Well-Being

Whereas the foregoing suggests a buzzing mass of confusion with respect to the mental and emotional pathologies said to occur more frequently in later life, the aspects of well-being that contribute to successful aging may be easier to specify.

Static concepts of the elderly that grow from a persistent search for pathologies and dysfunction, or for signs of the influence of theoretically based personality structures (for example, ego and superego), have tended to subvert legitimate concern with the role of the aged individual's contemporary situation and circumstances. What becomes hidden or lost is the older person's idiosyncratically devised coping styles and strategies, perceptions of environmental opportunities, self-direction into alternative or novel activities, and anticipation of and progress toward goal fulfillment. An older person's connectedness to current concerns is diagnostic of his or her state of well-being (Klinger, 1977). What is suggested is that meaningful involvement with incentives provides the structure for human activity. Without such customary involvement, humans become fragmented and despondent (Lefcourt, Martin, & Ebers, 1981).

Dysfunctional Elderly

It is currently estimated that approximately 10 percent of the total population of the United States (in excess of 23 million people) may have a "mental disorder." Unsettling as that vague statistic may be, it is even more unsettling to realize that to date no studies or surveys are available as a reliable guide for estimating the incidence of mental or emotional dysfunction among those aged sixty-five years or older. Some have placed the figure at 15 percent of the total population of older Americans, or about 3.9 million people. Other estimates suggest an even higher frequency (e.g., Redick & Taube, 1980). However, it must be noted that these widely cited figures are based on no hard data and are highly speculative, and thus remain open to challenge.

Admission and Discharge Data

Specific information is available with respect to the number of elderly patients residing in hospitals and admission rates of the elderly to selected mental health services. Table 3–1, for example, shows the number of patients sixty-five years of age and older in psychiatric hospitals in 1969 and 1973. What is most striking is the marked decline in the resident population aged sixty-five years and older in three types of hospitals over this five-year (inclusive) period (with the exception of nursing homes, of course). These data nicely illustrate the continuing trend of shifting the aged from primarily public facilities to private care centers, regardless of the ability of nursing home facilities to provide adequate and appropriate attention.

It remains unclear whether this trend signifies major migratory moves on the part of older persons (e.g., from rural to urban settings), or a change in funding patterns, or identification of nursing homes as cooperative if not wholly enthusiastic depositories for unwanted elderly patients.

What does seem evident is that, based on even modest estimates, the need for training of substantial numbers of competent professionals to serve a burgeoning older population is tremendous. A report to the Gerontological Society (Birren & Sloane, 1977) for use by the Department of Health, Education, and Welfare (now Health and Human Services) in assessing manpower and training needs in mental health and illness of the aged argues this

**TABLE 3-1.   Resident Patients 65 Years Old and Over in
Psychiatric Hospitals and with Chronic Condition of Mental
Disorder[a] in Nursing Homes, United States, 1969 and 1973**

Type of Facility	1969	1973	Percent Change 1969–73
State and county mental hospitals	111,420[d]	70,615[f]	−36.6
Private mental hospitals	2,460[d]	1,534[f]	−37.6
VA hospitals[b]	9,675[d]	5,819[f]	−39.9
Nursing homes[c]	96,415[e]	193,900[g]	101.0

Source: Redick, R.W., & Taube, C.A. Demography and mental health care of the aged. In J. E. Birren and R. B. Sloane (Eds.), *Handbook of mental health and aging.* Englewood Cliffs, N.J.: Prentice-Hall, Inc., 1980. P. 63.

[a]Includes mental illness (psychiatric or emotional problems) and mental retardation, but excludes senility.

[b]Includes VA neuropsychiatric hospitals and general hospital inpatient psychiatric services.

[c]Data on residents with chronic condition of mental disorder used rather than data on residents with primary diagnosis of mental disorder at last examination, since latter data were not available by age in 1969.

[d]*From* selected publications of Division of Biometry and Epidemiology, National Institute of Mental Health.

[e]*From* National Center for Health Statistics. "Chronic Conditions and Impairments of Nursing Home Residents: United States—1969." DHEW Publication No. (HRA) 74-1707. Washington, D.C.: Government Printing Office.

[f]*From* unpublished data, Division of Biometry and Epidemiology, NIMH.

[g]*From* National Center for Health Statitics, *Profile of Chronic Illness in Nursing Homes, United States: National Nursing Home Survey August 1973–April 1974.* Vital and Health Statistics ser. 13, no. 19, DHEW Publication No. (PHS) 78-1780.

case. Table 3–2 shows in some detail the mental health needs of the population at large, including those over sixty-five, based on certain assumptions of need.

Let us assume that 10 percent of the population aged sixty-five and older requires certain mental health services. As can be seen from the table, 220,354 are estimated to have received such care (column 3). But that leaves 1,996,646 persons sixty-five and older who presumably needed but did not receive such services (column 8). In other words, 90.1 percent of those estimated to be in need of such help did not receive it. Equivalent estimates for 1980 are 234,018 receiving care and 2,171,282 needing but not receiving care, again based on a 10 percent estimate of need.

The dimensions of need are further dramatized by one of the conclusions of Birren and Sloane's report. It recommended to the federal agency the training of the following numbers of professionals during the 1980s for work with the aged: 1,000 psychiatrists, 2,000 clinical psychologists, 4,000 social workers, 4,000 psychiatric nurses, 8,000 nurses aides and related personnel, and 10,000 paraprofessionals.

In conjunction with this issue is the astounding lack of physicians

TABLE 3-2. Extent to Which Needs for Psychiatric Services Would Be Met in Relation to Various Assumptions of Need: Assuming 1971 Use Rates Only, by Age, United States, 1975 and 1980

	Estimated General Population (in thousands)	Estimated Patient Care Episodes	Estimated Persons Receiving Care	Estimated Number of Persons Needing Care, Assuming			Number in Need Not Receiving Care, Assuming			% Unmet Need, Assuming		
				2% in Need	10% in Need	20% in Need	2% in Need	10% in Need	20% in Need	2% in Need	10% in Need	20% in Need
	(1)	(2)	(3)	(4)	(5)	(6)	(7)	(8)	(9)	(10)	(11)	(12)
1975												
Total, all ages	215,324	4,237,576	3,390,061	4,306,480	21,532,400	43,064,800	1,060,510	18,142,339	39,674,739	24.6	84.3	92.1
Under 18	68,109	809,377	647,502	1,362,180	6,810,900	13,621,800	714,678	6,163,398	12,974,298	52.5	90.5	95.2
18–24	27,780	716,150	572,920	555,600	2,778,000	5,556,000	0	2,205,080	4,983,080	0.0	79.4	89.7
25–44	53,835	1,504,340	1,203,471	1,076,700	5,383,500	10,767,000	0	4,180,029	9,563,529	0.0	77.6	88.8
45–64	43,430	932,267	745,814	868,600	4,343,000	8,686,000	122,786	3,597,186	7,940,186	14.1	82.8	91.4
65+	22,170	275,442	220,354	443,400	2,217,000	4,434,000	223,046	1,996,646	4,213,646	50.3	90.1	95.0
1980												
Total, all ages	228,676	4,500,344	3,600,275	4,573,520	22,867,600	45,735,200	1,030,028	19,267,325	42,134,925	22.5	84.3	92.1
Under 18	69,646	859,566	687,653	1,392,920	6,964,600	13,929,200	705,267	6,276,947	13,241,547	50.6	90.1	95.1
18–24	29,156	760,558	608,446	583,120	2,915,600	5,831,200	0	2,307,154	5,222,754	0.0	79.1	89.6
25–44	62,332	1,597,622	1,278,097	1,246,640	6,233,200	12,466,400	0	4,955,103	11,188,303	0.0	79.5	89.7
45–64	43,489	990,076	792,061	869,780	4,348,900	8,697,800	77,719	3,556,839	7,905,739	8.9	81.8	90.9
65+	24,053	292,522	234,018	481,060	2,405,300	4,810,600	247,042	2,171,282	4,576,582	51.4	90.3	95.1

Source: Kramer (1976).

Note: Column 1. U.S. Bureau of the Census, ser. D projection of the U.S. population (*Current Population Reports*, 1970, ser. P-25, no. 493)
Column 2. Total patient care episodes obtained by applying 1971 patient episode rate per 100,000 population (1968 per 100,000) to the projected 1975 and 1980 total U.S. population. Age distributions of patient care episodes obtained by applying 1971 percentage distribution of patient care episodes by age to the 1975 and 1980 estimated total patient care episodes.
Column 3. Represents a conversion of patient care episodes into number of persons accounting for these episodes by multiplying patient care episodes by a factor of 0.80. This factor was derived from findings of the Maryland Psychiatric Case Register that every person in that register had an average of 1.2 episodes of care per year.
Column 4 = Column 1 × 0.02.
Column 5 = Column 1 × 0.10.
Column 6 = Column 1 × 0.20.
Column 7 = Column 4 − Column 3 (Negative values assumed to be zero, i.e., the need for services would be met. Also the total is the sum of the parts.)
Column 8 = Column 5 − Column 3.
Column 9 = Column 6 − Column 3.
Column 10 = Column 7 ÷ Column 4.
Column 11 = Column 8 ÷ Column 5.
Column 12 = Column 9 ÷ Column 6.

trained or experienced in serving the elderly. A 1977 survey of physicians conducted by the American Medical Association revealed that less than 0.6 percent of those who responded indicated any interest in geriatric medicine. Moreover, physicians spend less time with older than with younger patients (on the average as little as twelve minutes per office consultation). The same survey was also able to identify fewer than sixty thoroughly competent, specialized geropsychiatrists in active practice in the United States. Thus, although the elderly use various types of medical care services extensively, these services are not tailored to their needs (Kane et al., 1980). Another survey could identify barely a hundred clinical psychologists who, by virtue of their training, could be regarded as having some appropriate qualifications for work with the aged (Storandt, 1977).

Underutilization of Services

Gerontologists continue to be preoccupied with the notion of the "underserved aged" or, conversely, with the underutilization of mental health services by the aged. A variety of explanations has been advanced (cf. Gatz, Smyer, & Lawton, 1980). Lawton (1979) has suggested that service underutilization results from the reluctance of older individuals to construe their problems in psychological terms. What this explanation suggests is the possibility of a lack of "fit" between the norms of a culturally diverse cohort of older persons and the norms that guide the judgments of professional helpers. In other words, the services offered may be viewed by the elderly as inappropriate or irrelevant to their perceived needs. What should not be overlooked in attempting to explain this phenomenon is the lack of experience on the part of the contemporary aged with using psychological services, the potential stigma associated with use of such services, and the cost of services, which may in itself be a primary deterrent to effective utilization.

CRITICAL DISCUSSION ▬▬▬▬

Senile Dementia—A Mask or the True Face of Old Age?

"Senility" is not, strictly speaking, a medical or psychological term, although it is commonly used as a synonym for "dementia" and is often loosely and indiscriminately applied to any eccentric, different, or unexplained behavior by old people. The same looseness of application is true of the word "dementia," which is used as a medical, psychiatric, and psychological diagnostic label.

Because terms like "dementia" and "dementing" can be defined only by means of behavioral description, their persistent use as labels when behavioral descriptions would better serve our understanding is most unfortunate, and certainly unjustified. "Demening" behavior, for most people (health professionals included), is connotatively equivalent to "demented" behavior, defined by Webster's Dictionary as "mad, insane." Thus, the question arises, is the use of the term "senile dementia" intended to indicate madness or insanity in older individuals? The most common clinical descriptions of behavior labeled senility or senile dementia include deterioration of previously acquired intellectual abilities, memory impairment, impairment of abstract thinking, impaired judgment, and personality change (Griffith, 1980). Other clinical features frequently cited are disorientation as to person, place, and time. One clinical geropsychologist has even invented the mnemonic acronym JAMCO—judgment, affect, memory, confusion, orientation (Peth, 1976)—to further add to the collection of labels for such behavior.

In reality, of course, none of these criteria are used to define psychotic behavior or other forms of "madness." The application of these norms with respect to the diagnostic entity of "senile dementia" is, at best, inappropriate and unfortunate. What serves to confuse the issue and further muddies our understanding of atypical behavior in older persons is the fact that "senility" and "senile dementia" are inevitably used to characterize the behavior of persons suffering from brain damage due to CVA (cerebral vascular accident, commonly called stroke) as well as deviant behaviors resulting from a host of other transient (and generally treatable) conditions. Included among the latter are a variety of toxic states from drug abuse or imbalance, electrolytic or endocrine imbalances, diabetes, vitamin and other dietary deficiencies, hypothyroidism, hypo- and hyperglycemia, tumors of the brain, fever, and infectious diseases. When deviant behaviors are long-standing, they are frequently but unjustifiably explained as resulting from organic brain syndrome, chronic type (often abbreviated to OBS or CBS). When the onset of atypical behavior is of recent vintage, they may be described as organic brain syndrome, acute type. In either case, the designation "organic brain syndrome" is vague and ambiguous, a "wastebasket diagnosis."

Many writers have pointed out that transient physical conditions can and do produce behavior in the old that cause them to be labeled "senile" or "dementing" (Goldfarb, 1974; Pfeiffer, 1977). The pernicious stigma and social destructiveness of this labeling process has been elaborated and documented elsewhere (cf. Rosenhan, 1973; Szasz, 1978). Further harm may be done when depression in an older person is identified as "senility" (Geschwind, 1975; Reichel, 1976).

Two unfortunate consequences of the inappropriate and inaccurate use of the terms "senility" and "senile dementia" should be noted. One is that older persons suffering from treatable diseases or modifiable environmental stresses that give rise to maladaptive or atypical behaviors are unnecessarily and wrongfully stigmatized. In more than a few instances they are shunted off to a low level of custodial care, which exacerbates their condition, making the misdiagnosis a self-fulfilling prophecy. The second consequence is that those who suffer from brain damage (as in the case of a CVA) are more often than not "written off." That is to say, because damage to the brain is irreversible, the assumption is made that the behaviors associated with such conditions are also irreversible. So families are told that nothing can be done, and nothing is. This, we know, is neither conceptually accurate nor it is practical. Much can be done. Other undamaged portions of the brain can, with care and skill, be retrained so that the speech of the aphasic can be restored and the paralyzed limb can become functional again. The case of actress Patricia Neal is a well-known example. Also, the insidious damage associated with physical, social, and emotional isolation of such unfortunate elderly individuals can be ameliorated and prevented (Ernst et al., 1978).

Common Problems of the Elderly

Surveys of older people repeatedly elicit two most common complaints: depression and loneliness. It is quite evident that these emotional reactions are closely related to a variety of stressful life circumstances. Among these are the psychological consequences of unrelieved multiple losses (social, physical, and vocational); inadequate and inappropriate physical environments that penalize the old and thus raise further obstacles to competent functioning; inadequate or inaccessible transportation, which creates barriers to mobility and discourages social contact; crimes (muggings, purse snatchings, rapes) that take advantage of the special vulnerabilities of the elderly and that, by increasing anxiety, tend to isolate older individuals; mandatory unemployment (retirement), which arbitrarily separates the old from a major source of satisfaction and self-worth; and demeaning and patronizing attitudes on the part of others (frequently middle-aged persons), as is evident in much of the humor about aging (Davies, 1977; Richman, 1977).

In certain respects, elderly persons are especially vulnerable to such stresses. In mid-1963, for example, approximately 292,000 elderly people with "mental disorders" were residing in either long-term psychiatric facilities, nursing homes, psychiatric hospitals, homes for the aged, or related facilities. Of the 23,480 who committed suicide in the United States in 1970, almost 7,400 (31.5 percent) were sixty-five years of age or older. Yet the elderly represent only about 10 percent of the total population. There is also a relatively high incidence of alcoholism among older persons. Obviously none of this happens in a vacuum; it is indicative of the severe emotional stress to which many elderly are exposed.

Intervention Strategies

This focus on depression and loneliness of the elderly should not be interpreted as denial or unawareness of other problems that face older persons. A complete list of relevant concerns and difficulties would only begin with such issues as marital and sexual problems, parenting problems, difficulties with interpersonal relations, housing and self-care crises, loss of interest and zest, and apathy, and would continue nearly ad infinitum. Depression and loneliness are exemplary of the problems that appear to be **endemic**[1] among the aged but yet are amenable to a wide variety of therapeutic intervention strategies, ranging from one-on-one counseling to legislative advocacy.

Virtually all interventions with respect to the aged may be subsumed under one of three broad classes of programs or strategies: treatment and cure, maintenance, or prevention. Although categorically discrete, these classes of intervention overlap considerably in practice.

Interventions often take the form of physical, social, and psychological compensations and supports. Intervention strategies with respect to physical losses are much better understood in our society because of the many precedents and models we have. Compensations for physical loss have become almost a matter of routine: a prosthetic limb for the amputee, eyeglasses for defective vision, hearing aids, heart pacers, false teeth, canes, "walkers," and so on. All these attachments to the body constitute compensatory devices. Their relevance to certain needs of the older population is beyond debate.

We have only begun to study and learn more about other compensating strategies and techniques and about the need for compensation for other than physical losses.

Study of the psychology of aging and clinical practice teach us at least this much about intervening in the lives of older persons:

1. A focus on intervention strategies that includes appropriate environmental design and conditions conducive to competent functioning is far more productive than mere descriptions of behavior, diagnoses of pathology, and palliative reassurances (e.g., "You have to learn to live with this, dear; it's just old age.").

2. Old age needs to be demythologized for the elderly, who must learn more about their range of options and the ways to use effective coping strategies.

3. When older people are properly motivated, that is, when they see the relevance and utility of an intervention, they are very responsive to intervention efforts.

4. The limits of helping must be recognized, so that under the guise of good intentions help does not become infantilizing, controlling, and patronizing.

Counseling of the Aged

Psychological therapies during the early part of the century were dominated by psychoanalytic theory, which was neither attuned nor available to people of advanced age. With the rise of the existential, reality, transactional, and "here and now" schools of therapy (derived in large measure from Sullivan's and Rogers' interpersonal formulations), individual and group coun-

---

[1]*endemic:* intrinsic to, common or characteristic of or among

seling of the aged and their families has begun to achieve legitimacy and is coming into widespread use.

This is not to say that counseling of older persons did not exist in the past. Much of it was conducted informally by professionals (most notably social workers and clergy) as an incidental service, and by volunteer helpers. Generally, such efforts were viewed as a supportive, kind gesture. Until recently, no serious effort was made to train counselor-therapists in a regular and systematic way.

Within the past half decade the picture has begun to change dramatically. Strong voices are being heard throughout the country (cf. Personnel and Guidance Association, 1976) arguing the validity and efficacy of counseling and therapy for the aged. A professional literature in this area, with particular emphasis on the family network, is now available (Herr & Weakland, 1979). More than that, a strong case is being made for the use of para- and nonprofessionals in counseling (Oden, 1974). Carkhuff and Truax (1965) have written extensively on the need for therapists to develop empathy, warmth, and genuineness, regarding these as necessary characteristics of the effective counselor. The importance of such traits, according to these investigators (including Oden), opens the door wide to nonprofessional and peer counselors of older adults.

Although training indigenous nonprofessionals is not a novel concept, training older persons to serve as counselors of their peers is a new wrinkle

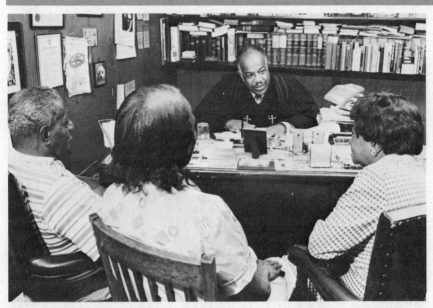

Clergy are potentially a good "frontline" resource for individual and family counseling of elderly people.

in an old strategy. This growing enterprise within gerontology is part of a nontraditional approach to therapy and counseling of the aged (Sargeant, 1980). Within the mainstream of this nontraditional approach, particular emphasis is put on training peer counselors, who in many instances have greater credibility and can more easily and quickly achieve rapport with an aged constituency (Schwartz, 1980).

Community Network Interventions

The amazing proliferation of varied therapeutic intervention programs in recent years makes this what business people might call a "growth industry." Older volunteer outreach groups (RSVP), nutritional programs (Meals-on-Wheels), legal counseling, Foster Grandparent programs, widow-to-widow counseling, day activities programs and multiservice centers, ombudsperson programs, hospices (centers that provide familial and emotional support to the terminally ill), adult education reentry and special interest educational programs: these are examples of community support and maintenance programs within a widening matrix of intervention strategies for older persons.

Prevention

The fact that this class of intervention strategies appears here after other intervention strategies should not be taken to mean that prevention is inferior or of less importance. Unfortunately, the concept of prevention has not been given the attention it deserves. Indeed, it has been suggested that the promotion of mental health is beyond the domain of health care per se. As Albee (1977) has pointed out, the mental health bureaucracy, despite its rhetoric, has a heavy investment in forestalling prevention. Even the rhetoric of prevention has, in most instances, been translated into yet another version of the treatment-and-cure approach, and is not truly prevention at all: "Come to us early and we will treat-and-cure you."

True prevention in the interests of emotional well-being aims at creating optimal conditions that will reduce the potential for (or eliminate entirely) maladaptive, maladjustive, or dysfunctional behaviors. For the aged this means, at best, to provide supportive, compensatory (prosthetic) environments; at a minimum, to provide environments that do not penalize the aged because of their disabilities or deficiencies.

This premise inescapably leads in the direction of a larger and more effective role for advocacy as intervention. In this respect, then, consciousness-raising in the private and public sectors is as credible and viable a helping intervention as individual or family counseling.

Bank managers and tellers, supermarket checkers, department store clerks, city bus drivers, women's dress designers, producers of cosmetics, architects and designers responsible for the construction of buildings, stairs, entries and exits, and living spaces—these and many other individuals should be seen as potential targets of consciousness-raising workshops, seminars, and instructional minicourses on the local community level. The purpose of such efforts should be to sensitize these service providers to the special needs of and special constraints on the elderly with whom they come into contact on the job, or who are consumers of their products.

The essence of such preventive measures is that they seek to insure that activities of daily living for aged people in their communities will be agreeable and successful, will be positive adventures rather than exhausting, frustrating, demeaning, and traumatic experiences that are to be avoided if possible.

Finally, among the many intervention strategies to be considered is the use of television and other media by gerontologists as influential forces in shaping public attitudes toward the aged. One of the pioneers in the use of TV on behalf of the aged is Richard Davis of the University of Southern California's Andrus Gerontology Center. His research efforts and his strong advocacy of the elderly have been instrumental in the development of public broadcasts and films on subjects of special interest to the aged, TV documentaries that present accurate as well as positive information about aging, and data on the impact of television as a teaching and evaluation medium.

Summary

Although treated as a separate topic in this chapter, it should be clearly understood that psychological aspects of aging are intrinsically interwoven with all other aspects of aging.

No single psychological theory of aging is capable of fully encompassing the broad range of behavior characteristic of the later years of life. The state-of-the-art continues to reflect our limited and somewhat fragmentary understanding of the cognitive, motivational, and personality factors that determine or otherwise affect the functional capability and competence of the elderly.

While early studies of cognitive processes in older people originally suggested the inevitability of declining capacity and aptitude with advancing age, the results of many of these investigations have been subject to much criticism in regard to the adequacy of their methodology and procedures (e.g., cross-sectional research designs, use of inappropriate tasks, lack of appropriate performance norms for older people). In fact the purported decline in cognitive functioning in the later years (which has provided the basis for many negative stereotypes about "senility" in the elderly) appear to be an artifact of cohort differences in education, training, and practice, rather than the result of changes in ability to perform. As Luria (1976) has noted:

> Higher cognitive activities remain sociohistorical in nature; . . . the structure of mental activity—not just the specific content but also the general forms

basic to all cognitive processes—changes in the course of historical
development [p. 8].

Thus "we may deduce that the natural course of aging in man does *not*
include cognitive decline" (Jarvik, 1973, p. 8).

Motivational factors may determine the extent to which the functional
capacity and competence of the elderly with respect to cognitive processes
and other forms of behavior are maintained throughout the later years. The
overwhelming majority of studies suggest that the key to functional competence resides in flexibility, adaptability, and a sense of personal control over
oneself and one's environment. To the extent that these key factors are limited, competent functioning may be impaired. Possible consequences of
such limitation may be learned helplessness and depression.

The study of personality in the aged suggests that behavior in the later
years, as earlier in the lifespan, is ordinarily not random but is consistent with
nomothetic (group) and idiographic (individual) behavioral laws. While
changes in personality across the lifespan are perhaps best characterized as
gradual and continuous, sometimes "sudden" discrete behavior changes
occur. In such instances, a careful analysis of life circumstances, motivations,
and other related factors may reveal that the change is actually the unmasking
of long-standing personality or behavior characteristics.

The assessment of the mental health status of elderly persons is ham-
pered by the lack of appropriate behavioral norms which describe typically
"healthy" individuals in the later years, as well as by inappropriate testing
and measurement methods. According to conservative estimates, approximately 15 percent of persons sixty-five years of age and older in the United
States today may be experiencing mental or emotional dysfunction. Unfortunately, relatively few skilled professionals have been specifically trained to
meet the needs of this older population. In addition, many older persons in
need of such help are reluctant to seek assistance due to the perceived inap-
propriateness of existing services, as well as the perceived negative stigma
attached to the use of these services. Cost factors, too, may inhibit help-seeking on the part of the elderly with such problems.

Intervention strategies providing treatment and care, maintenance, and
prevention of dysfunction in the elderly are greatly needed. Promising areas
in which services appropriate to the needs of the elderly are being developed
include counseling and community network interventions. While prevention
strategies have not to date been given the attention they deserve, advocacy
and consciousness-raising efforts in the interests of emotional well-being are
beginning to foster optimal conditions for the development of methods to
avoid dysfunction in the later years.

References

Albee, G. Preventing prevention. *APA Monitor,* May 1977, p 2.
Arenberg, D., & Robertson-Tchabo, E. Learning and aging. In J. E. Birren & K. W.

Schaie (Eds.), *Handbook of the psychology of aging.* New York: Van Nostrand Reinhold, 1977. Pp. 421–449.

Averill, J. R. Personal control over aversive stimuli and its relationship to stress. *Psychological Bulletin,* 1973, **80**: 286–303.

Birren, J. E., Bick, M. W., & Fox, C. Age changes in the light threshold of the dark adapted eye. *Journal of Gerontology,* 1948, **3**: 267–271.

Birren, J. E., & Renner, J. Concepts and issues of mental health and aging. In J. E. Birren & R. B. Sloane (Eds.), *Handbook of mental health and aging.* Englewood Cliffs, N.J.: Prentice-Hall, 1980. Pp. 3–33.

Birren, J. E., & Sloane, R. B. *Manpower and training needs in mental health and illness of the aging.* Report to the Gerontological Society of America for the Committee to Study Mental Health and Illness of the Aging for the Secretary of the Department of Health, Education, and Welfare, 1977.

Birren, J. E., Woods, A. M., & Williams, M. V. Behavioral slowing with age: Causes, organization, and consequences. In L. W. Poon (Ed.), *Aging in the 1980s.* Washington, D.C.: American Psychological Association, 1980. Pp. 293–308.

Boring, E. G. Intelligence as the tests test it. *New Republic,* 1923, **34**: 35–37.

Botwinick, J. Cautiousness in advanced age. *Journal of Gerontology,* 1966, **21**, 347–353.

Botwinick, J. Disinclination to venture response vs. cautiousness in responding: Age differences. *Journal of Genetic Psychology,* 1969, *115*: 55–62.

Botwinick, J. Intellectual abilities. In J. E. Birren & K. W. Schaie (Eds.), *Handbook of the psychology of aging.* New York: Van Nostrand Reinold, 1977. Pp. 580–605.

Botwinick, J. *Aging and behavior.* (2nd ed.) New York: Springer, 1978.

Braun, H. W., & Geiselhart, R. Age differences in the acquisition and extinction of the conditioned eyelid response. *Journal of Experimental Psychology,* 1959, **57**, 386–388.

Brehm, J. W. *Responses to loss of freedom: A theory of psychological reactance.* Morristown, N.J.: General Learning Press, 1972.

Brown, R., & Herrnstein, R. J. *Psychology.* Boston: Little, Brown, 1975.

Bugelski, B. R. Life and the laboratory. In I. Silverman (Ed.), *New directions for methodology of social and behavioral science: Generalizing from laboratory to life.* San Francisco: Jossey-Bass, 1981. Pp. 51–64.

Carkhuff, R. R., & Truax, C. B. Lay mental health counseling: The effects of lay group counseling. *Journal of Counseling Psychology,* 1965, **29**(5), 426–421.

Comalli, P. E., Jr. Cognitive functioning in a group of 80–90 year old men. *Journal of Gerontology,* 1965, **20**, 14–17.

Corso, J. F. Age and sex differences in pure-tone thresholds. *Archives of Otolaryngology,* 1963, 77, 385–405.

Corso, J. F. Aging and auditory thresholds in men and women. *Archives of Environmental Health,* 1963, **6**, 350–356.

Corso, J. F. Auditory perception and communication. In J. E. Birren & K. W. Schaie (Eds.), *Handbook of the psychology of aging.* New York: Van Nostrand Reinhold, 1977. Pp. 535–553.

Craik, F. I. M. The effects of aging on the detection of faint auditory signals. *Proceedings of the 7th International Congress of Gerontology, Vol. 6,* Vienna, 1966.

Craik, F. I. M. Age differences in human memory. In J. E. Birren & K. W. Schaie (Eds.), *Handbook of the psychology of aging.* New York: Van Nostrand Reinhold, 1977. Pp. 384–420.

Cunningham, W. R. Speed, age, and qualitative differences in cognitive functioning.

In L. W. Poon (Ed.), Aging in the 1980s. Washington, D.C.: American Psychological Association, 1980.

Davies, L. J. Attitudes toward old age and aging as shown by humor. *Gerontologist,* 1977, **17**(3), 220–226.

De Charms, R. *Enhancing motivation: Change in the classroom.* New York: Irvington Publishers, 1976.

Diggory, J. C. United States suicide rates, 1933–1968: An analysis of some trends. In E. Shneidman (Ed.), *Suicidology: Contemporary developments.* New York: Grune & Stratton, 1976. Pp. 25–69.

Eisdorfer, C., & Axelrod, S. Senescence and figural aftereffects in two modalities: A correction. *Journal of Genetic Psychology,* 1964, **104**, 193–197.

Eisdorfer, C., Axelrod, S., & Wilkie, F. L. Stimulus exposure time as a factor in serial learning in an aged sample. *Journal of Abnormal and Social Psychology,* 1963, **67**, 594–600.

Elias, M. F., & Elias, P. K. Motivation and activity. In J. E. Birren & K. W. Schaie (Eds.), *Handbook of the psychology of aging.* New York: Van Nostrand Reinhold, 1977. Pp. 357–374.

Ernst, P., Beran, B., Safford, F., & Kleinhauz, M. Isolation and the symptoms of chronic brain syndrome. *Gerontologist,* 1978, **18**(5), 468–474.

Estes, W. K. Is human memory obsolete? *American Scientist,* 1980, **68**, 62–69.

Farrimond, T. Prediction of speech hearing loss for older workers. *Gerontologia,* 1961, **5**, 65–87.

Feldman, R. M., & Reger, S. N. Relations among hearing, reaction time, and aging. *Journal of Speech and Hearing Research,* 1967, **10**, 479–495.

Fisher, J. Competence, effectiveness, intellectual functioning, and aging. *Gerontologist,* 1973, **13**(1), 62–68.

Furry, C., & Baltes, P. The effect of age differences in ability—extraneous performance variables in the assessment of intelligence in children, adults, and the elderly. *Journal of Gerontology,* 1973, **28**(1), 73–80.

Gajo, F. D. *Adult age differences in the perception of visual illusions.* (Doctoral dissertation, Washington University, St. Louis, Mo., 1966.) *Dissertation Abstracts,* 1967, **27**: 4573B, Ann Arbor, Mich.: University Microfilms, 1966. No. 67–7036.

Gatz, M., Smyer, M., & Lawton, M. P. The mental health system and the older adult. In L. W. Poon (Ed.), *Aging in the 1980s.* Washington, D.C.: American Psychological Association, 1980. Pp. 5–18.

Geschwind, N. Clinical pathology conference. *New England Journal of Medicine,* April 1975.

Gibson, J. J. *The senses considered as perceptual systems.* Boston: Houghton Mifflin, 1966.

Gibson, J. J. *The ecological approach to visual perception.* Boston: Houghton Mifflin, 1979.

Gilbert, J. G. Thirty-five-year follow-up study of intellectual functioning. *Journal of Gerontology,* 1973, **28**, 68–72.

Goldfarb, A. *Aging and organic brain syndrome* (manual). Bloomfield, N.J.: Health Learning Systems, Inc., 1974.

Gutmann, D. The cross-cultural perspective: Notes toward a comparative psychology of aging. In J. E. Birren & K. W. Schaie (Eds.), *Handbook of the psychology of aging.* New York: Van Nostrand Reinhold, 1977. Pp. 302–326.

Herr, J., & Weakland, J. H. *Counseling elders and their families.* New York: Springer, 1979.

Hoyer, W. J., & Plude, D. J. Attentional and perceptual processes in the study of cognitive aging. In L. W. Poon (Ed.), *Aging in the 1980s.* Washington, D.C.: American Psychological Association, 1980. Pp. 227–238.

Jarvik, L. F. Discussion: Patterns of intellectual functioning in the later years. In L. F. Jarvik, C. Eisdorfer, & J. E. Blum (Eds.), *Intellectual functioning in adults: Psychological and biological influences.* New York: Springer, 1973.

Jarvik, L. F., & Falek, A. Intellectual stability and survival in the aged. *Journal of Gerontology,* 1963, **18**, 173–176.

Jewett, S. P. Longevity and the longevity syndrome. *Gerontologist,* 1973, **13**(1), 91–99.

Kane, R., Solomon, D., Beck, J., Keller, E., & Kane, R. *Geriatrics in the U.S.: Manpower projections and training considerations.* Santa Monica, Cal.: Rand Corporation (R-2543-HJK) May 1980.

Kimble, G. A., & Pennypacker, H. S. Eyelid conditioning in young and aged subjects. *Journal of Genetic Psychology,* 1963, **103**, 283–289.

Kleemier, R. W. Intellectual changes in the senium. Proceedings of the Social Statistical Section. *American Statistics Society.* 1962. Pp. 290–295.

Kline, D. W., & Birren, J. E. Age differences in backward dichoptic masking. *Experimental Aging Research,* 1975, **1**, 17–25.

Kline, D. W., & Szafran, J. Age differences in backward monoptic visual noise masking. *Journal of Gerontology,* 1975, **30**, 307–311.

Klinger, E. *Meaning and void.* Minneapolis: University of Minneapolis Press, 1977.

Kobasa, S. C. Stressful life events, personality, and health: An inquiry into hardiness. *Journal of Personality and Social Psychology,* 1979, **37**, 1–11.

Korchin, S. J., & Basowitz, H. The judgment of ambiguous stimuli as an index of cognitive functioning in aging. *Journal of Personality,* 1957, **25**, 81–95.

Kuypers, J., & Bengston, V. L. Competence, social breakdown, and humanism. In A. Feldman (Ed.), *Community mental health and aging: An overview.* Los Angeles: University of Southern California Press, 1960.

Kuypers, J. A., & Bengston, V. L. Social breakdown and competence: A model of normal aging. *Human Development,* 1973, **16**(3), 181–201.

Labouvie-Vief, G. Beyond formal operations: Uses and limits of pure logic in life-span development. *Human Development,* 1980, **23**, 141–161.

Lawton, M. P. Clinical geropsychology: Problems and prospects. In *Master lectures on the psychology of aging.* Washington, D.C.: American Psychological Association, 1979.

Lazarus, R. S., & Launier, R. Stress-related transactions between person and environment. In L. A. Perrin & M. Lewis (Eds.), *Perspectives in interactional psychology.* New York: Plenum Press, 1978.

Lefcourt, H. M., & Martin, R. A., & Ebers, K. Toward a renewed integration of personality research and clinical practice. In I. Silverman (Ed.), *New directions for methodology of social and behavioral science: Generalizing from laboratory to life.* San Francisco: Jossey-Bass, 1981. Pp. 21–33.

Lowenthal, M. F., Thurner, M., Chiriboga, D., & associates (Eds.). *Four stages of life: A comparative study of women and men facing transitions.* San Francisco: Jossey-Bass, 1975.

Luria, S. M. Absolute visual threshold and age. *Journal of the Optical Society of America,* 1960, **50**, 86–87.

Luria, A. R. Cognitive development: Its cultural and social foundations. trans. M. Lopez-Morrillas & L. Solotaroff. Ed. M. Cole. Cambridge: Harvard University Press, 1976.

Maehr, M. L., & Kleiber, D. A. The graying of achievement motivation. *American Psychologist,* 1981, **36**(7), 787–793.

McClelland, D. Testing for competence rather than for intelligence. *American Psychologist,* 1973, **28**(1), 1–14.

Neisser, U. *Cognitive psychology.* New York: Appleton-Century-Crofts, 1966.

Neugarten, B. L. Personality and aging. In J. E. Birren & K. W. Schaie (Eds.), *Handbook of psychology and aging.* New York: Van Nostrand Reinhold, 1977. Pp. 626–649.

Noble, C. E. Age, race, and sex in the learning and performance of psychomotor skills. In R. T. Osborne, C. E. Noble, & N. Weyl (Eds.), *Human variation.* New York: Academic Press, 1978. Pp. 287–378.

Oden, T. A populist's view of psychotherapeutic deprofessionalization. *Humanistic Psychology,* 1974, **14**(2), 3–18.

Palmore, E. & Luikart, C. Health and social factors related to life satisfaction. *Journal of Health and Social Behavior,* 1972, **13**, 68–80.

Personnel and Guidance Association. *Special issue on counseling over the life-span.* Washington, D.C.: 1976.

Peth, P. Personal communication. In I. Burnside (Ed.), *Nursing and the aged.* New York: McGraw-Hill, 1976.

Pfeiffer, E. Psychotherapy and social pathology. In J. E. Birren & K. W. Schaie (Eds.), *Handbook of the psychology of aging.* New York: Van Nostrand Reinhold. 1977, Pp. 650–671.

Redick, R., & Taube, C. Demography and mental health care of the aged. In J. E. Birren & R. B. Sloane (Eds.), *Handbook of mental health and aging.* Englewood Cliffs, N.J.: Prentice-Hall, 1980., Pp. 57–71.

Rees, J. N., & Botwinick, J. Detection and decision factors in auditory behavior of the elderly. *Journal of Gerontology,* 1971, **26**, 133–136.

Reichel, W. Organic brain syndrome in the elderly. *Hospital Practice,* May 1976.

Richman, J. The foolishness and wisdom of age: Attitudes toward the elderly as reflected in jokes. *Gerontologist,* 1977, **17**(3), 210–219.

Riegel, K. F. Toward a dialectical theory of development. *Human Development,* 1975, **18**(1), 50–64.

Riegel, K. F. The dialectics of human development. *American Psychologist,* 1976, **31**, 689–700.

Robertson, G. W., & Yudkin, J. Effect of age upon dark adaptation. *Journal of Physiology (London),* 1944, **103**, 1–8.

Rosenhan, D. On being sane in insane places. *Science,* 1973, *179:* 250–258.

Rotter, J. B. Generalized expectancies for internal versus external control of reinforcement. *Psychological Monographs,* 1966, **80** (1, Whole No. 609).

Saltz, E. Higher mental processes as the bases for the laws of conditioning. In F. J. McGuigan & D. B. Lumsden (Eds.), *Contemporary approaches to conditioning and learning.* Washington, D.C.: V. H. Winston & Sons, 1973. Pp. 21–47.

Sarason, I . G., & Sarason, B. R. *Abnormal psychology.* Englewood Cliffs, N.J.: Prentice-Hall, 1980.

Sargeant, S. S. (Ed.) *Nontraditional therapy and counseling with the aging.* (Vol. 7 in Springer series, *Adulthood and Aging).* New York: Springer, 1980.

Schaie, K. W. Age changes in adult intelligence. In D. Woodruff & J. E. Birren (Eds.), *Aging: scientific perspectives and social issues.* New York: Van Nostrand Company, 1975. Pp. 111–124.

Schaie, K. W. The primary mental abilities in adulthood: An explanation in the development of psychometric intelligence. In P. Baltes & O. Brim (Eds.), *Lifespan development and behavior* (Vol. 2). New York: Academic Press, 1979, Pp. 68–115.

Schaie, K. W., & Labouvie-Vief, G. Generational vs. ontogenetic components of change in adult cognitive functioning: A fourteen year cross-sequential study. *Developmental Psychology,* 1974, **10**, 305–320.

Schaie, K. W., & Strother, C. R. A cross-sequential study of age changes in cognitive behavior. *Psychological Bulletin,* 1968, **70**, 671–680.

Schwartz, A. N. Planning micro-environments for the aged. In D. Woodruff & J. E. Birren (Eds.), *Aging: Scientific perspectives and social issues.* New York: Van Nostrand Company, 1975. Pp. 279–294.

Schwartz, A. N. Training of peer counselors. In S. S. Sargeant (Ed.), *Nontraditional therapy and counseling with the aging.* New York: Springer, 1980. Pp. 146–160.

Scott, W. A., Osgood, D. W., & Peterson, C. *Cognitive structure: Theory and measurement of individual differences.* Washington, D.C.: V. H. Winston & Sons, 1979.

Seligman, M. E. P. Fall into helplessness. *Psychology Today,* June 1973, 43–48, 51–54, 88.

Seligman, M. E. P. Depression and learned helplessness. In R. J. Friedman & M. M. Katz (Eds.), *The psychology of depression: Contemporary theory and research.* Washington, D.C.: V. H. Winston & Sons, 1974.

Seligman, M. E. P. *Helplessness: On depression, development, and death.* San Francisco: W. H. Freeman, 1975.

Silver, R. L., & Wortman, C. B. Coping with undesirable life events. In J. Garber & M. E. P. Seligman (Eds.), *Helplessness: Theory and applications.* New York: Academic Press, 1981.

Snyder, C. L. *A signal detection analysis of opticogeometric illusion susceptibility as a function of age.* Doctoral dissertation, University of Georgia. 1979.

Snyder, C. L. *Ecological perception and minority status: The castes of thousands.* Unpublished manuscript, 1981.

Stern, J. A., Oster, P. J., & Newport, K. Reaction time measures, hemispheric specialization, and age. In L. W. Poon (Ed.), *Aging in the 1980s.* Washington, D.C.: American Psychological Association, 1980. Pp. 309–326.

Storandt, M. Graduate education in gerontological psychology: Results of a survey. *Educational Gerontology,* 1977, **2**(2), 141–146.

Szafran, J. Psychophysiological studies of aging in pilots. In G. A. Talland (Ed.), *Human aging and behavior—recent advances in research and theory.* New York: Academic Press, 1968.

Szasz, T. *The myth of psychotherapy: Mental healing as religion, rhetoric, and repression.* New York: Anchor Books Doubleday, 1978.

Tanner, W. P., & Swets, J. A. A decision-making theory of visual detection. *Psychological Review,* 1954, **61**, 401–409.

Till, R. E. Age-related differences in binocular backward masking with visual noise. *Journal of Gerontology,* 1978, **33**, 702–710.

Wallach, M. A., & Kogan, N. Aspects of judgment and decision-making: Interrelationships and changes with age. *Behavioral Sciences,* 1961, **6**, 23–36.

Walsh, D. A. Age differences in central perceptual processing: A dichoptic backward masking investigation. *Journal of Gerontology,* 1976. **31**, 178–185.

Walsh, D. A., Till, R. E., & Williams, M. Age differences in peripheral visual processing: A monoptic backward masking investigation. *Journal of Experimental Psychology: Human Perception and Performance,* 1978, **4**, 232–243.

Wang, H. S. Dementia of old age. In W. L. Smith & M. Kinsborne (Eds.), *Aging and dementia.* New York: Spectrum Publications, 1977. Pp. 1–24.

Wapner, S., Werner, H., & Comalli. P. E. Perception of part-whole relationships in middle and old age. *Journal of Gerontology,* 1960, **15**, 412–416.

Weale, R. A. On the eye. In A. T. Welford, & J. E. Birren (Eds.), *Aging, behavior and the nervous system.* Springfield, Charles C. Thomas, 1965. Pp. 307–325.

Wigdor, B. T. Drives and motivations with aging. In J. E. Birren & R. B. Sloane (Eds.), *Handbook of mental health and aging.* Englewood Cliffs, N.J.: Prentice-Hall, 1980. Pp. 245–261.

FOR FURTHER READING

Baltes, P., & Schaie, K. W. Aging and I. Q.: the myth of the twilight years. *Psychology Today,* July 1974.

Gaitz, C. M., & Baer, P. Diagnostic assessment of the elderly: A multifunctional model. *Gerontologist,* 1970, **10**(1), 47–52.

George, L. K., & Bearon, L. B. *Quality of life in older persons: Meaning and measurement.* New York: Human Sciences Press, 1980.

Lazarus, R. S. The stress and coping paradigm. In C. Eisdorfer, D. Cohen, A. Kleinman, & P. Maxim (Eds.), *Theoretical bases in psychopathology.* New York: Spectrum Publications, 1980.

Lazarus, R. S. Stress and coping as factors in health and illness. In J. Cohen, J. W. Cullen & L. R. Martin (Eds.). *Psychosocial aspects of cancer.* New York: Raven Presss 1982. Pp. 163–190.

Selye, H. Secret of coping with stress. *U.S. News & World Report,* March 21, 1977.

Szasz, T. S. *The manufacture of madness.* New York: Dell, 1970.

The Sociology of Aging

Chapter 4

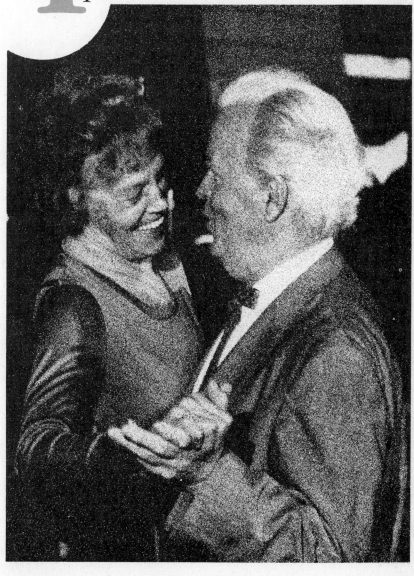

Do not go gentle into that good night,
Old age should burn and rave at close of day;
Rage, rage against the dying of the light.

And you, my father, there on that sad height,
Curse, bless, me now with your fierce tears I pray
Do not go gentle into that good night.
Rage, rage against the dying of the light.

Dylan Thomas

Sociology is the scientific study of people. The sociology of aging is the study of groups of older people, their characteristics, and how they interact, influence, and are influenced by individuals and other groups in society. Within its purview are included the ways in which status may be ascribed to the elderly and how, in turn, social status may affect the behavior (roles) of older individuals. It is also possible to examine age norms and age grading, and how these time-related social factors vary with attitudes and behavior. Of further interest is determining the ways through which continuity and change may complement each other with respect to the interaction of social norms and values in life.

Differences in generational experiences must be taken into account when we assess the genesis and development of intergenerational bias and conflict. Some of the more pervasive myths about the aging process, accepted at face value by older adults, may lead to self-fulfilling prophecies of lower self-esteem, poor self-concept, and reduce expectations and goals—all pernicious barriers to accurate evaluation of the real promise of the later years for present and future generations.

The following case illustration describes James North. His life history, briefly sketched here, is a good introduction to some of the social factors which are critical in the sociology of aging. It is important to keep in mind that his case, although somewhat representative, does not in any sense exhaust the experiences of men and women in their later years.

CASE ILLUSTRATION

"There Are No Brains in this Place"

James North is a sixty-eight-year-old Caucasian, currently in his third year as a resident in a retirement home in Los Angeles. Two senior counselors in gerontology were called in for consultations with the administrators of his retirement home because Mr. North was exhibiting a variety of disturbing behaviors: appearing at 4:00 A.M. by the bedside of other residents, introducing himself by strange names, refusing to eat for days at a time, and just sitting in a depressed stupor for extended periods. This was new and unusual behavior for Mr. North, and the cause of grave concern within the facility.

Mr. North's physical condition was addressed first. Nothing remarkable was in evidence; physiologically, all factors appeared to be within normal or acceptable limits. He had some difficulty with glaucoma and was incontinent on occasion, but no direct physical basis for his changed behavior could be discovered from medical records or consultations with his physician.

Assessment then focused on his psychological status. While he had been somewhat depressed in recent years, he had no history of extended bouts of depression. He had always been forgetful and sometimes distractable, yet during two months of consultation with the counselors he never missed an appointment. He did wander about at night, but only stood or sat by the bedside of fellow residents during that time. There was little from his prior psychological history to account for this and other instances of "deviant" behavior.

Evaluation of Mr. North's situation then focused on past and present social factors in his life. Noting the lack of any apparent physical or psychological antecedents to the change in his behavior, the consultants began to examine the ways in which he had previously related to other persons, in an attempt to formulate a sociological explanation.

Several elements relative to his social roles were identified as crucial to understanding his current behavior. Mr. North had been a high school principal in the same community for some forty years. In addition, he had vigorously pursued three other major roles. First, he had been a far-sighted community leader, having worked enthusiastically for his church, the Rotary Club's Eye Program, the Democratic Party, the Boys' Club, and other groups. Second, he consistently took courses at a nearby university and after many years had earned (with distinction) his Ph.D degree. His third role was that of husband and father.

All of these roles gave him a deep sense of personal value and satisfaction. But each of these important roles was abruptly terminated when he retired and moved into the retirement community, located far from either a school or an adequate library. His poor eyesight made reading difficult. There were no classes at the retirement center that challenged him, nor could he find individuals there who might have become intellectual friends. He underscored his plight when he rather succinctly stated, "There are no brains in this place."

The retirement community was run smoothly enough by an auto-crat who said he loved "older folks." But he appeared to love them only when he could control and manipulate them. Consequently, there was no resident council, no resident committee—no way for Mr. North or anyone else to participate meaningfully in decisions regarding programs that would affect the community's residents. All of Mr. North's years of training in community organizations and volunteer activities were ignored. Finally, his wife had died six months after they had moved into the retirement facility, and his children lived far away. So the forty-six years he had spent with his family in intimacy and warmth were lost as well.

If Mr. North sat silently in the retirement residence by the bed of a female resident, it had much to do with the fact that he very much missed the long-accustomed warmth and comfort of sleeping beside his wife. In his depression and bewilderment, it became apparent, he was reaching out. If he sat in a stupor and was depressed, it was because it was far more rewarding to contemplate his past intellectual and social interactions than to make any attempt to participate in a sterile and unrewarding life routine devoid of intellectual stimulation. If he refused to eat, it was a mute protest against a life that had no further challenge, as he saw it, and for which he had little taste. Those major social roles which had given him his sense of identity and satisfaction were now shrunken. Most of his usual sources of satisfaction were cut off.

As these facts began to emerge, Mr. North's behavior seemed less "strange," "bizarre," and incongruous. It was possible to understand what had happened to his social network and to his sources of past satisfaction, and what these events meant to him.

Sociological Theories of Aging

Just as Mr. North's behavior appears less bizarre when evaluated in the light of his life history, so the behavior of older adults in general may be more clearly understood in the context of the social events that have shaped and continue to affect their lives. Repeated observations, the development of propositions and hypothetical constructs, and the formulation and testing of hypotheses lead to the construction of theories which not only explain but may help to predict patterns of behavior (both adaptive and maladaptive) and their interrelationships with social forces throughout the lifespan. Social theory construction is a dynamic process which requires continuous reevaluation and reformulation of earlier explanations of behavior in the light of new observations and data, in order to provide a more reliable and valid view of aging and society over time. Although common reference is made to social theories of aging, most formulations of this type are as yet only frames of reference—that is, general statements made on the basis of observation without benefit of rigorous testing and validation. Nonetheless, these frames of reference provide a reasonable approximation to theory and have received a great deal of attention in the literature on the sociology of aging in recent years.

Historical Perspective

Before the turn of the century in the United States older persons enjoyed a different status and maintained different roles from those in evidence today. Life expectancy was shorter (about forty-five years) and fewer people survived into the later adult years than in modern times. At that point in history, the economic base was largely agrarian and prosperity depended heavily on the contributions of each person to the welfare of the extended family group. Whereas in contemporary society chronological age seems to be a significant determinant of task assignment and expectations for task performance, in earlier times chronological age mattered little in absolute terms. More important was a family member's age relative to the ages of other members; assignment of tasks to family members was based on the particular roles that each person was expected to perform as a function of experience, regardless of the number of birthdays she or he had celebrated.

Therefore older persons played a central role in the guidance, direction, and management of family activities and in determining the expenditure of time, money, and other resources within the family unit. The authority maintained by older persons was not conferred automatically, but grew from a lifetime of experience. The normative work roles of adulthood eventually shifted from the performance of more physically demanding tasks to advisory and supervisory activities. The elderly were thus a source of wisdom and knowledge, and in their later years reaped the benefits, rewards, and status generated by their collective labors. While adult children might be introduced to the management of the family enterprise (and thereby trained to assume their ultimate roles of leadership in the later years), the older individual, as head of the family unit, made all the major decisions. Older adults within the agrarian socioeconomic system did not depend on the largess of their children, or on outside sources of assistance; indeed, adult children were often dependent upon their elders for their own livelihood, income, and social position.

With the rapid growth of industrialization and technology in the United States after the turn of the century, the status and roles of older persons changed dramatically. Industrial innovations and technological advancements provided many benefits which ultimately resulted in increased longevity and the growth of the elderly population (in absolute as well as relative terms). Yet these increases in the "quantity of life" were rarely paralleled by increases in the quality of life for older persons.

In general, the transition from an agrarian to an industrialized society was not easy for older adults. The concept of family-centered work activities largely disappeared—and with it, the power and status afforded older family members as supervisors and managers of the family enterprise. While older adults tended to remain engaged in agriculture-related pursuits, younger adults began to seek employment in occupational fields beyond the confines and control of the extended family unit. The occupational continuity and residential stability which had characterized the extended family for many generations became disrupted, and semiextended and nuclear family structures began to replace earlier extended family patterns. Adult children were less likely to work in the same occupations as their parents, and more likely to live in or near the communities in which they worked, effectively reducing the control of older family members over the contributions of their adult children to the extended family unit. While this diminished control seemed to lead to a reduction in the roles and status of the elderly, their adult children enjoyed an increase in status provided by their new roles as wage- or salary-earning workers, as well as by their new independence and economic power. With the geographic and economic dispersion of the extended family network, many functions formerly performed by family members, particularly the elderly, were no longer centered in the family context. Education (both religious and secular), entertainment, social contact, health care, child care, and many other functions became institutionalized outside the family unit, further reducing the status of elderly family members as well as their power and control in shaping the lives of younger family members (Atchley, 1979).

These observations are consistent with the theoretical formulations of Cowgill and Holmes (1972) in their cross-cultural analysis of the status, roles, and treatment of the elderly as a function of modernization. Table 4–1 lists a number of characteristics associated with typical behavior patterns in agrarian versus modernized societies and their implications for the lives of the elderly.

Although the social picture for older persons residing in many modernized societies today may seem somewhat bleak in contrast to the apparently more positive and supportive context of agrarian life, in at least some societies the picture has been changing. The industrial revolution and its overwhelming emphasis upon the rapid, efficient, and inexpensive production of goods fostered considerable competition among people of all ages for survival in the system. As adults grew older, the experience and knowledge gained through their lifetimes became less important and less valued in industrial societies than their ability to produce goods quickly and in step with younger people. Because performance in this context was evaluated in terms of standards geared to production levels of younger and middle-aged adults, it often became the rule to retire older workers and hire younger, less experienced adults at lower wages. The social unacceptability of leisure time and of "retirement" in many cases led older persons to feel rejected. Not having anticipated and planned for the retirement years, and in particular not having normative support for the enjoyable use of leisure time, many older persons found that the transition to retired life very difficult indeed.

However, now that many countries, including the United States, a num-

TABLE 4-1. Aging and Modernization: Universals and Variations in Patterns of Behavior Across Cultures

Universals

1. The aged always constitute a minority within the total population.
2. In an older population, females outnumber males.
3. Widows comprise a high proportion of an older population.
4. In all societies, some people are classified as old and are treated differently because they are so classified.
5. There is a widespread tendency for people defined as old to shift to more sedentary, advisory, or supervisory roles involving less physical exertion and more concerned with group maintenance than with economic production.
6. In all societies, the mores prescribe some mutual responsibility between old people and their adult children.
7. In all societies, some old persons continue to act as political, judicial, and civic leaders.
8. All societies value life and seek to prolong it, even in old age.

Variations

1. The concept of old age is relative to the degree of modernization; a person is classified as old at an earlier chronological age in a primitive society than in a modern society.
2. Old age is identified in terms of chronological age chiefly in modern societies; in other societies onset of old age is more commonly linked with events such as succession to eldership or becoming a grandparent.
3. Longevity is directly and significantly related to the degree of modernization.
4. Modernized societies have older populations, i.e., higher proportions of old people.
5. Modern societies have higher proportions of women and especially of widows.
6. Modern societies have higher proportions of people who live to be grandparents and even great-grandparents.
7. The status of the aged is high in primitive societies and is lower and more ambiguous in modern societies.
8. In primitive societies, older people tend to hold positions of political and economic power, but in modern societies such power is possessed by only a few.
9. The status of the aged is high in societies in which there is a high reverence for or worship of ancestors.
10. The status of the aged is highest when they constitute a low proportion of the population and tends to decline as their numbers and proportions increase.
11. The status of the aged is inversely proportional to the rate of social change.
12. Stability of residence favors high status of the aged; mobility tends to undermine it.
13. The status of the aged tends to be high in agricultural societies and lower in urbanized societies.
14. The status of the aged tends to be high in preliterate societies and to decline with increasing literacy of the populations.
15. The status of the aged is high in those societies in which they are able to continue to perform useful and valued functions; however, this is contingent upon the values of the society as well as upon the specific activities of the aged.
16. Retirement is a modern invention; it is found chiefly in modern high-productivity societies.
17. The status of the aged is high in societies in which the extended form of the family is prevalent and tends to be lower in societies which favor the nuclear form of the family and neolocal marriage.
18. With modernization the responsibility for the provision of economic security for dependent aged tends to shift from the family to the state.
19. The proportion of the aged who are able to maintain leadership roles declines with modernization.

continued

TABLE 4–1.   Aging and Modernization: Universals and Variations in Patterns of Behavior Across Cultures (*continued*)

Variations   (*continued*)

20. In primitive societies the role of a widow tends to be clearly ascribed, but such role ascription declines with modernization; the widow's role in modern societies tends to be flexible and ambiguous.
21. The individualistic value system of Western society tends to reduce the security and status of older people.
22. Disengagement is not characteristic of the aged in primitive or agrarian societies, but an increasing tendency toward disengagement appears to accompany modernization.

Source: Cowgill & Holmes (1972), pp. 321–323.

ber of the Scandinavian countries, and Japan, have entered what has been called the "postindustrial age" (Bell, 1973), rapid social change and other salient factors which seemed central to the growth of industrialization have been deferred in recognition of other important concerns. As Hendricks and Hendricks (1977) remark, "It is only when humanity is not preoccupied with the necessities of survival that a humane treatment of nonproductive members can be realized" (p. 44). In contrast to industrialized societies, postindustrial societies are

> characterized by a technology based on theoretical rather than applied knowledge; an economy oriented toward performance of services rather than production of goods; and a stratification system based on the pre-eminence of the professional class [Pampel, 1981, p. 11; cf. Bell, 1973].

In postindustrial societies, government often plays a larger role in providing a more stable backdrop for the lives of elderly persons (Lakoff, 1976). Some of the more favorable prospects for older people in this context include:

1. major changes in the normative support for leisure;
2. continued growth of the economy [which] has created an economic surplus that has permitted institutionalization of retirement-income programs sponsored by the government and private organizations; and
3. the growth of public-interest groups supporting the aged [Pampel, 1981, pp. 11–12].

How do we explain and predict the behavior of the elderly in today's postindustrial society, given this historical perspective?

Disengagement versus Activity: The Social Context

During the 1960s, two contradictory frames of reference were developed to account for the social behavior of older persons, particularly following vocational retirement. Interestingly enough, the data which gave rise to these alternative views of social aging were drawn from the same series of investigations—the Kansas City studies, undertaken by a group of social scientists from the University of Chicago. The disengagement theory (Cumming

& Henry, 1961) and the activity theory (Havighurst et al., 1968), as these two divergent perspectives have come to be known, have stimulated a great deal of research and discussion because of their implications for social gerontology as well as for psychological aspects of behavior in later life.

Disengagement Theory

Based on their analysis of the data provided by the Kansas City Studies, Cumming and Henry (1961) described a process that they held to be a fundamental characteristic of senescence. Contrary to the traditional notion that society tends unilaterally to reject or isolate the elderly, these investigators interpreted their data to mean that the elderly themselves begin to limit their activities and thus literally begin to "disengage" themselves from the mainstream of living, presumably in preparation for and anticipation of the end of life. According to this theory, the process of disengagement is undertaken in mutual fashion by the elderly and the societies in which they live, as if by tacit agreement.

One conclusion drawn by Cumming and Henry with respect to the mutual disengagement process was that it produces personal satisfaction on the part of older people as well as an optimum level of continued functioning on the part of the social system. By means of a realignment of the relationships between the aged individual and society, the equilibrium between these entities developed in early adulthood and the middle years continues to be maintained in the later years in the form of what has been termed an "orderly transition of power" from older to younger members (Atchley, 1972). Primary features of this mutual withdrawal process are said to be its universality and inevitability.

The theory in its revised formulation allowed for variations in the rate and extent of the disengagement process, but maintained that the diminishing of social contacts and narrowing of interactive opportunities afforded by society occur regularly and in due time. The aging individual, according to this theory, sooner or later wishes the transition of power to take place, and society eventually demands it. At times, dissonance may occur when the process is not synchronous, that is, when society calls for some degree of disengagement and the individual clearly is neither ready nor willing to withdraw (e.g., forced retirement, as described by the retired professor from New York in Chapter 3).

The correlation between diminishing social contact (interaction) and increasing age is evident from Table 4–2, which depicts some of the data from which the theoretical perspective of disengagement was derived. It is obvious that as the number of roles diminish with age, high daily interaction is reduced. This phenomenon has been described as *social loss.*

The social role losses of older persons tend to be numerous and cumulative. Men and women who have worked as homemakers face their own early retirement when they reach the end of their child-raising careers. Not only do their children leave home, but all the roles ancillary to parenthood—PTA

TABLE 4-2. Roles of Interaction by Age and Sex

Sex and Age	Number Interviewed	Percent of Number Interviewed	
		Large Number of Roles	High Daily Interaction
Both sexes	211	41.7	47.9
50–54	36	61.1	72.2
55–59	34	61.8	58.8
60–64	34	58.8	58.8
65–69	31	38.7	45.2
70–74	50	22.0	34.0 ·
75 and over	26	7.7	15.4
Males	107	42.0	46.7
50–54	19	68.4	78.9
55–59	18	61.1	50.0
60–64	19	47.4	52.6
65–69	12	50.0	50.0
70–75	25	20.0	32.0
75 and over	14	7.1	14.3
Females	104	41.3	49.0
50–54	17	52.9	64.7
55–59	16	62.5	68.8
60–64	15	73.3	66.7
65–69	19	31.6	42.1
70–74	25	24.0	36.0
75 and over	12	8.3	16.7

Source: Cumming & Henry (1961).

member, Cub Scout board member, chauffeur to a dozen events, and many others—go with them. The man or woman who works outside the home likewise gives up daily associations and recreational linkages with fellow workers, as well as union or managerial ties. Many roles associated with work are forsaken: participant in the festive luncheon group, member of the work-associated recreation, such as the company softball or bowling team, the regular racquetball game, and others. And many times the end of a work career makes a serious impact on friendship networks previously tied to a specific occupation.

Shrinking Roles and Status

As a couple ages, their friendship network is also shriveled by the death and migration of neighbors and friends. Their coworkers and neighbors are transferred. Their clergyperson may be called to serve another congregation. Their physician or dentist may retire. Their siblings and other close relatives may die. All of the significant persons who were an integral part of their life support system may go. Sometimes financial and health factors contribute to narrowing the circle of friends and the range of interests. One potential price to be paid for extended survival is the disruption of family and friendship networks.

Along with a loss of social roles there must also be a loss of status. Older people in America ordinarily are not given the prestige or approval that was afforded them when they were middle-aged. If one asks older persons how old they are in the context of a survey, a very characteristic response is that they are "middle-aged." Then, if one asks how old their friends are, they typically say that they are all "old." This may well reveal much about their perceived sense of loss of position and status.

But one cannot change the evaluation of society by claiming membership in another age group. The older individual may lose a job, may lose positions as a leader in religious and political organizations, in service groups in the community, and even in some volunteer organizations as a result of too excessive an accumulation of birthdays. All of this spells lowered status and loss of power. Even an affluent older individual is likely to experience losses of roles and, more important, position and status. Indeed, some research indicates that the more affluent, influential older person is likely to encounter greater difficulty than the average person in adapting to status change (Shire, 1972). Alternatively, it may well be that if elderly individuals begin to form a reference group in a senior citizen center, a retirement community, or a Gray Panthers group, for example, the older individual may attain renewed or new status that is meaningful and relevant among such age peers.

Adaptation: A Congruent Fit

Adaptation to the conditions which produce loss of social roles and interactions does not, per se, imply withdrawal from life. Individuals who withdraw gracefully, who no longer have great expectations in their lives, may better adjust to life than those who try to hold on to a level of activity which was characteristic of and more appropriate to their earlier years. Thus, according to Cumming and Henry, to disengage is to move toward a congruent fit between one's capacities and one's possibilities for living. Disengagement may also serve as an adaptive mechanism for individuals with certain personality characteristics who require the self-protection from increasingly less desirable roles which mutual withdrawal provides (Lowenthal & Chiriboga, 1975).

There is a parallel between the notion of disengagement in later life and the last stage in the adjustment of individuals approaching death as described by Kübler-Ross (1969). In this final stage, "acceptance," those who are dying retreat from associations with intimates into their own world, so that the pain of separation will be reduced. In a sense, Kübler-Ross has reiterated in another context the same disengagement of which Cumming and Henry speak.

Disengagement: A Critical Appraisal

Following the appearance of the disengagement theory in the scientific literature (Cumming & Henry, 1961), the number of studies testing its validity was exceeded only by the number of discussions of what was then viewed as a most provocative contribution to theoretical frameworks of aging (cf. Henry, 1965; Maddox, 1964; Neugarten, 1964; Rose, 1964, 1965; Tallmer & Kutner, 1970). The ongoing debate about this perspective has raised serious questions about its universality and inevitability. It has been pointed out, for instance, that individual disengagement does occur, but that it occurs in selective fashion. The individual may disengage from certain social roles and their attendant responsibilities, but not disengage from other roles (Atchley, 1972).

Another criticism of this theory arises from its postulate of inevitability. The theory assumes that the desire to disengage develops and flourishes independent of any significant competing psychological forces or pressures. There is no evidence to support such an assumption. A common example of competing psychological pressure for engagement is observed in the continuing activity of many professional persons (educators, psychologists, physicians, nurses, politicians, writers, clergy, and musicians, to name but a few) who practice their art, craft, or trade and thereby receive great reward and satisfaction, even to the very last days of their lives.

Many studies of disengagement have been criticized on the basis of the methods used to collect information. Basically, the procedure is to count the number of social contacts currently reported by a sample of elderly persons and compare these with the number of contacts existing at an earlier time in their lives. The disparity between the two has been cited as primary evidence for disengagement. The vulnerability of this technique lies in its failure to take into account the kinds and quality of social contacts reported, the psychological responses to these contacts, and the significance of such interpersonal interaction in the overall perception of life events. Neither does this procedure give sufficient weight to other variables, which in specific instances may account for reduced frequency of social contacts: disruption of the family and friendship network through mobility or death, unavailable or inaccessible transportation, economic insufficiency, reduced energy, and presence of a disability or illness, among others.

Activity Theory

The activity theory of aging is essentially a direct contradiction of the disengagement premise, based on the same series of studies that gave rise to the disengagement theory. The rationale of the activity approach, which was developed by Robert Havighurst, is that even though some reduction in level of activity is to be expected in old age, the most successful agers are those

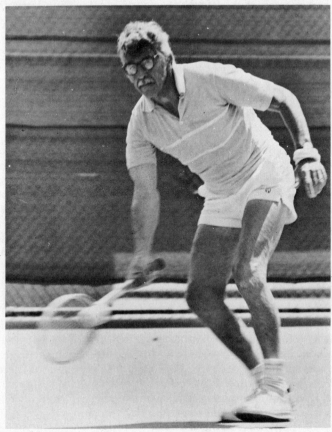

Variations in motivation, life style, health status, and personality influence the ways older people participate in community life and activities.

who maintain the highest possible degree of involvement and activity, particularly physical activity.

Social interaction, ego investment in social roles, and change in role activity were the major aspects of behavior measured in developing this perspective. "Life satisfaction" is thus an important dimension of activity theory. The older individual is presumed to experience a high degree of emotional well-being (life satisfaction) if he or she:

a. takes pleasure from activities of daily life
b. views his/her life as meaningful and is accepting of life circumstances;
c. has a positive self-image; and
d. ordinarily maintains happy and optimistic attitudes and moods [Havighurst, Neugarten, & Tobin, 1968].

To this list Jewett (1973) has added a sense of humor, or the ability to see things in perspective, and a life-style marked by consistent moderation. Lack of such characteristics appears to correlate highly with poor adjustment to aging.

CRITICAL DISCUSSION
"Fight or Flight—Bane or Blessing?"

Before addressing other social theories of aging it is important to evaluate the relative impact and relationship of the disengagement and activity theories.

Sociologists, like many other students of human behavior, have learned that any explanation based on a single factor is suspect. Both the disengagement and activity theories were formulated in an attempt to account for successful or well-adjusted aging by means of the unidimensional constructs for which they were named. Human nature, however, is much more complex than these theories imply; responses, although similar in nature or expression, may be the products of a variety of direct and indirect, antecedent and current factors, as is the case with life satisfaction.

An important study which illustrates this point was undertaken by Peterson, Hadwen, and Larson (1967) to investigate life satisfaction in retirement communities. Their findings showed that the high frequency of opportunities for activity in these places appealed to the majority of individuals living there. A significant percentage of residents, however, had moved to these communities not to engage in high levels of activity but rather to escape from excessive commotion and the difficult challenges of their previous housing situations. Surprisingly, there was no significant difference in life satisfaction between these two groups. In the case of those who wished for more activity than they were offered by their previous residential situation, participation was frequent and imparted much happiness. In the case of those who preferred to withdraw, the "wall" that separated them from an "involved" life seemed to provide the respite that they sought, and hence life satisfaction.

Antecedent events were important in determining the type of response preferred. Those who wanted to move into the community because they could not fully indulge their wishes for physical activity or social interaction in their previous circumstances were satisfied. Some remarked, "The only thing wrong with this retirement community is that we don't have enough time to do what we would like to do." These were the extraverts, whose life-styles had always reflected a high level of sociability and interpersonal interaction. In the minority were those incoming residents who had customarily pursued solitary endeavors. As introverts, they found satisfaction in aesthetic or intellectual pursuits or fantasy. These individuals resented the loud cries of children or the roaring sounds of cars racing around at the whim of adolescent drivers as intrusions upon their reveries. They felt no jealousy of nor any sense of challenge from others who spent their time in frequent social interaction, but they were just as happy.

There are various explanations as to why aging individuals develop different preferred life-styles and ways of coping. Some psychologists have speculated that introversion and extraversion result from genetic predispositions. As a consequence, according to this explanation some persons are "naturally" active participants in life's drama, while others just as "naturally" engage in passive observation. Psychoanalytic literature provides another explanation. Karen Horney, for example, proposed a dichotomy to describe how an individual might meet the challenges of life: fight or flight. One can observe both characteristic styles in older people. Some have been so buffeted by the "slings and arrows of outrageous fortune" that they simply turn their backs and "take flight." Others typically face the exigencies of life by fighting back. Still others may exhibit variable styles according to the nature of a given situation, taking action at times while withdrawing at others.

What is suggested here is that during the course of life, some individuals learn to cope by engaging in focused activity, while others retreat and withdraw. In other words, both the disengagement and activity theories are valid, but only when selectively applied to different individual life-styles. What is required is more refined, sensitive investigation in order to determine under what conditions and for whom disengagement or activity may provide the more satisfactory course. In one such study, Lemon, Bengston, and Peterson (1972) evaluated a number of hypotheses which resulted from the activity theory and discovered that most of the assumptions made by Havighurst in his original formulation were not supported. The conclusion of this study was that being an integral part of an informal friendship group was related to life satisfaction, but that frequency of interaction itself was not.

One conclusion to be drawn from this critical evaluation of the disengagement and activity theories is that they are not necessarily contradictory, but instead complementary. In addition, we do not as yet have sufficient data to conclude that either coping strategy is exclusively more efficient. Both theories require further specification and clarification before the validity of their implicit propositions can be determined. Nevertheless, they have contributed a great deal to our understanding of social aging by stimulating a number of studies and by demanding that social gerontologists look more carefully at the phenomena of differential coping styles in later life.

The Person-Environment Transactional Perspective

Although the social aging theories of disengagement and activity have received a great deal of attention in the literature, a number of alternative interpretations of aging in the context of society have been proposed. Among these are the person-environment transactional perspective and the exchange theory.

The person-environment transactional perspective (Schwartz, 1974), identified in Chapter 1 as providing the major conceptual focus of this book, places great emphasis upon the interaction and mutual influence of the individual and his or her environment, and attempts to underscore the potential for continuous and expanding growth and development throughout the lifespan.

Within this transactional frame of reference, positive self-regard (self-esteem) is viewed as the psychological foundation that provides the basis for competence throughout the lifespan. Multiple losses (or decrements) accumulating through the middle and later years are seen as working against the maintenance of self-esteem. According to this notion, successful aging is strongly associated with the ability to structure or modify the environment in such ways as to compensate the elderly for losses—physical, social, economic, and psychological. Given appropriate compensation, the senescent individual can continue to function quite effectively and with great satisfaction. This frame of reference proposes that the aging process itself, as well as services for the aged, should be assessed on the basis of what does—or does not—contribute to and enhance self-esteem. Whatever inhibits or is contrary to the maintenace of self-esteem in the provision of social services, for example, needs to be modified or eliminated altogether.

Rather than incremental or decremental steps or stages of life, this approach characterizes the life cycle as a continuous, dynamic process of adaptation and growth. In contrast to the decremental model, this view holds that the aging process consists of coexistent episodes of decline and renewal, given the compensations for loss required for continued competence throughout the lifespan. An essential psychodynamic aspect of the person-environment transactional view is that life cycle events are influenced by current situational events, through the achievement of positive goals, resolution of conflict, and maintenance of self-esteem factors, as much as they are by biomedical-genetic variables. With this in mind, Maddox (1976) has commented:

> Social scientists in the 1960s were apparently convinced that the phenomena they wanted to explain involved complex transactions between individuals and the sociocultural as well as physical environments within which and with which they interacted. Social scientists studying aging were not an exception; they found static, descriptive accounts of aging and the aged increasingly unproductive and uncongenial [p. 17].

In addition to its strong emphasis on interpersonal interaction and the mutual effects of the social and physical environments and the aging individual, the person-environment transactional perspective is dynamic and flexible, and lends itself to interdisciplinary analysis. Future investigations can be expected to further illustrate the validity of this perspective and its applicability to a wide range of contexts in the study of the sociology of aging.

Exchange Theory

The exchange theory entered the purview of social science by way of economics, where it has had a notable history. First introduced into sociology through the work of Homans (1961, 1974) and Blau (1964, 1974, 1977), Dowd (1975, 1978, 1980) has pioneered its extension into the field of aging. According to Dowd, the continuing relationship among "social actors" depends upon the relative costs and benefits of maintaining that relationship. When there exists an imbalance of power in the relationship—that is, when one actor benefits more than another in the context of social exchange—the "*power advantage* . . . can then be utilized to effect compliance from the exchange partner" (Dowd, 1975, p. 587).

Beyond middle age, exchange rates become increasingly less favorable for the aging individual and more favorable for social institutions and their actors. Emerson (1962) has suggested that a balanced and more equitable relationship can be restored by the less powerful exchange partner(s) through (1) *withdrawal* of the less powerful partner from the relationship (analogous to disengagement); (2) *extension of the power network* by the less powerful partner, who engages in attempts to expand his or her social roles and status (the basis of activity theory); (3) *emergence of status* occasioned by the revaluation of goods, services, skills, or other rewards available on a relatively exclusive basis from the less powerful partner; (4) *coalition formation* by the less powerful partner(s) to reduce the potential gain of the more powerful partner(s). Four constellations of power resources were identified by Blau (1964): money, approval, esteem or respect, and compliance. It appears that, because of the elderly's loss of roles and status in society and the resulting constriction of resources they face, the primary resource with which the elderly may enter into or maintain an exchange relationship is that of compliance (Dowd, 1975, 1978, 1980). While "there is nothing inherent in the aging process itself that necessitates a decline in individual power resources," it seems that "the nature and degree of power resources possessed by any group of older persons is a function of shared cohort experience in addition to individual attributes" (Dowd, 1975, p. 592). The reduced level of power observable in elderly cohorts today relative to their middle-aged counterparts is apparently, therefore, the result of the sociohistorical period in which they were educated and trained and the recent impact of technology on society. It is altogether possible that future aged cohorts may be able to enter and maintain more profitable and equitable relationships with social institutions and social actors by taking better advantage of power resources and balancing options to maximize their benefits and minimize their losses in society.

The exchange theory framework is very promising for the sociological study of aging because its propositions are easily transformed into empirical, testable hypotheses, and because it may be adapted to a number of areas of interest to social gerontologists, such as kinship patterns, political behavior, intergenerational relationships, and consumer behavior. As a result, it is likely that exchange theory will serve as the impetus of a great deal of research activity in future sociological studies of aging.

CRITICAL DISCUSSION

"Will You Myth Me When I'm Old?"

A number of negative myths about aging and older people still exist, despite growing evidence that should lead to more positive attitudes. Among the more pervasive of these misconceptions are:

1. *The Social Myth:* Social myths are defined as false beliefs about social groups. Such myths not only predispose society to adopt negative attitudes toward older people, but also undermine the real potential of the elderly by lowering their own expectations. The basic problem created by any social myth is its potential to make its victims act so that the myth becomes self-fulfilling. For example, if older persons accept the common belief that the aged lose the capacity to function well, they may act accordingly and begin to function below the level of their actual capacity or ability. If an older person is told repeatedly that sexual capacity is bankrupt after age sixty, for example, that belief may promote disinterest at best, male impotence or female frigidity at worst. If nothing else, it can cause elderly persons to avoid opportunities for satisfaction through sexual expression.

   Again, while attempts are made to lure older workers into earlier retirement, economic pressures continue to build for those with acceptable levels of health and skills to stay on the job and continue their careers. If society tells its oldest citizens that they have no further economic or political utility, they may withdraw from the economic or political scene. The same self-fulfilling process occurs when older individuals experience occasional forgetfulness (as we all do, regardless of age) and are taught to regard such behavior as a sign of senility, to which the response is intellectual retreat. It is worth discussing sexual, political, and intellectual myths in order to document the insidious and destructive nature of these myths of aging.

2. *The Economic Myth:* It is still widely believed that the majority of older persons are poor and economically dependent. "Not having enough money to live on" was judged a problem for older persons by 62 percent of the general public, but by only 15 percent of older people themselves (Harris, 1976). This myth has devastating consequences for any person approaching retirement, and can produce dread in adult children. The myth results in a distorted picture of our older population, gives them a poor public image, and makes adaptation to aging difficult.

3. *The Health Myth:* "Sans teeth, sans eyes, sans taste, sans everything" is Shakespeare's summary of the last stage of human life. Today this sort of portrayal of the "destroyed" older person is sheer myth.

Although there are in fact about one million older persons in some 25,000 nursing homes in this country, nonetheless this represents only about 5 percent of the aged (65 and over) population.

Chronic conditions like arthritis, rheumatism, high blood pressure, and depression are more common in the aging population than in younger cohorts, but nine of every ten older persons are not homebound and live mobile lives of comparative independence.

4. *The Myth of the Aging Mind:* One of the most devastating of all myths predicts that all older persons will gradually lose the acuity and resiliency of their thought processes. This myth is particularly insidious because it forms, in part, the justification for mandatory retirement, for suspicion of the political and social behavior of older persons, for relegation of "old ones" to insignificant life roles, and for stereotypic labels like "old crock" and "old biddy." It is generally believed that older persons think more slowly and less carefully than younger persons. It is true that the intellectual performance of elderly persons becomes much more deliberate, as evidenced in the results of many research studies. Clearly, too, the sensory deprivation experienced by many older persons can significantly affect their cognitive and intellectual processes. But despite these and other more equivocal findings, Schaie and his colleagues (among others) have concluded from extensive study that most of the so-called declines in intelligence are a myth (see Chapter 3), and that older persons can be as wise and insightful at age eighty as they were at age thirty, and perhaps even more so. What is important to note in this context is the damage to self-esteem, social usefulness, and political involvement and the waste of basic contributions and human potential that attend these myths.

These are a few of the social distortions and stereotypes about older persons that may impact upon their life satisfaction and aspirations. It is apparent that gerontology is faced with a major task of research and information dissemination: confronting these myths head-on and providing the evidence that will allow older persons to take a more optimistic view of themselves and to contribute more positively to their world.

A Demographic Basis for the Sociology of Aging

Demographers are social scientists who account for human behavior on the basis of analyses of the numbers of individuals in a society, their membership in various age groups, and, by implication, the social pressures those numbers exert on social change.

Demography deals statistically with changes in large, broad population groups, rather than with individual case studies. Demography does not pro-

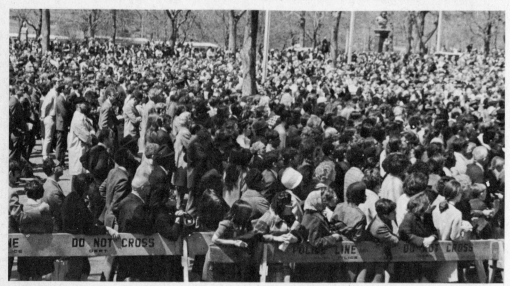

The elderly are constituent members of the total population. Demography helps us understand better how the aged "fit" into the population, how they affect it, and, in turn, how they are affected by it.

vide for individual variations. It can characterize populations in terms of percentages, means, medians, and modes. On this basis, it can "project" into the future (assuming all things remain equal). It cannot truly predict the future, nor does it claim to. Demographic projections, therefore, like all statistics, must be read with caution. They tell us what *could be,* not what *will be.*

Gerontologists are primarily concerned with populations aged sixty-five years old and older. Even though chronological age is neither a precise nor an optimal index of the aging process, sixty-five is nevertheless a widely used cutoff point to identify age cohorts in populations.

If these cautions are kept in mind, demography can be an important frame of reference in our effort to understand the sociology of aging.

Changing Trends in Life Expectancy

Human life expectancy has undergone a phenomenal shift since the time of the ancient Greeks. Then (about 1,000 B.C.), average life expectancy at birth was about 30 years; in 1970 it was 70.9 years; today, life expectancy approximates 73 years. Much of this increase has taken place within the past half-dozen decades or so. One remarkable fact is the advantage women have over men in average life expectancy and survival rates, an advantage that continues to increase (Cutler & Harootyan, 1975; cf. Figure 4–1).

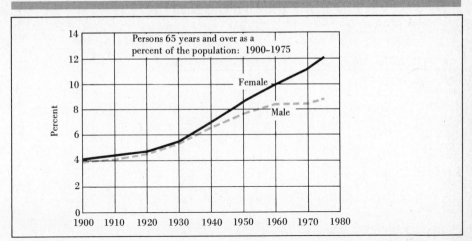

FIGURE 4–1. Persons 65 Years and Over as a Percent of the Population, 1900–1975

Source: U.S. Bureau of the Census, 1978

*The proportion of American women who are sixty-five years or over nearly tripled from 4.1 percent in 1900 to 12.1 percent in 1975. During the same period, the percentage of older men grew from 4 percent of the male population to 8.8 percent.

Some of the improvements in life expectancy, especially during the last century, may be attributed to the success of medicine in overcoming the usual childhood killers, particularly contagious and infectious diseases. Of greater significance as determinants of health, however, have been improvements in sanitation procedures and techniques, better nutrition, and birth control (McKeown, 1978). More persons are thus enabled to survive past childhood and middle age into the later years of life.

The present level of life expectancy at birth in the United States is paralleled in a number of other countries, as can be observed in Table 4–3.

What should be noted here about the countries listed in Table 4–3 is that they are so-called developed or industrialized societies. The picture is somewhat different for so-called less developed, less industrialized societies.

In Table 4–4 we see that life expectancy in most African countries, for example, is like that of our own country at the turn of the century. Furthermore, not only is the absolute number of elderly in countries like Haiti, Mexico, Brazil, and Venezuela much smaller than in the United States, but the elderly represent a much smaller proportion of the population as well (3.1, 3.7, 5.1, and 2.4 percent, respectively) in those societies.

Another aspect of life expectancy deserves attention. Life expectancy for humans, as for other species, is clearly related to age. A Swedish statistician of the early nineteenth century, Samuel Gompertz, is credited with the development of a mathematical formula describing the exponential increase in the probability of death as a function of increasing age—a formula which, incidentally, is applicable to the demise of water glasses, horses, and dishes, as

TABLE 4–3. Life Expectancy at Birth for Selected Countries

		Years	
Date*	Country	Male	Female
1973	Austria	67.4	74.7
1965–67	Canada	68.7	75.2
1970–71	Denmark	70.7	75.9
1966–70	Finland	65.9	73.6
1971	France	68.5	76.1
1970–72	Fed. Rep. Germany	67.4	73.8
1966–70	Iceland	70.7	76.3
1972	Israel	70.1	72.8
1972	Japan	70.5	75.9
1972	Netherlands	70.8	76.8
1971–72	Norway	71.2	77.4
1972	Sweden	71.9	77.4
1968–69	USSR	65.0	74.0
1968–70	United Kingdom	67.8	73.8
1972	United States	67.4	75.1

Source: United Nations (1975).

*Latest available figures.

well as to humans (see Hendricks & Hendricks, 1977). An illustration of this relationship between mortality rates and age is shown in Figure 4–2.

With this in mind, it is instructive to compare life expectancy in the United States at birth and at age sixty-five, as shown in Table 4–5.

This set of figures leads to an interesting conclusion. Although, as pointed out earlier, there has been a dramatic increase in life expectancy at birth since 1900, life expectancy at age sixty-five increased only slightly between 1900 and 1970. What this implies is that we may be seeing not so much an extension of the human lifespan as a greater possibility of survival to the longevity limits of our species. The reservation implicit in such a statement is that, given the present level of scientific knowledge, we cannot know with absolute certainty what those limits, if any, are for humans.

These life expectancy data are averages of the aging of individuals within a general population. They refer not to individuals but to total populations. What has already been referred to is a parallel demographic measure, namely, the probability of survival from one age category to another. This is known as *age-specific survival rate* (Cutler & Harootyan, 1975). These probabilities of survival at different ages are also averages derived from a given population (for example, the seventy-five-plus population). Both these measures of aging—life expectancy and survival rates—are largely a function of changes in mortality (death) rates within a population. Such information helps us to understand the age composition of a given population.

TABLE 4–4.   Life Expectancy at Birth and at Age 65 and Over for Various Countries

Country	Year	Life Expectancy at Birth		Population Age 65 and Over	
		Male	Female	Number (in thousands)	Percent of Total
North America					
United States	1970	67.0	75.0	20,101	9.9
Canada	1971	68.8	75.2	1,744	8.1
Haiti	1972 (est.)	—44.5—		157	3.1
Mexico	1970	61.0	63.7	1,791	3.7
South America					
Argentina	1972 (est.)	64.1	70.2	1,805	7.5
Brazil	1970	—60.7—		4,760	5.1 (age 60 +)
Venezuela	1970 (est.)	—63.8—		252	2.4
Asia					
China	1970 (est.)	—50.0—		—	—
Japan	1970	69.1	74.3	7,330	7.1
Iran	1971 (est.)	—50.0—		940	3.1
Syria	1970 (est.)	—52.8—		193	3.2
USSR	1970	65.0	74.0	28,514	11.8
Europe					
Austria	1970	66.6	73.7	1,047	14.2
Denmark	1969	70.8	75.7	590	12.1
France	1968	68.6	76.1	6,662	13.4
Hungary	1970	66.3	72.0	1,178	11.4
Netherlands	1971 (est.)	71.0	76.7	1,353	10.3
Sweden	1970	71.7	76.5	1,109	13.7
United Kingdom	1971	68.8	75.1	6,397	13.1
Africa					
Ethiopia	1968 (est.)	—38.5—		2,811	11.9 (age 45 +)
Ghana	1970	—46.0—		311	3.6
Kenya	1969	46.9	51.2	391	3.6
South Africa	1970	—49.0—		870	4.1
Uganda	1969	—47.5—		365	3.8
Zambia	1970	—43.5—		135	4.0 (age 60 +)

Source: United Nations (1973).

Proportion of Aged in a Population

Both the absolute (total) number and the proportion (percentage of the general population) of aged in the United States have been increasing dramatically. Based on past experience, demographers expect this trend to continue, but at a much more modest rate.

Table 4–6 shows the total number of those sixty-five and over within the general population and their proportional relation to the general population. By way of comparison, the table also shows the percentage of increase of

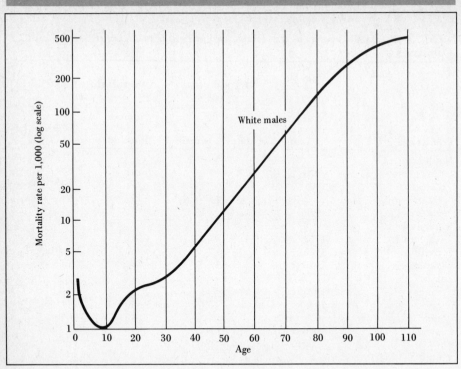

FIGURE 4-2. The Gompertz Curve: Mortality Rate as a Function of Age, United States, 1939-41

Source: B. L. Strehler, "Dynamic Theories of Aging," in N. W. Schock, ed., *Aging—Some Social and Biological Aspects* (Washington, D.C.: Association for the Advancement of Science, 1960), p. 286.

TABLE 4-5. Life Expectancy at Birth and at Age 65, by Race and Sex

Race and Year	At Birth		At Age 65	
	Male	Female	Male	Female
White				
1900–1902	48.2	51.1	11.5	12.2
1939–41	62.8	67.3	12.1	13.6
1954	67.4	73.6	13.1	15.7
1968	67.5	74.9	12.8	16.4
1976	69.7	77.3	13.7	18.1
Nonwhite				
1900–1902	32.5	35.0	10.4	11.4
1939–41	52.3	55.6	12.2	13.9
1954	61.0	65.8	13.5	15.7
1968	60.1	67.5	12.1	15.1
1976	64.1	72.6	13.8	17.6

Source: Jacob Siegel, "Recent and Prospective Demographic Trends for the Elderly Population and Some Implications for Health Care" (Presented to Second Conference on the Epidemiology of Aging, March 1977), table 7.

persons sixty-five and over, along with the percentage of increase of the total population for each succeeding decade from 1900, with projections to the year 2020.

Table 4–6 shows the proportion of persons aged sixty-five and older within the total population in 1900 as 4.1 percent, or slightly more than three million elderly. In contrast, the proportion of those aged sixty-five and older was almost 10 percent in 1970, representing somewhat in excess of 20 million elderly. By 1980 the proportion of older persons was greater than 10.5 percent, almost 23 million people aged sixty-five and over.

An analysis of the figures in Table 4–6 shows a small but steady rise not only in total numbers of older persons (column 1), but also in the proportion of elderly to the total population, moving from 4.1 to 9.9 percent from 1900 to 1970 (column 2). But while the numbers and proportions show a steady rate of growth, this is not the case when we examine the percent of increase by decades (column 4). There was a smaller proportionate increase in the 1930s (7.3 percent), followed by greater increases over the next two decades, and another relatively smaller increase during the 1960s (13.3 percent).

TABLE 4–6. Population Age 65 and Over in the United States for Each Decennial Year, with Projections to 2020: 1900–2020

	Population Age 65 and Over		Percent Increase from Preceding Decade	
Year	(1) Number (in thousands)	(2) Percent of Total Population	(3) Age 65 and Over	(4) Total Population
1900	3,099	4.1	—	—
1910	3,986	4.3	28.6	21.0
1920	4,929	4.7	23.7	14.9
1930	6,705	5.4	36.0	16.1
1940	9,031	6.8	34.7	7.3
1950	12,397	8.2	37.3	14.5
1960	16,679	9.2	34.5	18.5
1970	20,177	9.9	21.0	13.3
Projections		Series B[b] Series E[b]		Series B[b] Series E[b]
1980	24,051[a]	10.2 10.6	19.2	15.6 11.2
1990	27,768[a]	10.0 11.0	15.5	17.7 10.4
2000	28,842[a]	8.9 10.6	3.9	15.7 7.8
2010	30,940	8.1 10.6	7.3	18.3 7.2
2020	40,261	9.1 13.1	30.1	17.3 5.7

Source: U.S. Bureau of the Census (Nov. 1971; Dec. 1967).

[a]Revised data from United States Bureau of the Census. *Current Population Reports,* ser. P-25, no. 493, "Projections of the Population of the United States, by Age and Sex: 1972–2020" (December 1972).

[b]Assumptions of completed fertility (average number of births per woman upon completion of childbearing years):

Series B: 3.10 (high-fertility assumption).

Series E: 2.10 (low-fertility assumption, which mirrors present replacement level trend in the United States).

Two basic factors contribute to these changes, of course: mortality (death) and fertility (birth) rates. When fewer survive into later life (as during an economic depression or war), the proportion of the elderly is reduced. During a "baby boom" (for example, following World War II), the percentage of elderly in the population can also decrease. Balancing these periods may be another time (like the present period of replacement-level fertility) when the proportion of the elderly rises. We shall return to this issue shortly.

Another way to demonstrate this change in proportion of elderly in the population is to use the common age-sex population pyramid, which depicts the population profile by age and sex. Figure 4–3 shows these distributions at four times (1900, 1940, 1970, and projected for 1990). The distributions for males and females within each time frame are based upon five-year increments up through age seventy-five for the population profiles of 1900, 1940, and 1970, and similar-sized increments through age eighty-five for the projected population profile for 1990.

In 1900, when fertility and mortality rates were relatively high (32 births and 17 deaths per 1,000 people), the population pyramid was shaped much like a triangle. The shape of this profile changed markedly by 1940, reflecting the effects of low birth rates during the great economic depression of the post–World War I years. Further effects of changing birth rates are shown in the 1970 pyramid, as the population continued to age and the relative numbers of older persons increased. The projections for 1990 suggest that the "graying of America" will undoubtedly be the reality of the near future.

This "graying" phenomenon is reflected in other societies, too. It is interesting to note the parallels in countries such as Japan (see Figure 4–4) and the contrast in phenomenal growth in the aged population among Japan and such disparate countries as Sweden, Britain, France, the USA, and Brazil (see Figure 4–5). One can only speculate about the reasons for the disparity in rates of "graying" in these countries. But the fact that the aged population is increasing sharply at least in postindustrial societies once again draws attention to the need for cross-cultural research into needs and problems associated with such increases.

What do these demographic patterns mean? These data should begin to make clear the usefulness of demography as a tool for describing and assessing the age composition of a population as well as the attendant social implications. From these data, it is possible to observe the increasing probabilities of surviving into a good old age. The striking changes in the age composition of our population over the past four decades have had (and will continue to have) a marked impact upon the structure and values of our society. Our nation may be compelled to cope with issues it has never before had to face—issues with major implications for almost all sectors of society. Among those sectors in which the effects of demographic change will be particularly noticeable are the political system and public policy sector, the educational system, the legal system, and the economic system.

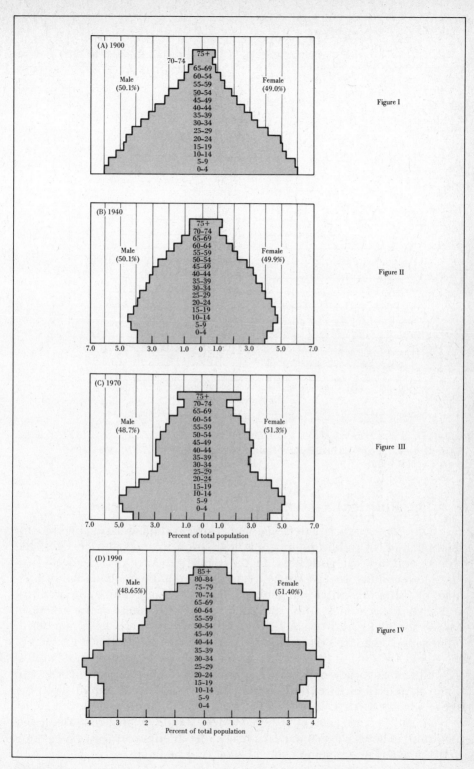

FIGURE 4–3. Age-Sex Population Pyramids for the United States; 1900, 1940, 1970, 1990

Source: U.S. Bureau of the Census. *Census of Population: Characteristics of the Population, 1940, 1970.*

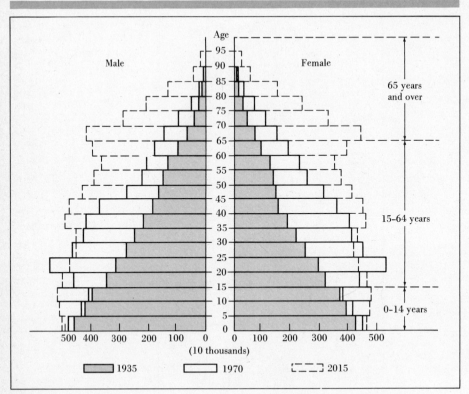

FIGURE 4–4. Population Pyramids of Japan for 1935, 1970, and 2015
Source: Yoshida (1974).

The Political System and Public Policy Sector

One consequence of demographic change is the increasing pressure for reformulation of public policy, new legislation to meet the needs of the elderly, and new categories of direct services to the aged. The elderly have become very much less passive and have learned to be more militantly articulate by using organizational strength. Consider, for example, the political and advocacy activities of the almost 13 million members of the American Association of Retired Persons (AARP). In addition there are a number of other active organizations of older persons, such as the National Council of the Aging (NCOA) and the National Council of Senior Citizens, as well as the militant advocacy of Maggie Kuhn and the Gray Panthers. These and other organizations of elderly persons have had a direct impact upon the entire health care delivery system with respect to definitions of health, delivery of health services, and how these services should be financed (Medicare/Medicaid). They have also played a major role in eliminating or liberalizing limits on mandatory unemployment—that is, retirement.

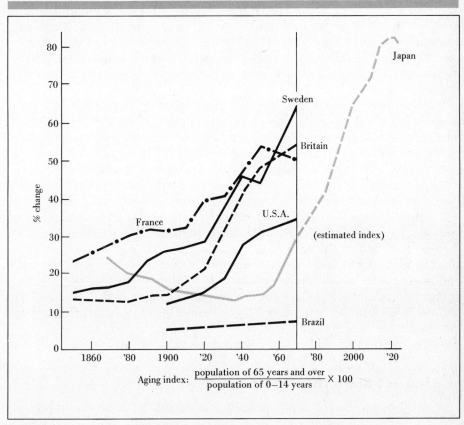

FIGURE 4–5. Annual Change of Aging Indexes of Several Nations
Source: Yoshida (1974).

The inevitable modification of mandatory retirement restrictions, namely, the recent change in federal law prohibiting mandatory retirement for those under seventy, is the result of a political process. This change comes as no surprise to those who are aware of the lobbying, voting, and other political activities of activist groups of elderly people. For the same reasons, we will continue to see further reforms of private pensions and Social Security, such as tying Social Security benefits to cost-of-living increases (see discussions of these and related issues in Chapters 5 and 6).

Impact on the Educational System

Our educational system also reflects these demographic changes. Not only are there more older people among us, but more of them are expressing their rising expectations regarding their adult educational needs; more are

going back to school. There is also the growing need for training in gerontology. Schools of every description, at the professional, preprofessional,
community college, and high school levels, are awakening to the need to
offer scientists, researchers, service providers (both professional and paraprofessional), clergy, teachers, and administrators more gerontologically
enriched curricula.

At the same time, school systems at the primary and advanced levels,
which were geared to anticipate the "baby boom" of the late 1940s, 1950s,
and early 1960s, are experiencing a recession from their formerly higher
crests of enrollment. This is especially evident at the university level. In
some areas, school systems have been forced to dismiss teachers, retrench on
existing curriculum offerings, or close entire schools. One aspect of the graying of America and the enrollment crunch in our educational system is the
determination and imaginative effort being shown by educators in their
attempts to encourage elderly citizens to return to school. This has also
focused attention on the necessity of sensitizing classroom instructors to the
special needs, apprehensions, and inhibitions of many elderly people who
are moving into an academic setting after a long absence. It has focused
attention on the need for training understanding counselors of the elderly
within the educational system, and the necessity for school administrators to
reduce the barriers to reentry into school by taking into account the special
physical, intellectual, and emotional needs of elderly enrollees.

Impact upon the Legal System

Nor has our system of jursiprudence been able to avoid the impact of
the changes in the nation's age composition. Increasing attention is being
focused upon legal advocacy for the aged, consumer protection, legal counseling, and the effects of crimes that particularly affect the elderly (e.g., mug-
ging, rape, fraud). A federally funded National Senior Citizens' Law Center
now serves as a clearinghouse for legal service to the elderly. A national
Bicentennial Conference on Justice and Older Americans that took place in
Portland, Oregon, in Sepetember 1976 was designed to synthesize research
and programs involving the legal and criminal justice systems and older
adults.

Over the past few years moves have been made to establish legal service
development offices in all fifty states and the U.S. territories. These offices,
generally associated with state offices or departments of aging, serve as focal
points for the expansion of legal programs for older persons and provide a
variety of free legal services as well. Given the large array of legal services
required, this may be viewed as too modest an effort. But it does reflect the
impact of changes in the demographic composition of America.

Impact on the Economic System

Some of the most profound effects of the graying of America are felt
within our economic system. The traditional American economic way of life

is increasingly affected by such issues as the legitimacy and utility of forced retirement. The encouragement of second or third careers, the reentry of older women into the work force, "parallel" careers, a reexamination and possible redefinition of the concept of "individual productivity," and pension arrangements including vested interests and portability have all become matters of public debate.

The Social Security system has received even greater attention in recent years, as was underscored by the 1981 White House Conference on Aging. Social Security provides at least a minimum income for the retired worker. Employers and employees pay into a fund out of which retired workers draw income following their retirement. When it was initially implemented in the 1930s, this system appeared to be consistent with the actuarial data upon which it was based; that is to say, most workers did not live (and thus did not draw funds) much beyond the retirement age of sixty-five years. Given these conditions, the Social Security system was able to maintain fiscal integrity. The ensuing decades have been accompanied by an increase in the standard of living, staggering inflationary increases, and, in some sectors, a reduction of retirement age. Because of these factors, combined with the increased longevity of our population, longer-living individuals who are drawing on Social Security funds for more extended periods than originally anticipated appear to be posing a major threat to the financial stability of the program (see Chapter 5 for more details).

Social Stratification and the Older Person

In all discussions of demographic profiles, chronological age is used as one of the most critical variables. Given the specific differences between, for example, those under age fifteen, those fifteen to sixty-four, and those sixty-five and older, students of gerontology can focus on the similarities and differences of persons in different age categories and determine how membership in the unique social structures associated with chronological age groups influences attitudes and behavior.

Stratification is a complex topic. The term as it is used in sociology refers to a special category of belonging: to a limited group (or *stratum*) that determines to some extent one's values and attitudes. At times, age itself puts constraints on individuals. The adolescent is "all hormones and pimples"; internal sexual promptings are novel and disturbing. Fifteen years later such feelings are accepted as normal. Fifty years later such drives may be more sporadic, and sometimes surprising. A child of six may want to wield an axe like its parent but can't quite manage it. Perhaps the child's grandparent walking up the road with a cane is feeling nostalgic for the days when that task could be undertaken with vigor. Childbearing may be a joy or a burden, but after the age of fifty, for most women is it no longer either an expectation or a threat.

Physical changes and decrements are factors that set limits and can

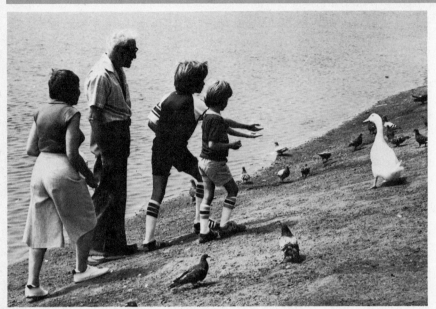

The experience of aging is enriched by contacts with children. Relatively few older persons prefer to limit their social contacts exclusively to peers.

influence behavior. No one would suggest that changes in strength, glandular secretions, vital capacity, sexual drive, vision, hearing, and the like are not often critical contributors to changes associated with age. But they are not necessarily the major component in determining specific responses. In the case of James North, described earlier in this chapter, an analysis eliminated physical states as particularly relevant in the assessment of his problems.

Position in the family often determines attitudes and values associated with behavior at given ages. In fact, the family is decisive in helping the upcoming generation adopt those values that are essential for smooth acceptance in their social class. Kohn (1969) explains the critical nature of the socialization process—how finely drawn are the influences of father and mother in this process and how the process is different for different social classes. From his national study, Kohn concludes:

> In both the middle class and the working class, mothers have their husbands play a role that facilitates children's development of valued characteristics. To middle-class mothers, it is important that children be able to decide for themselves how to act and that they have the personal resources to act on these decisions. In this conception fathers' responsibility for imposing restraints is secondary to their responsibility of being supportive. . . . To working-class mothers, on the other hand, it is more important that children conform to externally imposed rules. In this conception, fathers' primary responsibility is to guide and direct the children.

We will test the success of this socializing process in providing continuity of society's values and institutions and explaining intergenerational relationships later in this book. But family structures and functions are also sufficiently definitive that age-graded norms and roles are assigned and regulated. The child and early adolescent are not expected to support themselves independently; they are dependents. But young adults, on pain of disapproval, have to support themselves, their mates, and, later, their children. As individuals age in America, they must be industrious and frugal so that they can support themselves when their work days are over. And they must be over at a specified time, so that children and grandchildren may have job opportunities, too. This rite of passage into mandated unemployment—retirement—is another age-defined objective accompanied by a social role that determines the way to achieve, but the social environment in which this and other roles occur is changing rapidly and therefore strains the effort to achieve and be productive.

Summary

This chapter has focused on theoretical and demographic approaches to the sociology of aging. The disengagement and activity theories, based on the same series of studies of social adaptation to aging, were compared and were shown to be complementary rather than antagonistic in explaining the phenomena of aging in society. Other frames of reference, including the person-environment transactional view adopted by this book as well as the exchange theory, were highlighted in terms of their unique contributions to the study of aging and society. A number of myths about the aged and the aging process were examined with respect to the negative behavioral consequences they elicit at the expense of the dignity, functional capacity, integrity, and well-being of the elderly in our society.

The demographic study of aging was described as another means of studying aging and society. Demography focuses not on individuals, but on the composition of broad population groups over time, in order to describe not what will be, but what could be. The science of population dynamics was observed to rely heavily upon birth rates, death rates, and migration rates, which indicate how remarkably life expectancy has changed since the turn of the century. There has been an increase not only in the total number but also in the proportion of elderly persons in our society; this phenomenon, the "graying of America," is expected to continue for several years to come. These demographic changes have had a tremendous impact upon our country with respect to a number of dimensions: public policy, education, the legal system, and the economic system. Finally, the effects of demographic change may be observed to affect social stratification patterns in the near future, as social status and roles are redefined and reevaluated for different age groups in society.

References

Atchley, R. C. *The social forces in later life.* Belmont, Cal.: Wadsworth, 1972, 1979.

Bell, D. *The coming of post-industrial society.* New York: Basic Books, 1973.

Blau, P. M. Justice in social exchange. *Sociological Inquiry,* 1964, **34**, 193–206.

Blau, P. M. Parameters of social structure. *American Sociological Review,* 1974, **39**, 615–635.

Blau, P. M. *Inequality and heterogeneity: A primitive theory of social structure.* New York: Free Press, 1977.

Buckley, W. *Sociology and modern systems theory.* Englewood Cliffs, N.J.: Prentice-Hall, 1967.

Cowgill, D. O., & Holmes, L. D. (Eds.) *Aging and modernization.* New York: Appleton-Century-Crofts, 1972.

Cumming, E., Dean, L. R., Newell, D. S., & McCaffrey, I. *Disengagement: A tentative theory of aging. Sociometry,* 1960, **23**, 23–25.

Cumming, E., & Henry, W. *Growing old: The process of disengagement.* New York: Basic Books, 1961.

Cutler, N., & Harootyan, R. Demography of the aged. In D. Woodruff & J. E. Birren (Eds.), *Aging: Scientific perspectives and social issues.* New York: Van Nostrand, 1975, Pp. 31–69.

Dowd, J. J. Aging as exchange: A preface to theory. *Journal of Gerontology,* 1975, **30**, 584–594.

Dowd, J. J. Aging as exchange: A test of the distributive justice proposition. *Pacific Sociological Review,* 1978, **21**, 351–375.

Dowd, J. J. Exchange rates and old people. *Journal of Gerontology,* 1980, **35**(4), 596–602.

Emerson, R. M. Power-dependence relations. *American Sociological Review,* 1962, **27**, 31–41. Cited by J. J. Dowd, Aging as exchange: A preface to theory: *Journal of Gerontology,* 1975, **30**, 584–594. P. 589.

Harris, L., & Associates. *The myth and reality of aging in America.* Washington, D.C.: National Council on the Aging, 1976.

Harris, L., & Associates. *Aging in the '80s: America in transition.* Washington, D.C.: National Council on the Aging, 1981.

Havighurst, R., Neugarten, B. L., & Tobin, S. S. Disengagement and patterns of aging. In B. L. Neugarten (Ed.), *Middle age and aging.* Chicago: University of Chicago Press, 1968. Pp. 161–177.

Hendricks, J., & Hendricks, C. D. *Aging in mass society.* Cambridge, Mass.: Winthrop, 1977.

Henry, W. E. Engagement and disengagement: Toward a theory of adult development. In R. Kastenbaum (Ed.), *Contributions to the psychobiology of aging.* New York: Springer, 1965. Pp. 19–35.

Homans, G. C. *Social behavior: Its elementary forms.* New York: Harcourt Brace & World, 1961.

Homans, G. C. *Social behavior: Its elementary forms.* (Rev. ed.) New York: Harcourt Brace Jovanovich, 1974.

Jewett, S. P. Longevity and the longevity syndrome. *Gerontologist,* 1973, **13**(1), 91–99.

Kohn, M. L. *Class and conformity: A study in values.* Homewood, Ill.: Dorsey Press, 1969.

Kübler-Ross, E. *On death and dying.* New York: Macmillan, 1969.

Lakoff, S. A. The future of social intervention, In R. H. Binstock & E. Shanas (Eds.), *Handbook of aging and the social sciences.* New York: Van Nostrand Reinhold, 1976. Pp. 643–663.

Lemon, B. W., Bengston, V. L., & Peterson, J. A. An exploration of the activity theory of aging: Activity types and life satisfaction among in-movers to a retirement community. *Journal of Gerontology,* 1972, **27**(4), 511–523.

Lowenthal, M., & Chiriboga, D. Response to stress. In M. F. Lowenthal, M. Thurner, D. Chiriboga *et al.* (Eds.), *Four stages of life: A comparative study of women and men facing transitions.* San Francisco: Jossey-Bass, 1975.

Maddox, G. L. Disengagement theory: A critical evaluation. *Gerontologist,* 1964, 4(2), 80–82.

Maddox, G. L., & Wiley, J. Scope, concepts and methods in the study of aging. In R. H. Binstock & E. Shanas (Eds.), *Handbook of aging and the social sciences.* New York: Van Nostrand Reinhold, 1976. Pp. 3–34.

McKeown, T. Determinants of health. *Human Nature,* 1978, **1**(4).

Neugarten, B. L., et al. *Personality in middle and late life.* New York: Atherton Press, 1964.

Pampel, F. *Social change and the aged.* Lexington, Mass.: Lexington Books (D. C. Heath), 1981.

Peterson, J. A., Hadwen, T., & Larson, A. E. *A time for work, a time for leisure: A study of in-movers.* Los Angeles: University of Southern California Press, 1967.

Rose, A. M. A current theoretical issue in social gerontology. *Gerontologist,* 1964 4, 46–50.

Rose, A. M. The subculture of the aging: A framework in social gerontology. In A. M. Rose & W. H. Peterson (Eds.), *Older people and their social world.* Philadelphia: F. A. Davis, 1965. Pp. 3–16.

Schwartz, A. N. A transactional view of the aging process. In A. Schwartz & I. Mensh (Eds.), *Professional obligations and approaches to the aged.* Springfield, Ill.: Charles C. Thomas, 1974.

Shire, H. The corporate executive: Continuities, education, and schools of business and management. Master's thesis, Pepperdine University, Los Angeles, 1972.

Tallmer, M., & Kutner, B. Disengagement and morale. *Gerontologist,* 1970, **10**(4, part 1): 317–320.

United Nations. *Statistical Yearbook,* 1972 (24th ed.). New York: United Nations, 1973.

United Nations. *Statistical Yearbook,* 1974 (26th ed.). New York: United Nations, 1975.

Yoshida, S. Media for socio-medical service between home and institution in transitional Japan. Public Health Dept. Med. Faculty, Osaka Medical College, Japan. Aug. 1974.

For Further Reading

Beauvoir, S. de *The coming of age.* New York: Putnam, 1973.

Bengston, V. *The social psychology of aging.* New York: Bobbs-Merrill, 1973.

Bengston, V., & Haber, D. A. Sociological approaches to aging. In D. Woodruff & J. E. Birren (Eds.), *Aging: Scientific perspectives and social issues.* New York: Van Nostrand, 1975.

Bengston, V. L., et al. *A progress report: USC study of generations.* University of Southern California, Los Angeles, 1976.

Binstock, R., & Shanas, E. (Eds.) *Handbook of aging and the social sciences.* New York: Van Nostrand Reinhold, 1976.

Brotman, H. *Analytical and summary reference tables: The older population estimates for 1975 projecting through 2000.* Prepared for the National Institute on Aging, January 1976.

Brotman, H. Life expectancy: Comparisons of national levels in 1900 and 1974 and variations in state levels, 1969–71. *Gerontologist,* 1977, **17**(1).

Coale, A. J. The effects of changes in mortality and fertility on age composition. *Milbank Memorial Fund Quarterly,* 1956, **44**.

Kaplan, O., & Ontell, R. Social indicators and aging. In A. Schwartz & I. Mensh (Eds.), *Professional obligations and approaches to the aged.* Springfield, Ill.: Charles C. Thomas, 1974.

Manion, O. V. *Aging: Old myths versus new facts.* Eugene, Ore.: Retirement Services, 1972.

Neugarten, B. (Ed.) *Middle age and aging: A reader in social psychology.* Chicago: University of Chicago Press, 1968.

Reiss, I. *The family system in America.* New York: Holt, Rinehart & Winston, 1971.

Riley, M. M. et al, *Aging and society. Vol. I. An inventory of research findings.* New York: Russell Sage Foundation, 1968.

Rosow, I. *Socialization in old age.* Los Angeles: University of California Press, 1974.

Sachuk, N. N. Population longevity study: Sources and indices. *Journal of Gerontology,* 1970, **24**: 262–264.

Townsend, C. *Old Age: The last segregation.* New York: Bantam Books, 1971.

The Economics of Aging

Chapter 5

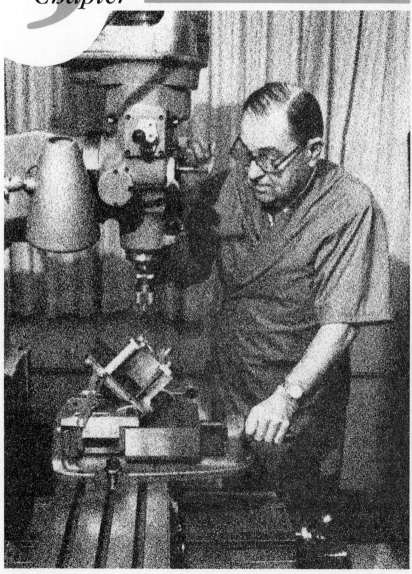

> If you wanted to punish a man . . . so severely so that even the most
> hardened criminal would quail, all you have to do is make his work
> meaningless.
> *Fyodor Dostoyevsky*

It is true, as the biblical saying has it, that humans do not live by bread alone. Yet our understanding of the aging process would be incomplete—and therefore deficient—were we to ignore the economic factors and contingencies that deeply affect the lives and aging of older people. Adequate shelter, food, clothing, transportation, health care, recreation, intellectual and social stimulation—all contribute to physical, emotional, and mental well-being. And all cost money.

For this reason it is important to understand the current economic circumstances of the elderly and the economic problems that impinge upon them. This chapter is designed to examine the adequacy of economic resources of older persons and to evaluate the probabilities that the economic foundation of the elderly will be maintained at a sufficient level to provide the basis for life satisfaction in the years ahead. Current controversies over many aspects of public policy, retirement, inflation, and intergenerational conflict will no doubt play a major role in determining the economic well-being of the elderly in the next several decades.

A basic question concerns the willingness of other segments of the population to allocate funds to those who are no longer viewed as "productive." At the turn of the century the vast majority of workers "supported" a relatively modest number of nonworking older persons. Today a growing number of retirees are becoming more and more financially dependent upon a smaller number of wage and salary earners. This phenomenon, illustrated in Figure 5–1, is described mathematically by means of the *dependency ratio*. To obtain this statistic, the number of "dependent" persons in the population is divided by the number of active wage earners. As it is frequently calculated, this ratio represents the number of retired or otherwise nonworking adults aged sixty-five years or older relative to the number of individuals aged eighteen to sixty-four years, inclusive, currently participating in the labor force. Sensitive to fluctuations in population size and levels of employment, the dependency ratio is a useful tool of demographic analysis for examining the ways society divides its "monetary pie" as a function of age.

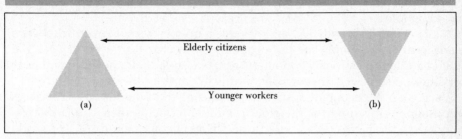

FIGURE 5–1.   The Dependency Ratio

Source: Schwartz (1979).

Table 5–1 shows the dependency ratios obtained in this manner by decades for the years 1930 to 1970, with projections for the years 2000, 2020, and 2050. Note that these ratios increase steadily through 1970, then begin to taper off. Hauser (1972), in fact, predicted a decline in the dependency ratio from 1970 to 1980, followed by a slight increase by 1990 and another decline by the year 2000. These patterns appear to be consistent with the observation that the rapidly increasing number of older dependent persons is being offset to varying degrees by the entrance of the baby boom generations of the 1940s and 1950s into the labor force. The lower birth rate which characterizes our present situation, however, will ultimately result in a smaller work force during the first decades of the next century, leading to an increase in the dependency ratios once again from 2000 to 2050. These predictions are based on the assumption that current trends in fertility, longevity, and employment status of the American population will not undergo significant change over the next several years as the result of major shifts in demographics or public policy. If this assumption proves invalid, however, these projections will require revision.

Throughout this chapter we will be analyzing the constraints on and attitudes of the employed and retired sectors of the population and the ways in which they affect and are affected by the relative allocations of economic resources. Included among the important issues to be addressed are:

1. From what sources do elderly persons draw their economic support?

TABLE 5–1.   Old-Age Dependency Ratios for the United States, 1930–2050

1930	1940	1950	1960	1970	2000	2020	2050
.097	.118	.133	.167	.177	.177	.213	.257

Dependency ratio = 65+/18–64.

Source: Years 1930–40 from U.S. Bureau of the Census (1942), table 8, p. 26; years 1950–70 from U.S. Bureau of the Census (1972), table 37, p. 32; year 2000 based on Series E projections from Brotman (1973), p. 3; years 2020 and 2050 based on Series E and Series W projections respectively, prepared by Dr. David M. Heer, Population Research Laboratory, University of Southern California, February 1974.

What provisions, specifically, are made by the private and public sectors for older people?

2. What do trends in employment, particularly those with respect to early retirement, imply for the economy, and what do they mean for the elderly? Can the national economy adequately support an increasing number of older persons who are partially or fully unemployed?

3. Can the economy sustain the impact of all of the various public sector programs in support of the elderly without reducing their standard of living—or the standard of living of those whose incomes are taxed to provide such public support?

4. How has inflation influenced the income of the elderly? What are future expectations with respect to the effects of inflation on the economic sufficiency of older people?

5. What is the nature of patterns of consumption by the elderly relative to other age groups in this country? How much economic clout do the elderly really have?

The following two case illustrations illustrate two unique perspectives on the economics of aging, as we prepare to address ourselves to these various concerns.

CASE ILLUSTRATION
"I Know What I Don't Want"

Mr. C. M. F. is a seventy-year-old man. In June 1973 he retired, after many years as a successful attorney practicing in Chicago. By August of that year he and his sixty-six-year-old wife sold their suburban home and fulfilled a longtime dream by moving to Southern California. They had no children and had sufficient income from investments to be financially comfortable. They found a suitable apartment not far from the ocean.

In spite of their involvement in a number of community activities and a growing circle of new acquaintances, Mr. F. found himself restless and dissatisfied. He knew what he *didn't* want to do (continue along the lines of his earlier career), but seemed to have great difficulty in focusing upon what he *would* like to do. The answer came through some consultations with a counselor.

Mr. F. had always been a skillful "Mr. Fixit." He enjoyed and was talented at repairing small appliances, clocks, bicycles, and the like. With some encouragement, he turned their spare bedroom into a small workshop, passed the word among friends and neighbors, and is now happily occupying his spare time with as much business as he chooses. And he finds that this second career provides a welcome supplement to his income.

CASE ILLUSTRATION

"So You Think It's Getting Better?"

Mrs. G. is an older woman, probably between sixty-nine and seventy-nine years old. During a visit to a senior counseling supervisor she stood before his desk and challenged him: "Don't give me that crap! You come with me to my apartment and *then* tell me how much the lot of older people has improved. Are you afraid? Why won't you come?"

Mrs. G. lived in central Los Angeles, near MacArthur Park. While studies of the park and its relationship to nearby residents had been conducted by the supervisor's colleagues, he still knew relatively little about her particular situation, so he accompanied her to her home.

She went slowly, experiencing great difficulty in walking. Her left hip had been broken years ago, and she had never received proper treatment. Mrs. G. and the counseling supervisor finally arrived at her building, where she slowly led the way up six flights of stairs (the elevator didn't work) to her apartment.

She had two rooms: small, untidy, cramped. The wallpaper hung down in a fold where it had peeled off the wall. The counseling supervisor was tempted to tear it down but didn't, for fear that the landlord would accuse Mrs. G. of destruction. The faucets didn't drip, they ran—resisting all of the efforts of the supervisor to tighten them. The place was dark, but when he offered to buy light bulbs, she laughed—evidently the wiring was defective.

They talked about her social contacts. There were none, except the owner of a local store. Whenever she didn't hobble down the six flights of stairs to his store, he would bring her a can of soup, bread, and milk. After rent and doctor bills were paid she didn't have any change left for streetcar fare to the senior center or church.

In some desperation, the counseling supervisor told Mrs. G. that he would take her to a social service center, where they could talk with a social worker. Again, she laughed. She'd been there. They would not listen. There were forms and more forms to fill out, but she couldn't understand them and the workers were impatient. She was hungry and they seemed to be indifferent—so she left.

The counseling supervisor assigned a bright, enthusiastic graduate student to follow Mrs. G.'s case, but Mrs. G.'s suspiciousness and excessive demands in the context of difficult environmental and social barriers proved too much. No one seemed able to succeed in surmounting the obstacles to promoting Mrs. G.'s well-being. Some months after their initial meeting, the counseling supervisor returned to her apartment to talk with her again, but Mrs. G. had disappeared.

We cannot ignore the substantial numbers of elderly persons living in poverty. On the other hand, gerontologists are aware that in the last thirty to forty years basic economic trends show some improvement for older persons, improvement which can be expected to continue into the future. Table 5–2 projects the number of families and singles aged sixty-five years and over and their income levels, based on twenty-five-year demographic projections (Olson, Caton, & Duffy, 1981). These projections assume no change in government policy with respect to the elderly from 1980 to 2005. Although this may be an unrealistic assumption, it is apparent that income levels may indeed increase substantially for older persons, all other conditions remaining relatively stable.

Economic conditions are improving for older Americans as a result of a number of factors. One contributor has been the growth of private pension plans (Atchley, 1979). Until recently, relatively few persons benefited from such plans because they were neither vested nor transferable. The Employee Retirement Income Security Act (ERISA) of 1974 improved the financial return to the worker from private pensions (Lowy, 1980). A second contributor is the inclusion in the Social Security system of many self-employed groups, such as farmers; now approximately 90 percent of the working population is eligible for retirement benefits through this source (Brown et al., 1979). A third contribution has come from recent legislation linking Social Security payments to the inflation-sensitive Consumer Price Index (CPI), so that real benefits are not lost due to rising prices. However, this is a current topic of debate in the federal legislature and may require modification in the future to lessen the financial burden placed on dwindling Social Security resources.

Basic to all of this has been the continued rise in the Gross National Product. The nation's increasing economic productivity is also reflected in the provision to the elderly of medical benefits through Medicare and Medicaid, and the Supplementary Security Income (SSI) program. This program, instituted in January 1974 to augment the income of those below the poverty level, has helped to improve (at least to some extent) the financial status of millions of elderly persons, along with allowing them to benefit from the Food Stamp program and federal housing subsidies. Finally, a 1978 amendment to the Age Discrimination in Employment Act (ADEA) has made it pos-

TABLE 5–2.   Numbers and Income Distributions for Families and Singles Aged 65 and Over
(Percentage within real 1980 income classes)

Income Distribution	Families of Two or More			Singles		
	1980	1990	2005	1980	1990	2005
$0 to $2,500	0.126	0	0	7.505	2.325	0.088
$2,500 to $5,000	7.254	2.931	0.260	43.774	44.109	32.110
$5,000 to $7,500	15.725	13.313	8.498	21.847	23.340	28.539
$7,500 to $10,000	15.312	15.200	14.240	10.679	11.536	14.554
$10,000 to $20,000	36.580	39.283	42.297	12.334	13.948	18.357
$20,000 and over	25.003	29.272	34.705	3.861	4.742	6.352
Number (thousands)	8,632.528	10,036.230	10,656.407	7,912.373	9,901.898	11,016.897

Source: Olson, Caton, & Duffy (1981).

sible for workers in jobs or occupations which feature mandatory retirement policies to work until age seventy (previously the age for mandatory retirement was sixty-five), thus increasing the opportunities for older persons to earn additional income for a longer period of time, if they so desire.

Resources among the Elderly: Past, Present, and Future

In Chapter 4 we sketched a brief history of America's metamorphosis from an agrarian to an industrial and, ultimately, a postindustrial society, and the implications of social change for the lives of elderly persons. Although many of the features of agrarian life, including the cohesive, supportive extended family network and the relatively prestigious position afforded elderly relatives within that network, may seem somewhat idyllic, it must be pointed out that not all older persons enjoyed such psychological, social, and economic advantages.

During the period prior to 1900, some older persons who were alone and dependent were provided economic assistance and support by private charitable institutions. Most, however, were sent to county poor farms. In 1871 there were twenty-four county hospitals and almshouses designated for this purpose in California alone. These institutions, often poorly ventilated and poorly maintained, were little more than warehouses for the elderly poor, dependent children, and the disabled, "feeble-minded," and "insane." After the turn of the century, many counties developed welfare boards which made some attempts to improve the living conditions and care of impoverished older persons and other dependent or indigent groups.

As the numbers (both relative and absolute) of older persons began to increase and the social structure began to evolve in step with the growth of industrialization, more attention was focused on the elderly, particularly those with insufficient economic support. As early as 1915, states began to pass legislation that earmarked public funds for "Old Age Assistance"; by 1929, ten states and the territory of Alaska had enacted such measures. Five years later, a total of twenty-eight states and two territories had adopted similar plans to support their elderly constituencies, and by December 1934 a total of 235,000 older persons received financial support under these "pension plans." Because some states elected to provide "optional plans," permitting the establishment of state support at the discretion of local county jurisdiction, however, only those elderly residents of participating counties were eligible for benefits. Eligibility for economic support thus ranged from 28 percent of older persons in states with optional plans to 91 percent of older persons in states featuring mandatory plans. Where state support was unavailable, counties were often enjoined to provide economic security for their aged residents, yet in many cases it was difficult for these smaller administrative units to assume the additional burden imposed by such welfare plans. In addition, subversion of state and local requirements stipulating that responsible relatives of elderly pension candidates contribute to the support of their elders was not uncommon, thus making the welfare of the old an even greater public liability.

During the Depression of the 1930s, state and county resources were hard pressed to meet the burgeoning cost of supporting increasing numbers of indigent people, including the elderly. In 1935 the U.S. Congress passed the Social Security Act, which offered individual states the opportunity to share the costs of Old Age Assistance with the federal government through Title I (Stein, 1980). Nonetheless, the amount of money available through this source was very limited. In California, the legislature was regarded as extremely beneficent for increasing monthly maximum payments from $40 to $50 in 1943. This was the most generous allocation of any state in the nation at that time. The federal government subsequently increased its contribution to the state's program so that an additional $5 could be added to maximum benefits in 1946, and again in 1947, thus increasing the total sum in California to $60.

The period immediately following World War II (1945 through 1947) was a time of unrest and controversy with respect to economic support of the elderly. Social agitation increased nationwide. A particularly outspoken fig-ure was George McClain, friend of the elderly, who organized older persons in California and demanded $75 a month in Old Age Assistance and $85 a month in Aid to the Blind. At the same time the Democratic Committee of Los Angeles County asked for $80 per month and urged the elimination of the "relative responsibility" clause. It is probably significant that McClain's father had gone bankrupt during the Depression and had been forced to apply for Old Age Assistance himself. The senior McClain was granted a sum of $18 a month, but an inquisitive social worker soon discovered that he was a Christian Scientist and concluded that he had no need for medical expenses. Consequently his monthly stipend was reduced to $15 per month!

McClain won an early election for the state senate the first time he ran, but lost his second bid. Although he tried repeatedly to regain his senate seat, it was apparent that he had lost his support. Nevertheless, a precedent was established in California, where older persons have ever since been strong advocates of financial support to elderly citizens.

The Social Security legislation passed in 1935 provided for a contribu-tory scheme of pensions through progressive taxation of employment income (Old Age Insurance, Title II), as well as a variety of public assistance pro-grams, including Old Age Assistance. When the legislation was enacted it was widely predicted that increasing numbers of persons would be covered by the insurance component while dependence upon public assistance would decline. This has indeed proved to be the case. As the Social Security Act has been amended over the years, more people have become eligible for benefits under its umbrella of financial support and fewer people have required Old Age Assistance. In 1974, Supplemental Security Income (SSI) was introduced as part of the Social Security program to replace Old Age Assistance and provide more comprehensive economic support to disadvantaged elderly persons.

In a recent appraisal of the income status of the elderly in this country, *U.S. News and World Report* (July 26, 1982) observed:

> *Older Americans,* by and large, are winning the war on poverty. In 1960, 1 in 3 persons over 65 was poor. Now the official figure is 1 in 6. Counting medicare, medicaid, food stamps, housing aid, the number is 1 in 20.
>
> Reason for the progress: Oldsters are winning the battle of the budget.
>
> They make up 11.4 percent of the population and receive 26.9 percent of all federal expenditures. Their share totals 195 billion dollars. It includes Social Security, medicare, other benefits to which they have contributed.
>
> In 1940, federal spending for each elderly person was $21 a year. Now it's $7,520. In five years, if present trends continue, it will reach $9,982.
>
> That means the elderly, 12 percent of the population by 1987, would be getting 283.3 billion dollars, or 28.9 percent of all federal outlays [p. 12].

There is considerable evidence, then, to support the conclusion that the past century has seen increasing attention to financial support for older persons in the United States. *U.S. News* reports hard evidence that the economic lot of the old is improving. What about present and future trends? Is the light at the end of the tunnel a sign of hope, or is it the headlight of an oncoming train?

Income Status of the Elderly

Older Americans presently rely on a variety of sources of financial support. In addition to Social Security benefits there are lifetime or current wages and salaries from employment, asset income (e.g., savings accounts, checking accounts, stocks, certificates of deposit, bonds, mutual funds, real estate), private pensions, government benefits such as Railroad Retirement, Civil Service Retirement, Veterans' Benefits, and Workers' Compensation, and intrafamily income transfers (Brown et al., 1979; Duffy et al., 1980; Kreps, 1976; Pampel, 1981; Stein, 1980). Table 5–3 indicates the relative contributions of various sources to the overall income of Americans aged sixty-five or older.

In addition, most older Americans may take advantage of at least some of the benefits provided through the following resources, which are estimated to contribute the equivalent of approximately 10 percent in in-kind income to elderly recipients (Moon, 1977):

1. Medicare and Medicaid
2. Housing subsidies
3. Food stamps
4. State planning, services, and information provided under the Older Americans Act, including meals served by the Nutrition Program
5. The national nutrition program for the elderly

TABLE 5–3. Largest Source of Household Income Base: More than One Source[1]

		Age				Age × Income				Age × Employment Status	
						65 and over				65 and over	
	Total	65 and over	65–69	70–79	80 and over	under $5,000	$5,000–$9,999	$10,000–$19,999	$20,000 and over	Labor Force	Retired
Base	2674	1619	596	748	275	344	416	334	203	112	1276
	%	%	%	%	%	%	%	%	%	%	%
Social security benefits	15	61	53	64	69	89	75	53	17	34	63
Supplemental security income (SSI)	*	1	1	1	1	3	*	—	—	—	1
Earnings from own current job	40	5	9	3	1	1	4	6	13	48	2
Earnings from spouse's current job	25	3	8	1	—	1	1	5	9	2	3
Railroad retirement	1	2	1	2	3	1	2	3	2	—	2
Veteran's assistance	1	1	1	1	1	—	1	—	1	1	1
Other government pension	1	2	3	2	1	—	2	5	1	2	3
Company pension or pension from federal, state, or local government employer	3	10	12	11	4	1	7	18	17	1	12

Savings	1	2	2	3	2	*	3	2	2	6	2	2
Investments	2	7	6	7	9	1	3	2	26	5	6
Insurance	1	1	*	1	—	1	—	*	—	1	*
Rent from renters or boarders	1	1	1	1	2	1	1	1	2	1	1
Inheritance	*	*	*	*	*	*	1	—	—	—	*
Money from parents, children, or other relatives	7	2	2	1	4	*	1	1	2	1	2
Aid for families with dependent children (AFDC)	1	*	*	—	*	—	—	—	—	—	*
Child support/alimony	*	*	*	*	—	*	—	—	—	—	*
Union pension	—	—	—	1	—	—	—	—	—	—	*
Other	1	1	1	1	*	1	*	*	3	*	1
Not sure	2	2	1	2	4	1	1	1	2	2	2

Source: Harris et al (1981).

[1]This table is based on answers to the following question: Which one source supplies the largest part of the income for this household?

*Less than 0.5%.

6. Operation Mainstream (older worker manpower program)
7. Research programs
8. Veterans Administration services [Schulz, 1976, p. 573].

These benefits will be discussed in the context of public policy issues in Chapter 6.

Income from Wages and Salaries

Currently income from wages and salaries comprises slightly less than one-fourth (23 percent) of the aggregate income of persons sixty-five or older (Harris, 1981). This figure is not surprising in view of the fact that only 13 percent of older Americans are presently included in the labor force: roughly 20 percent of older men, 8 percent of older women (Work in America Institute, 1980). While the participation of older women in the labor force has varied little, from 8 to 10 percent, since 1900, participation of older men has declined markedly during this period, as indicated by Table 5–4 and Figure 5–2.

In addition, relatively few older workers are employed on a full-time, year-round basis. Recent estimates suggest that approximately one-third of older employees work under such conditions, and that about one-half (44 percent of men and 56 percent of women) are employed part-time (Harris, 1981).

While income from salaries and wages has a relatively minor impact on the majority of older persons, the annual median income of those who work beyond age sixty-five is significantly enhanced by employment. Older workers are estimated to have a median annual household income of $14,200, in comparison to $8,700 reported for their nonworking peers (both figures include additional retirement income from other sources as well). In other words, the average annual income for nonworking elderly persons is only

TABLE 5–4. Men Sixty-Five and Over in the Labor Force, 1900–1978.

	Percent	Total
1900	63.1%	987,000
1947	47.8%	2,376,000
1950	45.8%	2,453,000
1960	33.1%	2,287,000
1965	27.9%	2,131,000
1970	26.8%	2,164,000
1975	21.7%	1,906,000
1976	20.3%	1,816,000
1977	20.1%	1,845,000
1978	20.5%	1,923,000

Source: Bureau of Labor Statistics, U.S. Department of Labor.

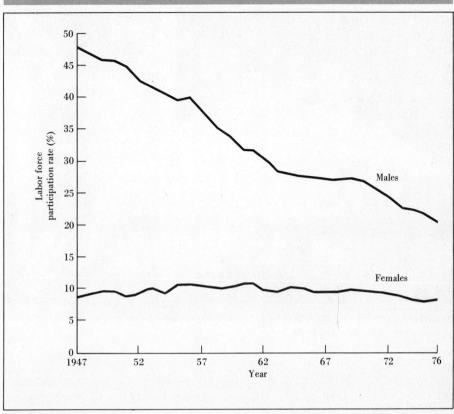

FIGURE 5–2.   The Labor Force Participation Rate of Males and Females Aged Sixty-five and Over

Sources: Employment and Training Report of the Presidents; Olson, Caton and Duffy (1981).

about 61 percent of that received by older workers, all other benefits taken into account (Harris, 1981).

Decline of Work Force Participation

Despite the obvious financial benefits of continuing employment in the later years, current trends suggest that increasing numbers of elderly persons will continue to leave the labor force unless major shifts in public policy occur to reverse this trend (see Chapter 6). While mandatory retirement regulations are often painted as the villains forcing the unwilling exodus of elders from their jobs, such regulations in fact have very little to do with the withdrawal of the elderly from the workplace (Parnes & Nestel, 1981). Indeed, congressional action in 1978 amended the Age Discrimination in

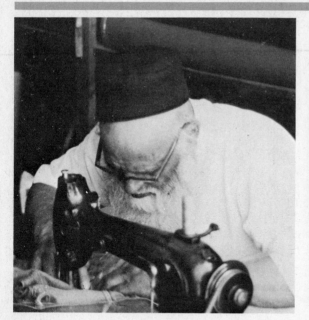 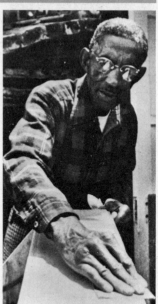

Vocation helps us to define ourselves. Continuing in a work role is important to the aged in maintaining self-esteem.

Employment Act (ADEA) to abolish mandatory retirement in federal government jobs, as well as increase retirement age from sixty-five to seventy elsewhere. The majority of mandatory retirement plans in effect today operate in conjunction with pension programs in the private sector. Yet, despite the ADEA revision, the trend among these pensioned workers is to retire from their jobs at even an *earlier* age than before—usually between the ages of fifty and sixty-two (Harris, 1981; National Committee on Careers for Older Americans, 1979; Parnes & Nestel, 1981; Schulz, 1976; Work in America Institute, 1980).

It has also been argued that increasing liberalization of Social Security legislation since 1935, including the indexing (or overindexing) of benefits to the inflation-sensitive Consumer Price Index (CPI) in 1972, actually encourages older people to remove themselves from their jobs. Often cited in behalf of this position is the fact that older workers were leaving the labor force and receiving Social Security benefits at age 62.9 in 1975 and at age 63.5 63.5 in 1981, in contrast to the expected norm of retirement and benefit receipt at age 65 (Harris, 1981).

Nonetheless, neither the existence of private pensions nor of Social Security as economic incentives to retire is sufficient to explain the marked decline in labor force participation of older individuals (especially men) over the past forty years, according to Pampel (1981). In *Social Change and the Aged,* Pampel examined the relative contributions of "compositional" and "processual" factors to decreasing frequency and intensity of labor force participation among older persons. Compositional factors as defined by Pampel are related to "changes in the characteristics of persons brought about by cohort replacement, or to the entrance of new persons into the aged population as they grow old and the exit of other persons out of the aged population through death," while processual factors are related to "changes in the process by which background characteristics of aged persons determine the social indicators of the aged" (pp. 3–4).

Based on extensive analyses of cross-sectional and aggregate time series data, Pampel concluded that, in general, compositional factors such as educational attainment, type of occupation, and level of socioeconomic status as reflected in levels of retirement benefits through Social Security and private pensions were of little explanatory value in accounting for changes in employment patterns among the elderly. Rather, it appears that "there has been a normative change in the meaning of retirement . . . the demand for leisure time may have increased" (p. 61). In other words, the positive changes which have accompanied postindustrial development in America have led to greater economic security in general, and more rational, equitable treatment of the elderly, for whom leisure pursuits are now considered legitimate in their own right. Thus, continued employment in the later years is no longer perceived as a necessary element in the definition of economic well-being or ascription of status for older persons.

This normative acceptance of retirement and the subsequent decline in labor force participation among the elderly will have major implications for public policy, particularly with respect to the economic status of the "baby boom" generations as they approach their sixth and seventh decades. Will current trends continue? Some estimates in fact predict that by 1990, the elderly will comprise only 2.4 percent of the national labor force, in comparison to their current 3 percent participation level (Work in America Institute, 1980), although the increasing impact of inflation on the real value of retirement income during the 1980s may modify this estimate significantly. Lowy (1980) comments,

> In light of the demographic, economic, and elderly labor-force-activity trends, it would make good sense for the government to permit and encourage greater labor-force participation on the part of older persons and for older persons to take advantage of the employment incentives and opportunities created. Increased elderly employment activity would generate additional tax revenue for use at all levels of government. The economy in general would benefit from the added production of goods and services and from improved productivity levels. The elderly would benefit from being able to supplement their income from other sources with income from employment, thus increasing their ability to maintain, if indeed not enhance, their standard of living and do it with a form of income (wages) that has better prospects for keeping up with inflation than other forms of income.

Finally, any share of that income that can be generated through the work effort of willing and able elderly individuals represents a share that need not be borne by other workers through taxes [p. 75].

We shall examine labor force participation trends in greater detail in the context of our discussion of public policy issues in the next chapter.

Income from Social Security

Perhaps the most dramatic trend in the economics of aging has been the complementary shift in the relative contributions of employment and family support versus Social Security and related retirement benefits to the income of older persons over the past several decades. Figure 5–3 shows the growth in the population aged sixty five years or older receiving Social Security benefits from 1940 (when benefits were first paid) through 1976. The increased percentage of older persons eligible for such benefits is particularly striking when one takes into account the general growth of the elderly population overall; with each successive year, every percentage point represents a larger number of people than in the past.

Benefit eligibility for Social Security is determined by the period of time (number of quarters) an individual has contributed earnings to the system through payroll taxation, and benefit levels vary with age of retirement. For example, while workers retiring at sixty-five are entitled to full benefits, those retiring at sixty-four receive only 93.4 percent of benefits; at sixty-three, 86.8 percent of benefits are payable, and at sixty-two (the lowest retirement age at which benefits may be obtained), retirees are entitled to only 80 percent of full benefits. These adjusted rates, furthermore, are constant through the lifetime of the benefit recipient; no modifications in payment rates are permissible once the decision to retire early has been made. At the present time, approximately 31.7 million persons receive retirement benefits through the Social Security program (which also includes disability and health insurance; Hildreth & Louise, 1982). These benefits are estimated to comprise approximately 38 percent of the aggregate money income of the elderly (Harris, 1981).

Title II of the Social Security Act of 1935 provided for the establishment of Old Age Insurance, a national pension plan to which both employer and employee contribute monthly. The trust fund generated by these contributions eventually pays the employee upon his or her retirement from work. When the program was being designed in 1934, government planners undoubtedly had no idea that it would ultimately grow to encompass such a large proportion of the federal budget; yet, 1982 figures suggest that as much as 28 percent of all federal expenditures are presently allocated to the payment of Social Security benefits in the form of Old Age, Survivors, and Disability Insurance (OASDI; *U.S. News & World Report,* June 7, 1982). Table 5–5 depicts the tremendous growth of the program with respect to maximum

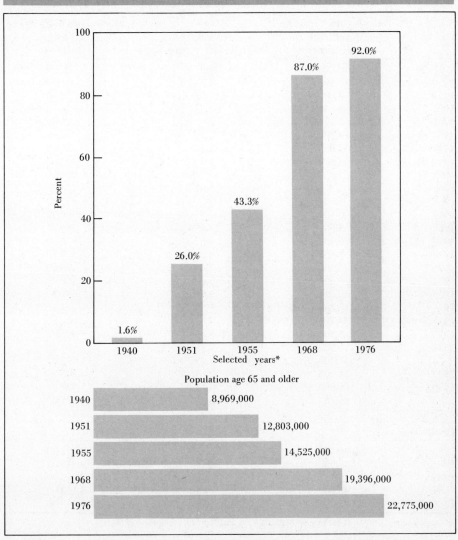

FIGURE 5–3.   How the Over-Sixty-five Population Receiving Social Security Benefits Has Increased

Sources: Social Security Administration; Bureau of the Census 1979.

* 1940 was first year in which Social Security monthly benefits were paid. Other years are those in which major extensions in Social Security coverage became effective.

taxable earnings and maximum tax dollars contributed jointly by employers and employees from 1937 to 1982, with projections through 1987.

   Although it is obvious from inspection of Table 5–5 that individual tax contributions to the Social Security program are considerably greater now than when taxation began in 1937, eligible retirees are currently receiving

TABLE 5–5.   Growth of the Tax Base: Social Security (OASDI), 1937–1987

	Maximum Taxable Earnings (dollars)	Tax Rates (employer-employee)	Maximum Employee Tax (dollars)
1937–49	3,000	1.0	30.00
1950	3,000	1.5	45.00
1951–53	3,600	1.5	54.00
1954	3,600	2.0	72.00
1955–56	4,200	2.0	84.00
1957–58	4,200	2.25	94.50
1959	4,800	2.5	120.00
1960–61	4,800	3.0	144.00
1962	4,800	3.125	150.00
1963–65	4,800	3.625	174.00
1966	6,600	4.2	277.20
1967	6,600	4.4	290.40
1968	7,800	4.4	343.20
1969	7,800	4.8	374.40
1970	7,800	4.8	374.40
1971	7,800	5.2	405.60
1972	9,000	5.2	468.00
1973	10,800	5.85	631.80
1974	13,200	5.85	772.20
1975	14,100	5.85	824.85
1976	15,300	5.85	895.05
1977	16,500	5.85	965.25
1978	17,700	6.05	1,071.00
1979	22,900	6.13	1,404.00
1980	25,900	6.13	1,588.00
1981	29,700	6.65	1,975.00
1982	32,400	6.7	2,170.80
Projections:			
1983	35,100	6.7	2,352.00
1984	37,500	6.7	2,513.00
1985	40,500	7.05	2,855.00
1986	43,800	7.15	3,132.00
1987	47,100	7.15	3,368.00

Sources: Munnel (1977); U.S. Congress, House Ways and Means Committee (1977).

benefits well in excess of those initially paid in 1940. When the first Social Security retirement benefits were paid, the average monthly allocation was $22.60 (LeBreton, 1974). In 1974, the average payment (including cost-of-living adjustments, or COLAs, based on the Consumer Price Index) amounted to $181 per month for the typical retired single worker and $310 per month for the retired married couple. Just six years later, in 1980, these payments had almost doubled; retired single workers at that time received an average of $341 per month, while retired married couples were paid a monthly average of $513 (Harris, 1981). As a result of the 1977 amendments to the Social Security Act, minimum monthly benefits have been established at a constant sum of $121.

Social Security: Special Problems

Social Security is the backbone of the income of a majority of aged couples and nonmarried persons alike. Many people, however, rely on sources of income in addition to Social Security in their later years, such as savings (33 percent), investments (22 percent), intrafamily transfers (5 percent), private pensions (32 percent), and employment (13 percent; Harris, 1981). While Social Security recipients may amass income from savings and investments and from family gifts of money or in-kind income without suffering any loss of federal benefits, the system presents special problems to those elderly beneficiaries who collect Social Security following retirement and receive a private pension or decide to return to work. Although such individuals have paid their premiums during their working life and would seem to

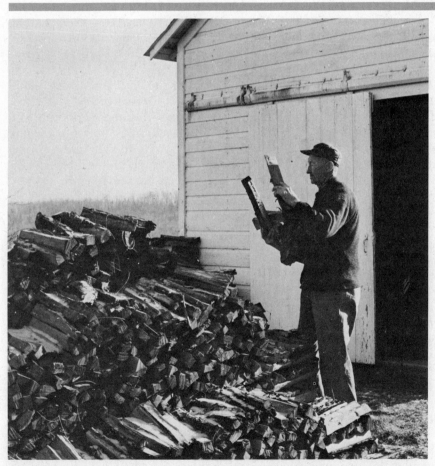

Whether through re-cycling or continuation of life-time careers, evidence increasingly supports the "use-it-or-lose-it" principle as the basis for well-being in later years.

be entitled to their monthly Social Security benefits, they can be penalized by a reduction in these benefits either for collecting deferred income through private pensions or for working for additional income in excess of specified dollar amounts. However, these penalties are considerably less stringent today than in previous times.

The precedent for imposing benefit penalties for additional income from employment during the retirement years was established in 1939, when older persons reentering the labor force following a period of retirement were allowed to earn no more than $14.99 per month in addition to Social Security payments. Employment income of $15.00 or more per month effectively jeopardized the right of an older worker to receive Social Security (Stein, 1980). In 1982, regulations stipulated that retirees under sixty-five may earn $4,200 annually, while those sixty-five to seventy may earn $6,000 annually without loss of Social Security benefits. Income in excess of these figures results in a downward adjustment of benefits: for every two dollars of income earned above the specified amounts, one dollar is deducted from monthly payments. Individuals seventy or older are currently exempt from such regulations and may now earn unlimited amounts of additional income through employment without penalty to Social Security benefits (Lowy, 1980).

These regulations, collectively referred to as the "retirement test," have often been criticized as disincentives restricting the initiative and productivity of older persons who might like to become active in the labor force but are concerned about loss of benefits. This criticism applies, however, only to those elderly individuals who for various reasons are limited in their earning power. For such persons, the fact that reentering the labor force for relatively little pay will provide no real net financial gain may prevent them from seeking employment.

While few would condemn the motives behind the development of the Social Security program, its structure and operation are currently topics of extensive and heated legislative debate. The government-sponsored trust funds which permit the payment of benefits to retirees (as well as to the disabled) are presently "paying out about 1 million dollars per hour more in benefits than they collect from payroll taxes" (Hildreth & Louise, 1982, p. 35). Despite the fact that the maximum taxable earnings, tax rates, and maximum employee taxes are presently higher than ever before in the history of the Social Security program (see Table 5–5), and that as of 1977 the proportion of taxable payrolls was increased from 85 to 91 percent (Stein, 1980), there are now only approximately three active workers per beneficiary.

Early in 1981, President Reagan proposed a number of sharp cuts in Social Security benefits as a move to slow the drain of trust fund resources. In a rare display of solidarity, the Senate voted 92 to 0 against this proposal, thus preserving the basic benefits guaranteed to date by law. Recognizing that the present system of financing is incapable of supporting the system indefinitely, the president subsequently appointed a task force to look at possible alternatives to current Social Security financing.

The precarious economic state of the Social Security program is due to a number of factors. First, the Social Security Act, developed hastily as part of the New Deal to provide financial relief at the earliest possible date to older persons in need, was based on the deficit spending model of Keynesian economics—a reasonable short-term solution, but a long-term disaster (Stein, 1980). Second, the demographic data employed in the development and projection of the program have changed significantly since the 1930s. Not only are many more people surviving to the age of eligibility for retirement benefits, but increased longevity means that greater numbers of individuals will be surviving to depend upon Social Security resources for considerably longer periods of time than in the past. For example, as of 1978, men retiring at sixty-five can expect to live an additional fourteen years, while women retiring at the same age will likely survive an additional twenty-two years past the date of their retirement (Harris, 1981). Add to that the additional years of survivorship for persons taking advantage of early retirement, and the prospects for collapse of the system are greatly increased. An even greater threat to the system's integrity is the maturation of the "baby boom" generations, which will be entering their retirement years during the first decades of the next century. Without some creative and highly effective alternative financing strategies in the immediate future, intergenerational support for the elderly will soon become past history. The details of at least some of the plans currently being discussed in Congress will be presented in the context of public policy issues and the elderly in the next chapter.

Supplemental Security Income

In 1974, the Supplemental Security Income (SSI) program was established by Congress under Title XVI of the Social Security Act, subsuming the functions of Old Age Assistance (OAA), Aid to the Blind (AB), and Aid to the Totally and Permanently Disabled (ATPD) programs. According to Lowy (1980):

> It was hoped that the program would result in poor people having more cash to spend; a national minimum income for the aged, blind, and disabled; uniform eligibility conditions instead of conditions that differed widely from state to state under OAA [and] a start in unraveling the administrative snarl enveloping welfare programs [p 58].

Eligibility requirements for SSI are quite specific. To be eligible for these benefits in 1977–79, for example, single individuals and married couples had to have less than $189.40 and $284.10, respectively, in "countable income." These figures corresponded to the maximum monthly benefits payable by the federal government to SSI recipients in those years, although all but eight states provide additional state supplements to these federal funds. SSI recipients living in institutional settings in which Medicaid payments covered at least half the cost of residential care were limited to benefits of only $25 monthly ($50 for married couples), less countable income. No SSI benefits were payable to individuals or married couples residing in institutions without access to Medicaid. Regular payments were also reduced by one-third for individuals or married couples living in another person's home and receiving major maintenance and support within such a setting.

A new term used in determining payments is "disregards." This means that for given levels of income, certain resources are not included as "countable income." For example, if an older person earns income from work or business, the first $195 per quarter plus one-half the remainder of earned income is not counted in determining the amount of SSI payments. Other disregards may include gifts, income from occasional work, property tax refunds, and tuition. The limits on salable property are fixed at $1,500 for single individuals and $2,250 for married couples. Such properties as a home, reasonable amounts of household goods, a car, and a life insurance policy with a cash value of less than $1,500 are not included in the calculation of SSI benefits. Older persons with resources in excess of those specified may sell them and use the money from their sale to buy excludable resources in order not to jeopardize maximum SSI payments. This can create some difficult situations for older persons with very limited means who have small accumulations of additional cash or other countable income. For example, if an older man has essentially no regular income but has more than $4,000 in cash through savings, he is ineligible for SSI benefits. Should he spend his nest egg, in order to qualify for a higher monthly income from SSI, or would it be better to reserve that money as "insurance" against catastrophic illness or some other potential crisis?

The major differences between Social Security and SSI are their sources of funding and their underlying philosophies. Social Security was conceived as an *insurance* program, making payments to retired (as well as disabled) workers based on contributions from employer-employee dyads through payroll taxes. SSI, in contrast, was designed as a *public assistance* (welfare) program to benefit older and disabled persons with insufficient income, and is funded through general federal and (in the majority of states) state revenues (Stein, 1980). As economic conditions improve for the elderly and as the Social Security program continues to underwrite larger numbers of longer-living beneficiaries, progressively fewer individuals are receiving SSI or Old Age Assistance payments, as Figure 5–4 indicates.

Income from Assets

According to the most recent Harris poll (1981), assets held by elderly Americans comprise approximately 19 percent of the aggregate money income received by this group on an annual basis. In 1978, 57 percent of elderly persons receiving Social Security benefits also received some form of asset income, which may have included interest from accumulated savings and checking accounts, as well as investments in stocks, bonds, certificates of deposit, mutual funds, and real estate (sales and rentals).

A number of recent developments associated with pension reform (see

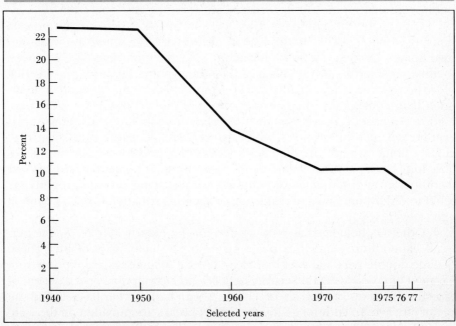

FIGURE 5–4. Decline in the Proportion of the Aged Population Receiving Public Assistance, 1940–77

Sources: Statistical Abstracts of the United States; 1975 *Annual Statistical Supplement to the Social Security Bulletin* (1976); HEW *Monthly Benefit Statistics,* December 1976; *Social Security Bulletin,* April 1978.

next section) and tax benefits may help to increase asset holdings within the elderly population over the next several decades. For example, in 1974 the Employee Retirement Income Security Act (ERISA) mandated the development of Individual Retirement Accounts, IRAs, as an alternative to private sector pension plans. These IRA trust funds act as tax-free savings accounts. The maximum deposit is equal to no more than 15 percent of annual salary or wages up to $2,000 per person. Income taxes are payable upon withdrawal of money from an IRA, with penalties imposed for withdrawal of funds prior to the investor's sixty-fifth birthday. For older persons living on restricted budgets, the need for liquid assets which must be removed from an IRA can present a very unpleasant financial situation; it is anticipated that at least initially, most persons participating in this type of savings plan will be representative of middle-class or higher economic status. Given the trends over the past few decades, however, it is not unreasonable to assume that the rise in economic prosperity of the elderly may continue long enough for people of less substantial means to become involved in such savings plans. Although the full impact of IRAs will likely not be felt by older persons for several years, since those who will most probably benefit from long-term involvement in IRA plans are now in their early and middle adult years, these investments will no doubt provide an important source of income for older people in the future and thus perhaps help to relieve at least some of the burden on public retirement funds in the years ahead (Stein, 1980).

One of the more important assets held by older persons is equity in housing (Atchley, 1979). Better than 60 percent of older Americans own their own homes, in comparison to only about 12 percent of those aged eighteen to fifty-four (Harris, 1981). This is an important point, because it means that older homeowners have relatively more disposable income to spend on items other than housing, in comparison to much of the rest of the American population. An unsettling consequence of inflation and rising costs, however, is ever-increasing property taxes, which can seriously jeopardize the security of elderly homeowners. In some instances, older persons whose mortgages have long been paid in full are forced to give up their homes because of their inability to pay property taxes. Fortunately, most states provide property tax relief to older homeowning residents, so that this situation is not a common one (Lowy, 1980).

Other tax benefits that are provided for the elderly help to reduce personal expenditures and thus boost assets in the later years of life. These include double personal exemptions on federal income tax, exemption from payment of taxes on Social Security benefits, and exemption from payment of capital gains taxes on the sale of a home after a homeowner has reached the age of fifty-five. In addition, a number of tax breaks are provided on the state level (Lowy, 1980). While these are essentially "hidden assets," not often taken into account in determining the income levels of the elderly, they do indeed help to improve the standard of living for older persons.

Private Pensions

In addition to providing for the establishment of IRAs and analogous Keogh retirement investment plans for self-employed individuals, ERISA in 1974 also specified regulatory standards for retirement pension plans offered through private sector employers (Stein, 1980). Nonetheless, these reforms affect a relatively small proportion of today's elderly population. Although approximately 43 percent of private sector employees were enrolled in ERISA-regulated pension plans in 1978, only 31 percent of married and 14 percent of unmarried persons sixty-five or older received pension benefits that year. This is consistent with the fact that about 9 percent of the aggregate money income of older people in 1978 was attributable to private pension payments (Harris, 1981).

Since the ERISA reforms, the major criticism of private pension plans is that they are often not inflation-proof, in contrast to Social Security and SSI. However, prior to 1974, most private pensions were neither portable (transferable), nor did they feature equitable vesting provisions. In other words, if a worker decided to change jobs before completing a certain number of years with an employer (i.e., before becoming fully vested), the years of work credit earned on the first job would not count toward potential pension benefits with the new employer. To illustrate this situation, Schulz (1970) quotes one Labor Department official's comments to the Senate Special Committee on Aging:

> If you remain in good health and stay with the same company until you are sixty-five years old, and if the company is still in business, and if your department has not been abolished, and if you haven't been laid off for too long a period, and if there is enough money in the fund, and if that money has been prudently invested, you will get a pension.

Despite the fact that many of the effects of the complex ERISA legislation have yet to be realized, "ERISA is shaking the worst out of the [private pension] plans" (Stein, 1980, p. 85). Given the problems inherent in the present funding structure of Social Security, mentioned earlier in this chapter, revised private pensions may ultimately come to offer a more substantial proportion of retirement support to older persons than has been the case thus far.

Income from Relatives

At the beginning of this chapter (and in Chapter 4) it was pointed out that elderly persons who resided with the members of their extended families at the turn of the century and before were part of a psychosocial and socioeconomic support network. From our discussion of changes in family structure and function and the rise of public support for the elderly, it is perhaps obvious that the economic interdependency of older persons and their family members—especially their adult children—has declined apace. Stein (1980) points out, "No state may treat adult children as legally responsible for the well-being of their parents" (p. 46), a fact which certainly was not true for most states less than a hundred years ago. Recent estimates suggest that the level of intrafamily transfers of income to the elderly are very low— likely no more than about 2 percent of the total income received by the elderly population is derived from family members (Harris, 1981).

In *The Measurement of Economic Welfare,* Moon (1977) discussed the relative contributions of various income sources, including intrafamily transfers, to the economic welfare of aged families in 1966. One important finding was that only about half of these transfers shifted income from younger to older family members. While some 15.64 percent of aged families received an average of $1,632.31 from younger family members in 1966, another 12.66 percent of aged families gave away an even greater sum—$2,049.43, on the average—to their younger relatives. In conclusion, Moon commented, "Intrafamily transfers alter the well-being of only 28 percent of aged families, and the average across all aged families is very small" (p. 66). Although this conclusion was based on analysis of 1966 data, the state of intrafamily income transfers is little different today. Older persons generally receive only minor *economic* support from the members of their extended families.

CRITICAL DISCUSSION

Poverty—An Age-Old or an Old-Age Problem?

"One of the most basic rights of older persons is the right to an adequate income to ensure that the last years of life are lived in comfort and dignity" (Brown et al., 1979). It cannot be denied that the postindustrial era has ushered in better times—at least in terms of access to economic resources and material well-being—for older Americans in general. Nonetheless, there are many people not unlike Mrs. G. (described in a case illustration earlier in this chapter) whose daily struggle against poverty attests to the fact that an adequate income for at least some segments of society is less of a right than a privilege.

Is poverty an age-old problem, as Jesus suggested nearly 2,000 years ago? Or is it an old-age problem—something that occurs as an inevitable consequence of growing older? Or both? Lowy (1980) notes:

> There are the poor who become old and the old who become poor. The latter must cope with a vastly altered life-style, which may have negative social, psychological, and personal consequences. For the former, old age is the final insult and hardship added to what may have been a lifetime of inadequate income, inadequate health care, and demoralization [p. 27].

The Poor Who Become Old. In 1981, 15.3 percent of the population sixty-five or older lived in poverty (defined by the government as having an annual income of $4,000 or less if single and $5,000 or less if married and living with a spouse). This proportion roughly parallels that of the nation in general (14 percent), thus supporting Lowy's contention that "the economic well-being of older persons is intimately linked to the economic well-being of all people in any society" (1980, pp. 82–83).

At least some of the elderly poor are members of traditionally disadvantaged minority groups whose precarious economic foundations have created the climate for lifespan poverty. For example, while 11.1 percent of all white Americans were described as "poor" in 1981, 26.5 percent of Hispanics and 34.2 percent of blacks fell into this category (*U.S. News and World Report,* August 2, 1982), regardless of age. Not surprisingly, similar group differences obtained with respect to the annual median income reported for elderly members of these three groups in 1980. While elderly whites received $9,100, Hispanics and blacks received only $5,600 and $5,000, respectively (only about 55 to 60 percent of the income of their white counterparts)—confirmation of a lifespan phenomenon in this country (Harris, 1981). Minority elderly rely on public assistance, most notably Supplemental Security Income (SSI), to a larger extent than do white elderly; more than 20 percent of black and Hispanic older persons identify SSI as a source of income, in comparison to 5 percent of white elderly. However, it must be kept in mind that only about 10 percent of elderly persons are minority members; the relatively small proportion of 5 percent of white elderly translates to almost 1.2 million people (Harris, 1981).

The latest Harris poll (1981) indicates that only about 10 percent of Hispanic and black elderly persons feel they have sufficient economic resources to "get by," in contrast to 52 percent of white elderly respondents. These results echo Lowy's description of old age as "the final insult and hardship" for those who, after a lifetime of poverty, enter what are presumably their "golden years."

The Old Who Become Poor. Morgan and associates (1974) reported that the risk of living in poverty does indeed seem to increase with advancing age. The results of their study suggested that the chances of being poor for any given year during a five-year period were about 30 percent for persons aged twenty-five to fifty-five, 40 percent from ages sixty-five to seventy-four, and 50 percent for people seventy-five or older. In general, it appears that the risk of poverty is less for those who are still married (particularly if both partners worked or otherwise contributed to their income prior to retirement, or are still working), and greatest for those who are widowed and alone.

Given the statistics on survivorship of elderly persons, it is not surprising to find that older women are at considerably greater risk of becoming impoverished in their later years than older men are. Whereas approximately three-fourths of all older men (sixty-five and over) are married, only one-fourth of older women presently enjoy such a relationship. This discrepancy is magnified when it is recalled that older women greatly outnumber older men; nearly two-thirds of the population sixty-five or older is female. More than half of older women (57 percent) live alone, while fewer than one-fifth (17 percent) of older men report such living arrangements. Given the fact that older women have annual incomes which, on the average, are the equivalent of about 57 percent of the annual incomes of older men, it is understandable that older women indicate more frequently than their male peers that they have great difficulty making ends meet and are barely able to manage on the basis of their present financial resources (Harris, 1981). For many elderly women who never worked but relied solely on their husbands' incomes for economic support for so many years, their spouses' deaths mean not only the loss of continued companionship but also a major reduction in their standard of living, at a time in their lives when they may be ill-prepared to make such an adjustment. For those who have never had to cope with a small, fixed budget it can be a devastating experience.

The Double Whammy: The Poor Who Become Old Who Become Poorer. A number of authors have remarked on the plight of those whose economic situation in the later years reflects the joint disadvantages of lifetime poverty and the economic constraints which can accompany old age. "Double jeopardy" describes the situation of female elderly individuals who are members of a disadvantaged minority group. Despite Pampel's (1981) observation that the progressive tax system which underlies Social Security seems to be closing the gap between the income levels of whites and those of minority groups, and of men and women, in the later years, the gap still exists. And, according to Cyril Brickfield, executive director of the American Association of Retired Persons (*Modern Maturity,* June–July, 1982), it is not likely that the situation will improve significantly in the near future: "There is mounting evidence that inflation has begun to wipe away the progress made by older Americans in the last decade. . . . Millions of elderly remain in a precarious economic position" (p. 7). Particularly for those facing their later years in double jeopardy, this is not encouraging news. Chapters 6 and 8 discuss the political and social sides of this economic dilemma.

Life-Styles and Patterns of Economic Consumption

As we have seen, older people comprise one of the more rapidly expanding sectors of the American population today and will continue to do so well into the next century. Despite this fact, relatively little information exists to describe two very important facets of the lives of the elderly which society cannot afford to overlook much longer. The first has to do with "the orientation to self, others, and to society that each individual develops and follows . . . derived from personal beliefs based on cultural context and the psychosocial milieu related to the stages of the individual's life" (Schutz, Baird, & Hawkes, 1979, p. 4). This orientation is referred to as one's life-style. The second facet is the impact of the behavior of older persons as consumers of goods and services upon society (and vice versa). Although a number of older persons must cope with severely restricted economic resources, the financial status of the elderly has improved over the past several decades. Indeed, the combination of relatively greater buying power and the sheer weight of numbers of elderly persons in this country cannot help but make an impression on business and industry; the aged will be a force to be reckoned with in the years ahead.

In response to the growing need for information about the life-styles and patterns of economic consumption of older persons in America, Schutz, Baird, and Hawkes (1979) conducted an investigation "to define lifestyle patterns existing among older Americans empirically and to relate lifestyle quantitatively to consumer behavior in the following areas: consumer problems, buying style, store choice, income management, health care, food and nutrition, transportation, housing, and clothing" (p. v). Their study consisted of preliminary and large-scale surveys of older people living in Northern California in 1976. "Life-style" was defined for purposes of this study in terms of respondents' temporal investments, affective or emotional investments, and levels of interaction with their social and physical environments, in the contexts of their roles as workers, homemakers, parents, spouses, friends, community workers, and leisure-time consumers. "Consumer behavior" focused on

buying style, which included frequency of actual shopping, brand loyalty, credit use, venturesomeness, planning, impulsiveness, price orientation,

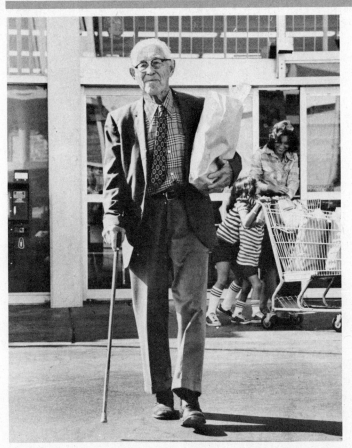

The needs of the elderly are often similar to the needs of people of all ages, depending primarily on life-style and personal preferences that have been redefined and refined over a lifetime.

information sources, and degree of family involvement in purchase decisions; store relations, or types of stores shopped at and mode of transportation; budget allocations; inventory; alienation; attribute importance; and store choice [p. 46].

In contrast to myths which suggest that "older people are all alike," Schutz et al. discovered that no single life-style was typical of elderly persons, and that consumer behavior varied as widely among the elderly as it does among individuals of any other age group. In other words, specific life-style and consumer behavior variables that characterize an individual at one point in the lifespan will probably continue to do so, with minor modifications, at a much later point in time. Just because a person has passed a certain birthday, there is no automatic shift in tastes, preferences, attitudes, or opinions to usher in membership in a new age group. Schutz and associates comment:

> In employment, leisure and social activities, marital roles and relationships, and personal habits and health, older Americans' needs are not different from those of their younger counterparts. The differences that do appear are related to lifestyle, or how the elderly person copes with the unique set of circumstances he or she experiences and creates, and not to age. . . . The portrayal of the elderly as a separate market segment . . . is unfounded; they are actually part of the larger, general market. . . . Consumer behavior, per se, is one of the most stable conditions in the lives of older Americans, and . . . lifestyles or role experiences, relationships, level of activities, and involvement in or away from home have more of an effect on the elderly than age, sex, or income [pp. 153, 158, 159].

Summary

The economics of aging is a complicated topic. We have looked at the various sources of support for retired and aging persons. The general outlook is encouraging, in that the number of individuals who exist below the poverty line has been lowered. A second encouraging factor is the change in public policy that now ties Social Security payments to the cost of living, thus alleviating to a certain extent the erosion of income by inflation. Some of the major areas of rising costs, such as taxes and medical expenses, have been blunted in their impact by special consideration of the tax obligations of older persons and the institution of Medicare and Medicaid. All in all, the treatment of older persons in our society has improved (Pampel, 1981).

References

Atchley, R. C. *The social forces in later life.* (3rd ed.) Belmont, Cal. Wadsworth, 1979.
Brickfield, C. F. This stereotype is false image. *Modern Maturity,* June–July 1982, **25**(3), 6–7.
Brown, R. N., Allo, C. D., Freeman, A. D., & Netzorg, G. W. *The rights of older persons—the basic ACLU guide to an older person's rights.* New York: Avon Books, 1979.
Duffy, M., Barrington, E., Flanagan, J. M., & Olson, L. *Inflation and the elderly.* Report to National Retired Teacher's Association and American Association of Retired Persons. Lexington, Mass.: Data Resources, 1980.
Harris, L., & Associates. *Aging in the '80s: America in transition.* Washington, D.C.: National Council on the Aging, 1981.
Hauser, P. Extension of life—demographic considerations (mimeographed). Paper presented at 25th annual Conference on Aging, Ann Arbor, Mich., 1972. Cited in J. Kreps, Intergenerational transfers and the bureaucracy. In E. Shanas & M. Sussman (Eds.), *Family bureaucracy and the elderly.* Durham, N.C.: Duke University Press, 1977. Pp. 21–34.

Hildreth, J. M., & Louise, R. Your social security benefits—the outlook now. *U.S. News and World Report,* June 7, 1982, **93**(1), 35–37.

Kreps, J. The economy and the aged. In R. H. Binstock & E. Shanas (Eds.), *Handbook of aging and the social sciences.* New York: Van Nostrand Reinhold, 1976. Pp. 272–285.

LeBreton, E. *Plan your retirement now—so you won't be sorry later.* Washington, D.C.: U.S. News and World Report Books, 1974.

Lord, L. J. (Ed.) Currents in the news. *U.S. News and World Report,* Aug. 2, 1982, **93**(5), 6–8.

Lowy, L. *Social policies and programs on aging.* Lexington, Mass.: Lexington Books (D.C. Heath), 1980.

McBee, S. (Ed.) Tomorrow: A look ahead from the nation's capital. *U.S. News and World Report,* July 26, 1982, **93**(4), 11–12.

Moon, M. *The measurement of economic welfare: Its application to the aged poor.* New York: Academic Press, 1977.

Morgan, J. N. et al. *Five thousand Americans: Patterns of economic progress.* Vol. 1. Ann Arbor: University of Michigan, Institute for Social Research, 1974.

Munnel, A. H. *The future of social security.* Washington, D.C.: Brookings Institution, 1977.

National Committee on Careers for Older Americans. *Older Americans: An untapped resource.* Washington, D. C.: Academy for Educational Development, 1979.

Olson, L., Caton, C., & Duffy, M. *The elderly and the future economy.* Lexington, Mass.: Lexington Books (D.C. Heath), 1981.

Pampel, F. *Social change and the aged.* Lexington, Mass.: Lexington Books (D.C. Heath), 1981.

Parnes, H. S., & Nestel, G. The retirement experience. In H. S. Parnes (Ed.), *Work and retirement: A longitudinal study of men.* Cambridge, Mass.: MIT Press, 1981. Chapter 6.

Schulz, J. H. Income distribution and the aging. In R. H. Binstock & E. Shanas (Eds.), *Handbook of aging and the social sciences.* New York: Van Nostrand Reinhold, 1976. Pp. 561–591.

Schutz, H. G., Baird, P. C., & Hawkes, G. R. *Lifestyles and consumer behavior of older Americans.* New York: Praeger, 1979.

Stein, B. *Social security and pensions in transition: Understanding the American retirement system.* New York: Free Press, 1980.

Work in America Institute. *The future of older workers in America: New options for an extended work life.* Scarsdale, N.Y.: Author, Special Task Force to the Secretary of Health, Education, and Welfare, 1980.

For Further Reading

Best, F. *Flexible life scheduling: Breaking the education-work-retirement lockstep.* New York: Praeger, 1980.

McCluskey, N. G., & Borgatta, E. F. *Aging and retirement: Prospects, planning, and policy.* Beverly Hills: Sage, 1981.

Monk, A. More on the economics of aging. In E. F. Borgatta & N. G. McCluskey (Eds.), *Aging and society: Current research and policy perspectives*. Beverly Hills: Sage, 1980. Pp. 42–46.

Morrison, M. H. *Economics of aging: The future of retirement*. New York: Van Nostrand Reinhold, 1982.

Muller, C. F. Economic roles and the status of the elderly. In E. F. Borgatta & N. G. McCluskey (Eds.), *Aging and society: Current research and policy perspectives*. Beverly Hills: Sage, 1980. Pp. 17–41.

Sinick, D., & McKibbin, G. B. *A study of the need for and nature of aging employment clearinghouses*. Monograph of the Western Gerontological Society. Prepared for The Regional Education and Training Program of the AOA, 1982.

Social Policy: Its Implications for the Aged

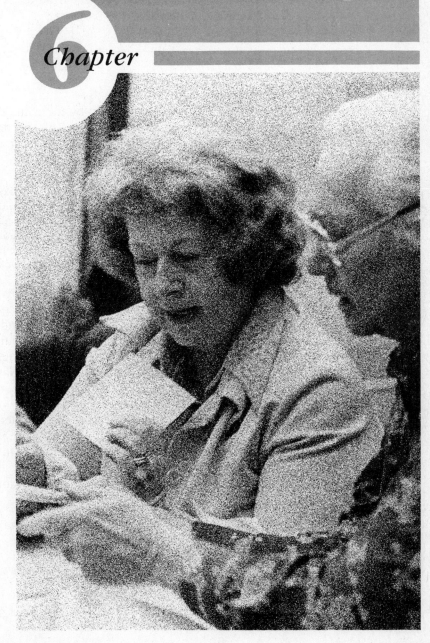

Chapter 6

All would live long, but none would be old.
Proverbs

On November 8, 1977, a seventy-three-year-old widow by the name of Isabella Cannon was elected mayor of Raleigh, North Carolina. This was her first political outing, as they say. The *New York Times* reported her victory the following day:

> Mrs. Cannon, a retired library administrator, defeated the incumbent mayor in a stunning upset vote. She said that she had no idea the campaign would be so strenuous, but that she had thrived on the very demanding schedule. Asked whether her age or sex had been any handicap with the voters, Mrs. Cannon said that she had rarely gotten a question related to her age or sex. She felt that was more a concern of the media than it had been for the average citizen.

Isabella Cannon is but one of many older persons who are involving themselves in the arena of public policy and politics in their later years. The old age lobby has a loud voice in Washington, D.C., and at the state and local levels, illustrating the growth of "gray power" as a political force in our society. National, state, and local chapters of organizations such as the American Association of Retired Persons (AARP, formerly combined with the National Retired Teachers' Association) and the Gray Panthers are beginning to have a noticeable impact on the formation of our nation's social policy.

But what is the impact of social policy on the aged? Which decision makers most affect the lives of elderly persons in this country? How are policy decisions affecting older Americans developed and implemented? On what basis is social policy formulated, and what must administrators and service providers know in order to provide and carry out effective and relevant programs for the elderly?

Approaches to Social Policy

Kerschner and Hirschfield (1975) have described a four-fold approach to the analysis of public policy formulation, implementation, and outcomes. Their approach has been schematized in Figure 6–1.

188

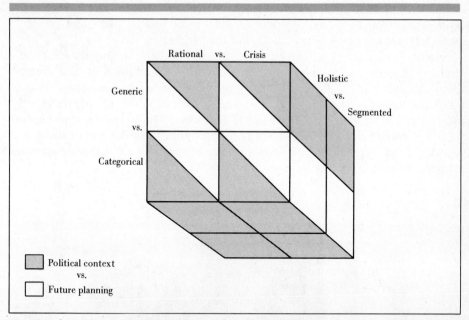

FIGURE 6–1. Schematic Representation of Model Public Policy Dichotomies
Source: After Kerschner & Hirschfield (1975).

In the schematic representation of their approach to public policy, Kerschner and Hirschfield identify four salient dimensions for analysis:

1. nature of the population to be served *(categorical versus generic)*
2. degree of specificity of policy content or issues *(holistic versus segmented)*
3. reason(s) for public policy formulation *(crisis versus rational)*
4. relevance of public policy over time *(political context versus future planning)*.

Categorical versus Generic

Determining the nature of the population to be served by a given social policy has proved to be a highly challenging task for policymakers. Should public policy be oriented to the specific needs of a limited, relatively well-defined category of individuals—such as the elderly—or should it serve the needs of the overall (generic) population, regardless of individual or group characteristics? We have observed throughout this text that the elderly have special needs. But to what extent do we truly want to treat the elderly as different from the remainder of the population? Given what has been said thus far about the disruption of lifespan continuity by the arbitrary imposition of a chronological marker at age sixty-five signaling the departure from middle age and entry into "the later years," exactly how should public policy differ, if at all, for persons immediately on either side of this transparent boundary line? When do older people need to be treated like older people, and when are they best assimilated into the larger population?

Not unlike their fellow citizens, older people have needs for food, clothing, shelter, companionship, transportation, entertainment, and countless other items and services that have at one time or another served as the focus of major social policy debates. These are not needs of *just* the aged, but of people in general. Lowy (1980) remarks, "The aging process represents a continuum: being old is not being different from the rest of the population. Therefore, the basic needs of older individuals will be more similar to rather than different from other age groups" (p. 153).

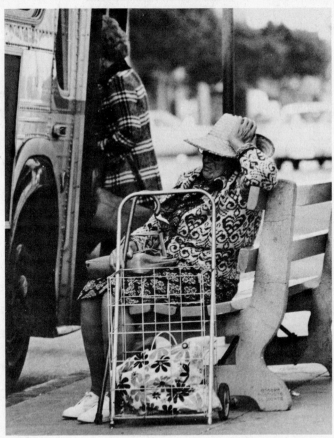

The availability and accessibility of convenient and cheap transportation is a major problem for many older people. Although they are apprehensive about using public transportation, it is generally their only means of shopping and reaching activities and friends.

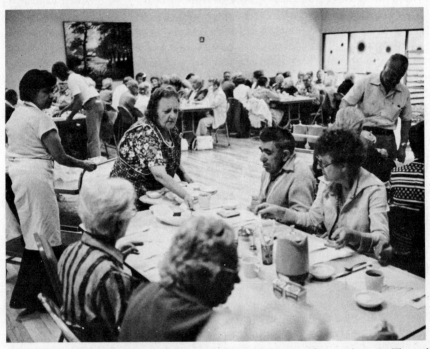

Nutrition programs for the elderly provide good, hot meals—and more. They also provide opportunities for social exchange, which for most people is an important element in the enjoyment of food.

As was pointed out in the last chapter, the satisfaction of many of these needs is contingent upon the availability of financial and other resources to the needy. For example, transportation across town for an elderly woman confined to a wheelchair is no problem if she has enough money to hire a driver, rent or buy a specially equipped van or truck to accommodate her chair, recruit people to help her in and out of her vehicle, etc. In this case, neither age, nor gender, nor physical handicap prevents this person from the satisfaction of her need because she has the economic resources to provide for herself. Without those resources, whether provided privately or publicly, her need would probably not be satisfied. The root of this evil does indeed seem to be money.

It is important to keep in mind that while the needs for food, shelter, transportation, and so on exist throughout the lifespan—from birth, not just the sixty-fifth birthday, and for as long as life continues—the economic means of satisfying those needs often do not. In our discussion of retirement and related issues in Chapter 5, we referred to the findings of the most recent Harris poll (1981), which indicated that in 1980 the average age of retirement for American men and women was 64.3 and 62.9, respectively. Early retirement (i.e., prior to age sixty-five) not only results in a decrease in annual income for older persons, but—more important—extends the period of time during which the retiree must depend on that decreased income to provide for the satisfaction of these needs. The fact that only one-fifth of men and one-twelfth of women in this country continue to work beyond age sixty-five suggests that a large proportion of elderly persons may be at risk—not because of their age per se, but because of age-related employment and retirement practices that may threaten the satisfaction of these generic needs.

Social policy analysts who evaluate the costs and benefits of categorical versus generic approaches to planning, implementation, and outcomes often argue that the generic approach may overlook and ignore the needs of the elderly, who only comprise about a tenth of our national population. Yet if the policies being planned, implemented, and evaluated pertain to the satisfaction of needs the elderly have in common with other segments of the population, there should be little difficulty in serving the needs of the aged along with the needs of others. Another argument against categorization has to do with the fact that policies designed and tailored to suit the needs of a specific subpopulation must be based on a highly specialized, detailed, and accurate assessment of these needs and of the particular nature of the subpopulation to be served. As Kerschner and Hirschfield (1975) note, the use of insufficient or inaccurate information as the data base for categorical planning "may well be destructive to the well-being of the user population" (p. 354). In addition, efforts to base categorical planning and implementation of social policy on groups arbitrarily distinguished by their age cohort overlook salient differences within age groups that would provide for more realistic policy formulation. In *The Aging Enterprise,* Estes (1980) writes:

> A pervasive and powerful American ideology sets the aged apart from the rest of society as a group with needs that require special policies and programs. The adoption of this ideology has been deemed necessary by the more sincere advocates for the aged, but its application has been at the expense of the aged themselves. . . . The stigmatization of the aged may also cause them to be seen as responsible for their own problems and therefore undeserving of public action to ameliorate their disadvantaged status. . . . This . . . view of aging emphasizes the similarities (and negative image) of all older persons. . . . Deemphasized are the differences across sex, ethnic, and class boundaries within the same age group [pp. 17, 18].

An excellent illustration of this point is the subpopulation of the ethnic elderly (see Chapter 8). Ethnic minority elders differ in a number of important ways from white majority elders. To be truly responsive to the needs of this subpopulation, social policy planners and decision makers must be fully aware of the characteristics and nature of the ethnic experience of growing old. Yet there is a paucity of information on the interactions of ethnicity and aging. Furthermore, not all ethnic groups are alike—and in addition to significant group differences because of cultural and ethnic heritage, the variability within any given ethnic group can be tremendous. The heterogeneity of the ethnic elderly can play havoc with efforts to plan, implement, and evaluate a social policy that is designed to serve the needs of all.

Some poignant facts illustrate the problem. Because the average black man's life expectancy is about seven years shorter than that of his white counterpart, it is less likely that a black man will collect any benefits from the Social Security or pension contributions he has made over the years (Jackson, 1972 a & b). Mexican-Americans often work as highly mobile migrants and in occupations that are not included under the Social Security umbrella. Women of both these minority groups may share a fate similar to that of the migrant worker if they have entered the labor force as domestic workers—another job category which heretofore has fallen outside the range of eligibility for Social Security coverage and benefits. The inequities of the Social Security system with respect to ethnic and female workers were apparent years ago (cf. Burns, 1936), although they were regarded more as a curiosity than an injustice demanding action. For Pacific Asians, problems of language, social isolation, and cultural difference are particularly important as they encounter retirement, which is a phenomenon novel to their heritage. Benetiz (1973) summarizes some problems of the ethnic minority elderly:

> For all the minority groups . . . there is little positive modeling of roles for the young with whom they come in contact. When there is a break in intergenerational continuity it is hard, sometimes impossible, for the elderly to see what will transcend them. Many are left not with a sense of immortality through the existence of the next generation, but with a sense of loneliness and despair. . . . Benefits could be given earlier and other social policies could be devised to include alternatives particularly suited to the unique situations of [ethnic] minority elderly.

Given the problems inherent in providing an accurate and up-to-date description of the characteristics and needs of successive elderly cohorts over the next several decades, generic planning, implementation, and evaluation look even more attractive as a model public policy option.

Holistic versus Segmented

The degree of specificity in the content of social policy provides another dimension for analysis. Should policies be oriented to particular, circumscribed issues or needs, or should they be broader and encompass a larger, more integrated set of issues and needs?

At present, the elderly are served in a highly segmented manner. Dozens of specialized agencies serve housing, health, income, and nutritional needs. A more holistic approach would integrate these various services so that older persons would not have to patronize a large number of different agencies in various geographic locations.

There may be certain administrative advantages to the provision of segmented services to the elderly (not to mention the rest of the population). This approach may provide checks and balances against abuse of the system.

Nonetheless, abuse continues to occur. Further, the distances separating various service agencies may provide a disincentive for their use among those
with limited access to transportation, resulting in a reduced drain on public
resources. Yet it is those very individuals who are in greatest need of social
or public assistance who are most likely to suffer from this "assembly line"
or "progressive dinner" approach to service provision. In addition, segmen-
tation in the planning and implementation of services frequently "is supported by many providers . . . who stand to benefit by the further entrench-
ment of pluralistic market approaches to services that assure costly, often
profit-making, fragmentation" (Estes, 1980, p. 17). Any advantages to the provision of social services in segmented form certainly appear to be out-
weighed by the advantages of the holistic approach to social policy and its
more comprehensive, integrated perspective to service provision.

Crisis versus Rational

An examination of the reasons for social policy development in our
country suggests very strongly that the crisis approach is by far the more dominant rationale for planning, implementation, and evaluation. The crisis orientation is, essentially, a "knee-jerk reponse" to the most pressing social
problems on the part of social policymakers. While a crisis-based response
may provide a temporary solution to a difficult problem, the response is generally such that it may ultimately create even more problems in the future.
Sound social policy is best developed from a careful analysis of as much
information about present and expected future circumstances as possible.
From this data base, a rational, well-conceived, well-organized strategy for
social policy formulation may emerge that not only addresses present issues
and concerns, but provides a preventive outline for avoiding further related
problems in the future. The distinction between crisis and rational
approaches to social policy, according to Kerschner and Hirschfield (1975),
is similar to that between curative or palliative versus preventive strategies in
the treatment of disease. If we consider social policy as the remedy for social
ills, we can elect to provide episodic care, which deals with problems only
when their malignant effects become obvious, or we can anticipate these
problems and develop a strategy for "wellness" that insures the continued
integrity of the social system and mobilizes resources to maintain its "good
health" over an extended period of time.

This dimension of social policy is currently the topic of discussion with
respect to the future of the Social Security system in America. Developed in
response to the crisis of the Depression, the Social Security system was built
upon the model of deficit spending advocated by economist John Maynard
Keynes. While the system was effective in providing benefits at a rate well
within its fiscal capacity for many years, the shifting demographic composition of the American population and the changes in federal and state funding
priorities have produced an increasing financial strain on the system. At present, the financial outflow from the system far exceeds incoming revenues

from the taxation of workers. A financial crisis is expected in the foreseeable future as a result, unless measures with long-range effects are taken immediately to devise an alternative strategy for generating additional revenue for the system, to revise the benefit structure of the program, or both.

Critics argue that public policy specialists have been aware of the impending Social Security crisis for years, and should have focused their efforts on the development of preventive strategies for avoiding this situation long ago. Periodic palliative measures adopted to minimize financial strain have been largely ineffective to date. Those defending the crisis orientation adopted to maintain the system's integrity in recent years reply that valuable rational planning time has been preempted by the need to address other policy crises (e.g., defense spending for nuclear armaments). The patchwork nature of the crisis approach, however, has created more problems than it has solved. The "Catch-22" result of this situation, of course, is that time has run out for anything but additional crisis-based responses to the problems of the Social Security system. In sum, preventive, rational planning may require more time and resources in its initial stages, but is far superior to crisis-based approaches to social policy which can only produce a fragmented, disintegrated response to social needs.

Political Context versus Future Planning

The time frame within which social policies are planned, implemented, and evaluated is the final dimension presented for analysis by Kerschner and Hirschfield. Should social policy be formulated and carried out on the basis of short-range or long-range expectations and objectives, and to what extent should the present political context of planning be allowed to impact upon policies whose effects range far into the future? These authors comment:

> Social legislation, at the time of its enactment, reflects the values of the society it represents. In other words, public policy is a reflection of what the times, or better yet, the market will bear. Legislation consistently is based on prevailing social standards and conditions of the present, and rarely on the anticipated needs of the future. . . . The tragic elements of this approach, from a public policy perspective, are that most legislation in aging evolves not from a group of policy scientists drafting programs for the future, but rather from some pragmatic assumptions about what will be tolerated by the dominant forces in society [pp. 355–356].

Behavior scientists often assure us that the best predictors of the events of the future are the events of the past. Nonetheless, the implications of demographic projections about the future of aging and the elderly in America based on current and past information should not be accepted uncritically. In general, we expect that the numbers and proportions of the elderly in our society will burgeon by the turn of the century. But people who will be sixty-five or older in the year 2000 are members of different cohorts from those to which today's elderly belong. Should long-range public policies be based on

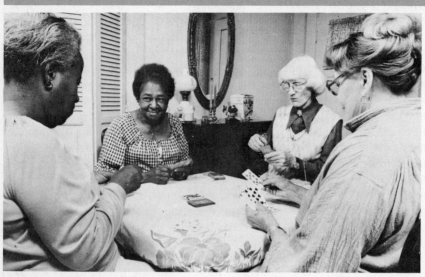

Women tend to outlive men. Being single requires women to cope with loneliness, reach out for companionship, and create a social support network. The problem is often exacerbated for minority elderly women.

the assumption that the elderly today and in the future share common needs and preferences that "go along with the territory" of old age? Or is it more realistic to look at today's middle-aged and younger cohorts, assume that there is more continuity than discontinuity over the lifespan, and base our future policy on the present status of those who will be old years from now? Should we try to maintain the status quo in our current attempts to develop policy issues for the future, or should we try to formulate our policy models with major social change in mind? What are the priorities for policymaking with respect to the elderly at present—and what will they be in the future— relative to other priority areas for our country? Indeed, social policy often seems to be limited in its impact by legislative bargaining and selective interpretation of what is acceptable to a given constituency at a particular moment in time; careful studies of long-term needs may be ignored or rejected in favor of popular but inaccurate notions of what these needs may (or should) be. The result of attempts to make future-based policy palatable to modernday constituents may be a watered-down plan that bears little if any resemblance to the original prototype and, as suggested earlier, may do more damage than good in the long run.

In conclusion, Kerschner and Hirschfield state:

> We are suggesting here that given the resultant stalemates of the dilemmas created by categorical versus generic approaches, holistic versus segmented programming, current political context versus future planning designs, and crisis versus rational planning, aging legislation has been caught in a morass

fragmented approaches is that in most cases involving major aging legislation, policy makers have abdicated moral responsibility by passing laws based on flimsy and often inaccurate data [1975, p. 357].

The Fifth Dimension: Who Pays?

There is another special policy issue fundamental to our understanding of policy decisions in the United States, beyond those noted by Kerschner and Hirschfield above. In their discussion of approaches to policy, no mention was made of the funding sources, fiscal responsibility, and authority for social policy formulation, decision making, or implementation. The fifth dimension to be considered in this context is, simply, private business and industry versus the public sector: who pays? For example, Kane and Kane (1976) reported the results of a study in which they compared the long-term care policies adopted by six different countries in order to identify some useful policy issues for consideration in the United States. Among their conclusions was the realization that there was little control over the long-term care industry in this country compared to the others studied. Furthermore, private enterprise, stimulated by the profit motive, was identified as basic to the system in this country but not the others. These conclusions were interpreted to mean that any improvement in care in the United States should be tied to the "entrepreneurial ethic"—no other type of motivation or control beyond the profit system was viewed as effective in the provision of long-term care in this country. Kane and Kane proposed, however, that within this context quality of care could be enhanced by rewarding settings that best serve the needs of their elderly residents and penalizing those that do not.

A Final Consideration: Who Plans?

One last but nonetheless important consideration in the discussion of social policy and the elderly is the extent to which older people are themselves involved in decision making and policy formulation on their own behalf. Lowy (1980) notes that "older persons perceive themselves as entitled to public participation as a group and as individuals, although they do not appear to have as yet developed a political self-image" (p. 189). Various aging advocacy groups, such as the Gray Panthers and the American Association of Retired Persons, are becoming increasingly influential in shaping the course of social policy regarding the elderly—but until more older persons become directly involved in the process of policy formulation through elected participation, the clout of these lobby-type organizations may not fully be realized.

Kuypers and Bengston (1973) have pointed out that in order to avoid the "social breakdown syndrome" occasioned in the later years by negative labeling and stigmatizing of the elderly, it is imperative that

> those who would envision themselves as serving the elderly must define as one of their major goals the systematic deinvestment of their power and

control. They must, at all the subtle junctures of decision-making, policy formation, and administration, acknowledge the experiential value to their clients of individual power and control. Self-government, resident directorship, political advocacy, and aging group consciousness are all part of the beginning vocabulary of practitioners which underscores this view, i.e., self-determination and individual control of policy and administration is the foundation for competent aging [pp. 196–197].

These authors conclude their observations by proposing that this approach to the avoidance of social breakdown

would begin to transfer the locus of control to its rightful place, would enhance the effect of the elderly to define their own existence, and would provide society a source of exciting and relevant efforts to improve the condition of the elderly [p. 198].

In other words, for social policy to be most responsive to the needs of the elderly, older people must have a strong voice in its formation, implementation, and evaluation. Logical as this may be, the number of nonelderly individuals who currently find themselves enmeshed in political struggles as advocates of the elderly is large, and growing every day. The likelihood that all these persons will cheerfully hand over their jobs, their power, their salaries, and all the other benefits that accrue to their positions to a cadre of

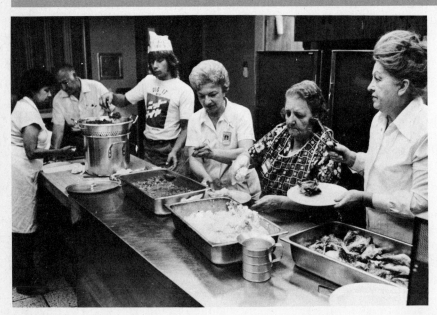

Many elderly women who are excellent cooks welcome the opportunity of having someone other than themselves to cook for. Opportunities to do so was one of the many concerns of the recent White House Conferences on Aging.

aging self-advocates is certainly not great. As Estes (1980) points out, the overwhelming bureaucratization and politicization of "the aging enterprise" too frequently results in the exploitation of the very group whose interest is presumably at stake.

Thirty Years of Social Policy Development in America

We now turn to a brief history of national program efforts and legislation in support of elderly Americans in order to provide a better understanding of the issues raised above.

There have been four major national conferences designed to focus attention on the elderly and to define social policy issues relative to aging over the past three decades. The first was held in August 1950 under the auspices of the Federal Security Agency during President Truman's administration. The objectives of this precedent-setting conference were:

1. To provide a forum for persons concerned with aging;
2. To reevaluate the potentialities of older people;
3. To stimulate the exchange of ideas among interested people with a view to solving problems of aging;
4. To define the nature and extent of the problems;
5. To promote research in the various phases of aging; and
6. To transmit the findings to interested groups as guidelines for the development of policies with regard to older people.

Following the first conference, the National Committee on Aging produced a report on the proceedings, and a Special Staff on Aging was created in 1956. In that same year, President Eisenhower established a special coordinating body, the Federal Council on Aging, whose task it was to make recommendations concerning the needs of older persons. All of these efforts pointed to the fact that there was a growing need for unification and direction as well as increased activity in the field of aging. In response to this situation, President Eisenhower called the second national conference on aging in 1960. The 1960 conference was the first federally financed White House Conference on Aging. In anticipation of the conference, each state was requested to perform a detailed analysis of the needs and circumstances of its aged constituencies. This careful preparation led to increasing awareness of state and local programs as well as a greater public focus on older people and their problems. The conference also recommended that a strong federally based agency on aging be established and charged with the following directives:

1. A statutory basis and more independent leadership;
2. Adequate funds for coordination and other assigned functions through line item appropriations;

3. Responsibility for formulation of legislative proposals for submission to Congress; and
4. Responsibility for periodic reviews and reports on the various federal programs, departments and agencies working in behalf of older persons to achieve effective coordination and operation [Senate Special Committee on Aging, 1961].

As a direct result of this conference, Congressman John E. Fogarty introduced a bill in Congress that would create such an agency in the Department of Health, Education, and Welfare (now the Department of Health and Human Services). The agency was to help older persons through grants to states for community planning, training, and research. First proposed in 1963, the Older Americans Act became law in 1965. Among the major provisions of this act was the establishment of the Administration on Aging (AoA), which functioned in an independent capacity until August 1967, when it was subsumed under the Social and Rehabilitation Service.

Among other major outcomes of the first White House Conference was the adoption of amendments to the Social Security Act which provided for and authorized Medicare and Medicaid, and the enactment of the Age Discrimination Act, limiting the age of mandatory retirement to sixty-five years, in 1967.

In 1971, a third national conference on aging—the second White House Conference—was held in Washington. The need for the conference stemmed from the fact that, despite major gains over the previous decade, "progress was at best sporadic and its momentum slowing. There was still no comprehensive set of national policies on which all levels and parts of government were working together to articulate" (*White House Conference on Aging,* 1971). The objectives outlined for the 1971 conference were:

1. To initiate the development of specific, thoughtful guides and recommendations for policies and actions in aging at community, state, and national levels.
2. To draw these guides and recommendations from cross-sections of older people, providers of service, specialists on aging, key decision-makers, and youth, in order that they may represent a broad and effective consensus.
3. To broaden the understanding, at community and state levels, of the needs of older people, and strengthen the willingness to act on the policy proposals that will emerge from the White House Conferences on Aging at all levels [*White House Conference on Aging,* 1971, vol. 1, p. 7].

These objectives were to be accomplished according to a three-year plan, beginning in 1970. The first year, dubbed the Prologue Year, was identified as a period in which older persons across the country could present their needs through Older American Forums. More than 6,000 forums were held, with over 500,000 participants, during that year. In the second year—the Year of the Conferences (1971)—local and state conferences and national organizational task forces gathered to make policy recommendations to be addressed at the National White House Conference at the end of the year. Each state was responsible for planning, coordinating, and evaluating various services and programs within its purview, and further asked to make a "comprehensive study" of income, health, housing, social status, and other issues relevant to its elderly constituency. Finally, the third year (1972) was identified as the Year of Action. It was during this year that the recommendations of the national conference began to be implemented.

The 1971 White House Conference was highly successful in stimulating national response to the concerns of the elderly. Among some of the major achievements of the Conference were the establishment of the National Institute on Aging in 1975, the NIMH Center for Studies of Mental Health of the Aging in 1976, and the amendment of the 1967 Age Discrimination in Employment Act in 1978 to raise the age of mandatory retirement from sixty-five to seventy years.

In 1981, the fourth national conference on aging, the White House Conference on Aging III, addressed the theme, "The Aging Society—Challenge and Opportunity." The rationale for convening the third White House Conference stressed the importance of social policy planning for growing numbers of older Americans and

> the fostering of broad public awareness of great social issues arising from a demographic revolution: the fact that for the first time in history large numbers of human beings are reaching old age, not only in the United States but all over the world [*White House Conference on Aging,* 1981, vol. 2, p. 7].

Not unlike its predecessors, the 1981 White House Conference was the culmination of a great flurry of planning and organizational activities which began roughly two years in advance of the convention. In addition to the already established Older American Forums (conducted in more than 9,500 sites and involving in excess of 390,000 participants of various ages), state White House Conferences were held across the country; technical committees were formed to organize content areas, identify salient issues, and create preliminary recommendations for the national meeting; and miniconferences designed to explore the needs of special interest groups among the aged were convened. As a result of these activities the following goals were established for the national conference in 1981:

- To provide the elderly with the maximum opportunity to live an independent and healthy life and to encourage them to remain in the economic and social mainstream.
- To provide economic, medical and social support to the elderly who really need help.
- To encourage serious discussion of the choice we must make as a result of the very large baby boom generation that will become elderly in the 21st century [White House Conference on Aging, 1981].

A total of 2,200 delegates and 1,150 observers attended the 1981 White House Conference on Aging. Each of these individuals was assigned to one of fourteen committees helping to formulate the nation's social policy on aging for the ensuing decade. Participants, regardless of specific committee assignments, were asked to address themselves particularly to the following concerns in their attempts to develop recommendations for social policy and aging: (1) special needs of minority members; (2) needs of the low-income elderly; (3) differences in urban and rural needs; (4) needs of the elderly who are frail or disabled; (5) access to services; (6) private and public sector roles; (7) means of implementing conference recommendations; (8) the role of older Americans themselves in influencing change so as to realize their aspirations.

These were not the only agenda items submitted for discussion and action at the conference. A coalition of more than two dozen national organizations in service to the elderly—the Leadership Council of Aging—presented "Eight for the '80s," a list of policy issues deemed crucial to the well-being of their elderly constituency over the next ten years:

1. Safeguard current eligibility conditions, retirement ages, and benefit levels in Social Security.
2. Broaden opportunities for older workers to remain active voluntarily in the labor force.
3. Older persons should be assured an income sufficient to maintain a minimum income level of dignity and comfort.
4. Enact a comprehensive national health plan for all Americans.
5. Interim steps must be taken to improve health care for older persons. Medicare and Medicaid should fund a full range of community-based and in-home services and institutional care for older people, including health maintenance.
6. No fewer than 200,000 units of publicly-financed housing for the elderly should be made available for each year during the decade.
7. Comprehensive service delivery systems for older people at the community level must be completed in the 1980s.
8. Strengthen the federal commitment to gerontological research, education and training. It is essential to develop a base of knowledge and of knowledgeable personnel [American Psychological Association, 1982, p. 4].

Conference committees were organized to study current trends and future prospects for the well-being of older people in America, and to provide specific recommendations for policy formation and action consistent with the issues they were assigned to address. Of the fourteen committees, two focused on economic issues (implications for the economy of an aging population and economic well-being); three addressed health care of older persons (promotion and maintenance of wellness, health care and services, options for long-term care); two were concerned with the contributions of older persons to society (older Americans as a continuing resource, conditions for continuing community participation); and one each dealt with family and community support systems, housing alternatives, and educational and training opportunities. Another two committees were devoted to the "fifth dimension" referred to earlier in this chapter—that of fiscal responsibility and programs for the elderly (private sector roles, structures, and opportunities; public sector roles and structures); one spoke to the concerns of older women, their growing number and special needs; and the final committee was reserved for the discussion of research issues germane to the elderly in the formation of social policy.

A total of 668 recommendations were produced by the fourteen committees. The Gerontological Society of America (1982) summarized the most important recommendations, which appear in Table 6–1.

According to a survey of delegates to the 1981 White House Conference in late December of the same year, the five recommendations ranked most favorably were: (1) Eliminate all restrictions on older workers; (2) expand home health care and in-home services; (3) provide tax credits for families who care for elderly relatives in their homes; (4) organize a continuum of services for the elderly using the Older Americans Act as a focal point; (5) expand Medicare to provide reimbursement for preventive care and maintenance of wellness.

Conference observers responded in similar fashion, although the priorities assigned to the recommendations listed above were somewhat different. Observers also felt that the government should institute a comprehensive

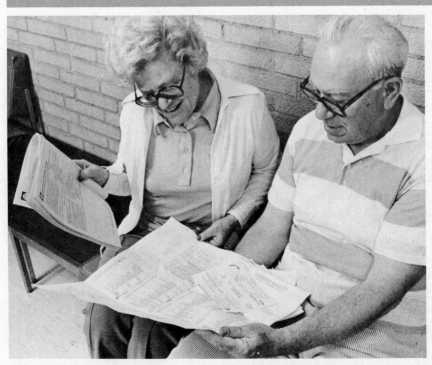

The elderly are more conscientious about voting then are the younger generations. They have also discovered how to make use of their political "clout."

TABLE 6-1. Major Conference Recommendations, 1981 White House Conference on Aging

Income Security

- Retain current levels of benefits for all Social Security recipients
- Restore the Social Security minimum benefit
- Determine eligibility for Medicare, SSI, and OASI for members of minority groups on the basis of life expectancy rather than chronological age
- Eliminate the earnings test for Social Security
- Require federal employees to contribute to the Social Security system
- Raise SSI payments to the poverty line, and determine SSI eligibility without regard to assets

Employment

- Increase workforce participation by the elderly via incentives for workers and employers
- Eliminate mandatory retirement

Health and Long-Term Care

- Expand Medicare and Medicaid coverages to include prescription drugs, eyeglasses, hearing aids, dental care, foot care, hospices, ambulatory care, lab tests, mental health services, home health, nurse practitioner and physician assistant services, and preventive care
- Establish a comprehensive national health program, which includes a long-term-care community-based health system
- Provide a prospective payment system for Medicare and Medicaid
- Maintain current levels of financing for Medicare and Medicaid
- Provide tax credits and cash payments to family caregivers
- Require education in geriatrics and gerontology for all health professionals
- Expand the ombudsperson program
- Shift Medicare and Medicaid to a system placing emphasis on competition among payers and among providers

Research

- Require federal aging programs to set aside 2 percent of their budgets for research, without jeopardizing service delivery
- Include in primary research an emphasis on long-term care, service delivery, and special subpopulation groups
- Conduct research in the areas of employment, retirement, living arrangements, and the role of the elderly in the changing American family
- Support basic research on the processes of aging

Education

- Give highest priority to educational programs to improve the economic status, health, social functioning, and life satisfaction of older people
- Expand and adequately fund gerontological and geriatric training
- Continue the shared responsibility between state and federal governments in meeting educational needs
- Provide for the education of the elderly, education and training for professionals working with the elderly, education of the public about aging, and funds for aging research by the federal government

Housing

- Provide a minimum of 200,000 units of housing each year for the elderly through government and private sectors, with no less than 20,000 units of Section 202 annually
- Expand congregate housing
- Base housing design on gerontological research
- Provide incentives to families providing housing to elderly kin

continued

TABLE 6-1. Major Conference Recommendations, 1981 White House
Conference on Aging (*continued*)

Housing (*continued*)

- Provide adequate funds for Sections 202 and 8, with continued administration of these programs by the Department of Housing and Urban Development.

Legal

- Make legal services avalable to older people through a combination of public and private
financing

Private Sector

- Urge corporations to contribute 2 percent of their pretax earnings to social service needs,
with some contributions for the elderly

Source: Gerontological Society of America (1982).

national health plan, including a long-term-care community-based health
system.

At first glance, it would appear that the goals established for the third
White House Conference were accomplished. Consideration was given to
eight special concerns of the "Eight for the '80s" agenda, as reflected in the
recommendations offered by delegates and observers. Yet these outcomes
must be evaluated in terms of the hidden agendas evident throughout the
national conference sessions.

Unlike earlier national conferences on aging, the 1981 Conference was
distinctly political in nature—"the aging enterprise" come home to roost, as
it were. The administration was accused of attempting to stage a political
coup by changing voting rules for the adoption and rejection of recommendations, "planting" unsympathetic government representatives on each committee in order to dilute the impact of committee resolutions and actions,
and other means. Despite the fact that at least some of the charges leveled
against the administration were ultimately documented, government officials
continued to deny their disruptive involvement in the conference proceedings. The 1981 White House Conference provided an excellent example
indeed of policy planning from a political (as opposed to future planning)
standpoint, inasmuch as recommendations were colored by what the "market" established by the national government seemed able to bear. Another
interesting observation about conference outcomes is that the major recommendations called for the promotion of mainly *indirect* services or measures
in support of the elderly; direct service provision was deemed of less importance to need satisfaction and problem solving for older Americans. The significance of this situation is that the provision of indirect services entails the
expansion of the aging network—those who provide the interface between
major agencies and organizations from which services originate and the
elderly recipients of those services. In other words, the recommendations
were primarily oriented toward the creation and provision of jobs for those

in service to the elderly, rather than toward the distribution of economic and other resources to the aged through the existing service provision network. Unfortunately, the increased emphasis on provision of indirect (as opposed to direct) services to the aged stands in direct contradiction to the prescription for competence in the elderly cited earlier by Kuypers and Bengston (1973). It is obvious that the 1981 White House Conference represents a turning point in national policy formulation for the elderly. The next ten years will reveal the extent to which older Americans are willing to allow others to decide their fate—and the degree to which they will set the precedent for unified action for peer support in the future.

While most contemporary analyses of public policy for the aged differ with respect to their assessment of the failures and successes of policy formulation, implementation, and evaluation, they do appear to reach a consensus with respect to three major considerations. First, there is a growing awareness that the elderly will no longer remain passive recipients of increasingly "brokered" services. Second, there is a mandate for full participation on the part of the elderly themselves in shaping the course of social policy. Third, and finally, there is the insistence that social policy for the aged be based upon solid, realistic, and precise information on this diverse constituency. These considerations must be taken into account before social policy can meet the criterion, not of political expediency, but of rational, informed, long-range planning.

Summary

In this chapter, four salient dimensions of public policy analysis were identified; categorical versus generic, holistic versus segmented, crisis versus rational, and political context versus future planning. One other dimension of analysis—sources of funding and locus of authority for social policy formulation, decision making, and implementation—was also discussed. Particular attention was directed to the need for up-to-date, sufficient, and precise information about the aged, the lack of which was shown to lead to inconsistent and inappropriate policy formulation. The interaction of ethnicity and aging is a special case and a pertinent example of this need.

Much of what passes today for social policy regarding the aged suffers from deficiencies arising from short-term perspectives about older persons, with little account taken of major social changes or of differences that may be anticipated between today's elderly and cohorts of aged in the future. A major weakness of social policy with respect to the aged would appear to be a direct result of policy formulation based on expediency and "what the market will bear" rather than on rational planning. Another glaring weakness in the formulation of such policies is the limited participation of the elderly themselves in the process.

The history of four major national conferences held over the past thirty years which specifically addressed social policy and the elderly in this country was briefly reviewed. Of special interest are the stated objectives of the White House Conferences on Aging and the various recommendations they produced. These activities, taking place within the wider political arena, have unquestionably given national visibility to the concerns, needs, and aspirations of older people in our society, and produced several sociopolitical changes of consequence.

Nevertheless, much of what has been presented as social policy proposals for the aged has continued to be little more than optimistic and rather pious rhetoric. Also noted was the concern of many participants and observers at the 1981 White House Conference on Aging about thinly veiled attempts by the political party in power to politicize what has been presumed by most to be a nonpartisan effort by and for the elderly.

References

American Psychological Association. (Division 20.) *Newsletter of Adult Development and Aging,* Winter 1982, 9(3).

Benetiz, R. Ethnicity, social policy, and aging. In R. Davis & M. Neiswande (Eds.), *Aging: Prospects and issues.* Los Angeles: Andrus Gerontology Center, University of Southern California, 1973.

Burns, E. M. *Toward social security: An explanation of the Social Security Act and a survey of the larger issues.* New York: McGraw-Hill, 1936.

Estes, C. L. *The Aging Enterprise.* San Francisco: Jossey-Bass, 1980.

Gerontological Society of America. *Gerontology News,* Jan.–Feb. 1982.

Harris, L., & Associates. *Aging in the '80s: America in transition.* Washington, D.C.: National Council on Aging, 1981.

Jackson, J. J. Aged Negroes: Their cultural departures from statistical stereotypes and rural-urban comparisons. In D. P. Kent, R. Kastenbaum, & S. Sherwood (Eds.), *Research planning and action for the elderly: The power and potential of social science.* New York: Behavioral Publications, 1972. Pp. 501–513. (a)

Jackson, J. J. Black aged: In quest of the phoenix. In *Triple jeopardy—myth or reality.* Washington, D.C.: National Council on Aging, 1972. Pp. 27–40. (b)

Kane, R., & Kane, R. *Long-term care in six countries: Implications for the United States.* Department of Health, Education, and Welfare (NIH) Publication No. 76-1207. Washington, D.C.: Government Printing Office, 1976.

Kerschner, P., & Hirschfield, I. Public policy and aging: Analytic approaches. In D. Woodruff & J. Birren (Eds.), *Aging: Scientific perspectives and social issues.* New York: Van Nostrand, 1975.

Kuypers, J. A., & Bengston, V. L. Social breakdown and competence: A model of normal aging. *Human Development,* 1973, 16(3), 181–201.

Lowy, L. *Social policies and programs on aging.* Lexington, Mass.: D. C. Heath, 1980.

Stein, B. *Social security and pensions in transition: Understanding the American retirement system.* New York: Free Press, 1980.

White House Conference on Aging. *Toward a national policy on aging.* Washington, D.C.: Government Printing Office, 1971. 3 vols.

White House Conference on Aging. *A national policy on aging.* Washington, D.C.: Government Printing Office, 1981. 3 vols.

For Further Reading

Clark, R. L., Barker, D. T., & Cantrell, R. S. Outlawing age discrimination: Economic and institutional responses to the elimination of mandatory retirement. Report to the Administration on Aging. Washington, D.C., September 1979.

Clark, R. L., Kreps, J., & Spengler, J. The economics of aging. *Journal of Economic Literature,* September 1978.

Neugarten, B. L., & Havighurst, R. J. (Eds.) *Social policy, social ethics, and the aging society.* Report prepared for National Science Foundation/ RANN, Research Applications Directorate, Division of Advanced Productivity Research and Technology. NSF/RA 76-000247. Washington, D.C.: Government Printing Office, 1976.

Schechter, I. *1980 chartbook of federal programs in aging.* Washington, D.C.: Care Reports, 1980.

Wachs, M. *Transportation for the elderly.* Berkeley: University of California Press, 1979.

Society, Its Structure, and Aging

Chapter 7

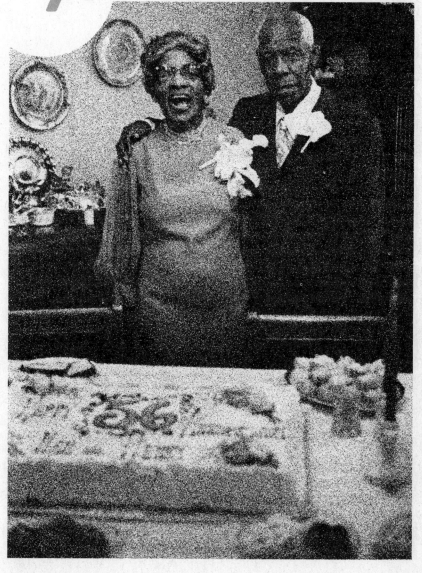

> If a man is moderate and contented then even age is no burden—if he is not, then even youth is full of cares.
>
> *Plato*

When I get older, losing my hair,
Many years from now.
Will you still be sending me a Valentine,
Birthday greetings, bottle of wine?
If I'd be out till quarter to three
Would you lock the door?
Will you still need me, will you still feed me,
When I'm sixty-four?
You'll be older, too,
And if you say the word, I could stay with you.
I could be handy, mending a fuse
When your lights have gone.
You can knit a sweater by the fireside,
Sunday mornings go for a ride.
Doing the garden, digging the weeds,
Who could ask for more?
Will you still need me, will you still feed me,
When I'm sixty-four?[1]

The haunting verse of this popular song becomes all the more poignant when we ponder a case study like the following.

CASE ILLUSTRATION ▄▄▄▄

"Nothing Left"

Don was referred for consultation because he had attempted to throw himself from a ten-story building. His story was simple. Two years earlier when he was 74 his wife had died. His two grown sons came for the funeral but stayed only three days. Then the demands of their work took them away again: one a thousand miles away, the other across the continent. Friends had hovered about for a week or so and then seemed to

[1]From the Beatles' album *Sgt. Pepper's Lonely Hearts Club Band.* Song: "When I'm Sixty-Four." Capitol Records, Hollywood, Cal. 1967.

forget him. His sons called him by phone but had little to say to him. Most of his friends were couples, and he felt he didn't "fit into his social life" anymore. His apartment was pleasant enough, but he had little interaction with his neighbors, who were mostly younger than he was. Sometime earlier he had fractured his hip, so he found it difficult to get to his church. He called, but no one came to visit him. He found it difficult to get to the market regularly, his diet suffered, he got little exercise and no mental stimulation. After a time he became increasingly depressed, concluded there was "nothing left for him," and decided to "join his wife." Hence his attempt at suicide.

Cases like this, which with many variations are repeated literally thousands of times, raise important questions for us about the effectiveness of family and friendship support for a great many older persons, and about family and community support and assurance for the isolated and the widowed. Before one can effectively help the "Dons" of our society, much needs to be known about their communities, their friendship networks, and their families. Our discussion, then, is about those basic institutions of society in which the older individual is enmeshed.

Societal Institutions

On May 8, 1982, a tiny newspaper item quietly reported, "The average U.S. life expectancy for persons born in 1981 reached an all-time high of 70.3 years for men and 77.9 years for women, according to preliminary life tables of the Metropolitan Life Insurance Company." As has been documented elsewhere in this text, America's population *is* aging. The question is, in what ways are society's institutions affected by this phenomenon, and how do these institutions respond?

One of the classic sociological descriptions of a societal institution is that it is both an idea and a structure. It is the structured and permanent way in which society organizes itself to meet human needs. That millions of individuals within a given geographical area manage to carry out and coordinate their multifarious activities with only a moderate degree of disarray and disorder is an almost incredible phenomenon. The answer lies in the function of that matrix of social groups which we call institutions. These "structures" establish and maintain a focus for the central concerns and activities of society. They develop and sustain norms, roles, and rituals (the culture) as a template for the behavior and activities of its members. From the very earliest moments of interpersonal interaction, the youngest members are socialized first into childhood roles, then into adolescence, young and middle adulthood, and at last into old age. In other words, we learn how to live successfully in our society by conforming (more or less) to the values and expectations expressed through its institutions.

The institutions that predominate in every society, primitive and advanced, are those of the family, religion, education, and government (which includes politics and commerce/economics). Governmental policies and economics are discussed in other chapters; this chapter will focus largely on the first three: the family, religion, and education. We will begin by examining the basic institutional and structural unit of society, the family.

The Family and Its Elders

One of the major controversies in family sociology over the past twenty years derives from failure to agree on the basic structure of the contemporary family. In spite of its status as the basic unit of society and its preeminence among social institutions, the family is difficult to define except in the most imprecise terms.

Theoretical constructs most appropriate to the bonding of aged persons and family units are those of social exchange and linkage (Sussman, 1976; cf. also Shanas & Sussman, 1977). Linkage denotes the relationships established by blood (being born into a family) and by legal process (marriage, adoption). The elements of exchange involve interactions based on profit and cost, reward and punishment, and the "generational stake" equation (cf. Dowd, 1975, 1980, Sussman, 1976).

Conventionally the "functionality" of kin relationships has been defined in terms of the nuclear family, consisting of parent(s) and child(ren), and the extended family. Kerckhoff (1965) has suggested the utility of proximity and help exchange as the principal elements of a structural classification of kin networks. He has proposed the following categories:

1. "nuclear-isolated," where family members are in close geographic proximity but have few or no contacts with each other;
2. "modified extended," where families are spatially dispersed but have a high degree of contact, exchange, and interaction; and
3. "extended," where units of the family are propinquitous and high in functionality.

Given all the talk in the recent past about the "changing American family," the most striking fact about it is that "the connectedness of most elderly with their families and kin network remains unbroken despite industrialization and modernization" (Sussman, 1976).

Corroborating the connectedness of the aged are the statistics regarding their living arrangements, as shown in Table 7–1.

Clearly the vast majority of elders, both white and ethnic live not in isolation or in institutions, but in families. Almost 80 percent of the men and 60 percent of all persons over sixty-five live in families, but these families generally consist of husband and wife. Less than a fourth of these individuals live with their children, and less than 3 percent are part of households com-

TABLE 7-1. Living Arrangements of Those Sixty-Five and Older by Race and Sex, 1970

Living Arrangement	Male		Female	
	White	Black	White	Black
In families	79.1	69.6	58.2	62.2
Primary individual[a]	15.1	21.6	33.7	31.2
Other[b]	2.1	5.5	2.1	3.3
Institutionalized	3.8	3.2	5.9	3.2
Total[c]	100.0	100.0	100.0	100.0

Source: U.S. Bureau of the Census, 1973.

[a]A household head living alone or with nonrelatives only.

[b]Includes lodgers, resident employees, and those living in group quarters such as convents or rooming houses.

[c]Totals do not add to 100 due to rounding error.

prised of parents, children, and grandchildren (i.e., modified extended families).

As of 1970 there were some 8,300,000 widows and some 1,700,000 widowers fifty-five years old or older. In addition there were 500,000 divorced men and 1 million divorced women who still had not remarried. While 22 million were married, a total of about 11.5 million were single and generally living alone or with nonrelatives (Peterson & Payne, 1975).

Table 7-2, a more recent tally, reveals more clearly the effects of the increased longevity enjoyed by women. The fact of their increased survivorship also inflates the number of those who, because of widowhood, are more likely to be found living alone, with children, or in an institutional setting. (For further discussion of this issue see Chapters 8 and 10).

If one wishes to compare familial living arrangements in the United States to those of another society, Table 7-3 shows analogous information for heads of families in the Netherlands.

We note that in the Netherlands, too, the majority of elderly (sixty-five and over) live in a family arrangement. Note the clear trend in the Nether-

TABLE 7-2. Percentage of Elderly Men and Women in Various Living Arrangements, 1970

Living Arrangement	Men	Women
Family	79	59
Head of household	71	10
Wife is head of household	x	33
Other relative is head of household	8	16
Alone or with nonrelative	17	37
Head of household	14	35
Living with a nonrelative	3	2
Institution	4	4

Source: Administration on Aging. *Facts and Figures on Older Persons,* no. 5 (Washington, D.C.: Department of Health, Education and Welfare Pub. [OHD] 74-20005), pp. 4-6.

TABLE 7–3. Number and Percentage of Married Couples in Various Living Arrangements, 1971

Age of the Head of the Family	Household Arrangement								
	Couple Alone	%	Couple with Unmarried Children and Possibly Others	%	Couple Without Unmarried Children, but with Others	%	Total	%
40–49	69,600	10.3	600,000	88.9	5,600	1.8	675,200	100
50–64	264,400	33.2	512,600	64.4	18,800	2.4	795,800	100
65–69	130,800	70.9	49,200	26.7	4,400	2.4	184,400	100
70–74	99,200	78.9	23,800	18.9	2,800	2.2	125,800	100
75 and over	87,600	81.3	17,600	16.3	2,600	2.4	107,800	100
Total	651,600	34.5	1,203,200	63.7	34,200	1.8	1,889,000	100

Source: Woningbehoeftenonderzoek, table 5 (The Hague: Central Bureau of Statistics, 1978).

lands, as in the U.S., toward smaller family units. The total number of households consisting of married couples living alone increases steadily as the age of the head of the family increases.

Coresidence: Aged and Children

This pattern of living arrangements provides no information as to *why* elderly individuals are not more often found living with their children. We do know that the vast majority of elderly persons seem to prefer what has been called "intimacy at a distance" (Treas, 1975), that is, the wish to have frequent contacts with children and to live in reasonable proximity to them, but not to live with them as part of the same household. This particular type of relationship between the elderly and their adult children may, in fact, contribute most to good life adjustment of the elderly (Treas, 1975). When Murray (1973) studied 11,153 individuals fifty-five to sixty-three years of age he found that those living with relatives in the same household were less happy. Kerckhoff (1966) reported that retired married couples' morale was inversely related to the propinquity of their children.

The reason most often advanced by older persons for not wanting to live with adult children is the fear that they, the elder parents, may prove to be a burden to their children. While this concern may indeed be a very real factor, a more powerful motivation is seen in the need older individuals have to maintain their privacy and sense of autonomy (Lopata, 1973; Pampel, 1981; Schutz, Baird, & Hawkes, 1979). After all, moving into another's home—even that of one's child—usually reduces one's status to that of a permanent visitor or guest, with all that that implies. Such coresidence arrangements are likely to prove satisfactory all around only in instances in which a warm, congenial, and tolerant relationship already exists and the "rules of the house," expectations, and roles are clearly defined and articulated, thoroughly discussed, and acceptable to all parties involved. Not surprisingly, cases in which this situation works harmoniously make up a negligible percentage of all instances.

Proximity and Contact

On the other hand, the finding reported by Shanas (1968) that over 90 percent of respondents over the age of sixty-five had seen at least one of their children in the past month corroborates the repeatedly expressed desire of older parents to have frequent contact with their children. The majority of older persons live less than an hour's drive from at least one of their children (Sussman, 1976). Living in the vicinity of their children helps maintenance of close contacts and exchange of various services. Piotrowski supports this observation with data from other countries: 80 percent of older people in Poland, 82 percent in Great Britain, 77 percent in the United States, and 75 percent in Denmark have children living no more than a half-hour's walking or driving distance. The postal service, telephone, and airplane further facilitate a sense of closeness or accessibility, even in a highly mobile society such as ours (Piotrowski, 1977).

Nature of the Relationship

The foregoing suggests that the following issues are relevant for this particular analysis:

1. What is the degree of satisfaction or adjustment in those 22 million older persons who are married?
2. What is the possibility of marriage for the 11.5 million persons who are single?
3. What is the degree of the relationship between parents, children, and grandchildren when they do not live together?
4. What are the special problems of widows and widowers?
5. What other community support systems beyond the family are important to older people?

How can the patterns of relations between parents and adult children, primary constituents of the nuclear family, be evaluated? The responses of elderly parents and adult children, when asked directly about the closeness of relationships, do not coincide. The elderly parents are more likely to perceive closeness in the relationship than their adult children are, and tend to rate the relationship higher (Johnson & Bursk, 1977).

Two early studies provide interesting data pertinent to the issue of the quality of the relationship when parents, children, and grandchildren do not live together. Although not recent investigations, they are of special interest because the study by Streib and Thompson (1965), using an Eastern sample, was replicated by a California study using the same measure (Peterson, Hadwen, & Larson, 1967). This kind of scientific replication using samples from two disparate regions of the country usually indicates the presence of a robust, reliable phenomenon. The results of these studies, surveying attitudes of older family members toward their children, are reported in Table 7–4.

TABLE 7–4.   Parental Norms Concerning Achievement, Content, and Living Arrangements of Children

Statement	Agreement with Statement	
	Streib-Thompson %	Peterson, Larson, & Hadwen %
Getting ahead in the world may be a bad thing if it keeps your family from being close.	49	67
When children are unmarried adults, it is nice to have them live at home with parents.	45	46
Children should not move away from their parents because of better financial opportunities elsewhere.	10	5
When parents get older and need help, they should be asked to move in with their married children.	8	14
Even when children are married, it is nice to have them living with parents.	5	2

Source: Peterson, Hadwen, & Larson (1967).

These findings from the East and West Coasts illustrate the extent to which "achievement motivation" has contributed to modifying parental expectations about living arrangements and care from their children. It may also be considered a measure of the degree of independence older people are asserting (cf. Pampel, 1981). Only 17 persons out of the more than 400 elderly in the California sample reported every having lived with their adult children. Fourteen of them went to great pains to point out that in their case it happened only because of a transitional period in the life of the parent and was regarded by all as temporary. When probe questions sought to discover under what circumstances any of the respondents would move in with their children, almost 100 percent said that under no circumstances would they ever consent to such a situation. These responses led the authors to generalize that for these two groups, the norms associated with the extended family are tenuous. Further analyses indicated that the persons in the California sample were not too enthusiastic about contacts with their grandchildren, preferring to see them only when they wished and for a limited time period. They seemed especially to resent being used as babysitters at the convenience of their own adult children.

A further analysis of the California sample (see Table 7–4) indicated that there was no statistical association between **familism**[1] and life satisfaction. Furthermore, about one-half of the children of the respondents in this sample lived far distant from them in California or in other states. The impli-

[1]*familism*—involvement with family relationships and family activities.

cations of these data are supported by an investigation by Solomon of a lower-class group which showed that most parents in this group take for granted separation and lack of intimate contact but rely on letters and telephone calls, so that their children may be called upon in case of emergencies. The children do not play a daily or major part in their lives, but they are viewed as a kind of insurance against the exigencies of tomorrow. Undoubtedly Hill and Sussman and others are right to stress the value of the kind of relationship that is expressed by older persons in terms of gifts, babysitting (when possible), and communication; but this may be negligible protection against loneliness.

Treas (1975) has summarized the controversy well and added some explanatory inferences which help to illuminate the issue:

> In reviewing all the evidence on contemporary kin relationships, Peterson finds considerable support for the thesis that family "relations do not offer substantial intimacy or emotional support to aging persons." For many older people, contact with kin is too infrequent to provide companionship. Money and services may be exchanged with only minimal affect and interaction. While families may fall short of providing day-to-day social sustenance to the aged, younger kin are sources of generative gratification and vicarious accomplishment. Parents view offspring as social heirs who extend their personal histories and validate their lives. Given this involvement, it is not surprising that older people feel their children should move away from them if better economic opportunities beckon (Peterson, 1970; Streib, 1958). This "developmental stake" in descendants encourages parents to minimize generational differences and to perceive greater closeness, understanding and communication between family members than do their young. Clearly, family satisfaction and solidarity survive even in a mobile and rapidly changing society such as ours [p. 97].

The "Sandwich Generation" and Role Reversal

Special problems in relationships between the elderly and their adult sons and daughters are evident in spite of the tendency to idealize the relationship. The recently coined expression "sandwich generation" nicely identifies the dilemma experienced by many middle-aged children. Many of the tasks of the middle years—letting go of one's youth, coping with responsibilities for adolescent children still living at home and confronting the prospect of the "empty nest," facing aging parents who want attention and increasing assistance and support—all these inherently increase the hazards to becoming truly a peer to one's aging parents and maintaining a relationship of mutual affection and respect. Feelings of guilt often become characteristic of such relationships (Silverstone, 1979), even though such feelings are inappropriate and based on misperceptions (Schwartz, 1977, 1979).

Why the guilt? "Whether . . . family . . . can in any sense be said to be failing hinges in large measure upon our ability to establish a clear and accurate identification . . . of the dependency needs of the aged. . . ." (Schwartz,

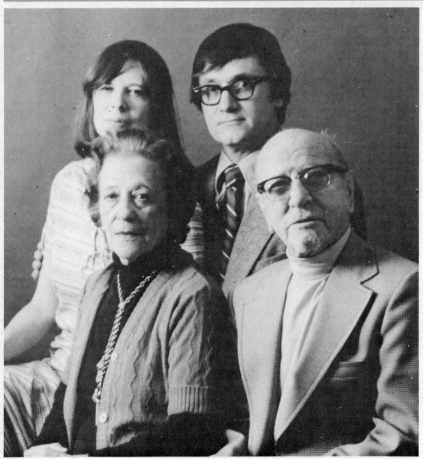

Middle-agers have become a "sandwich generation," needing to cope with the demands of their own children and those of aging parents.

1979, p. 119). The dependency needs of aging parents are a relative matter (both literally and figuratively). Aged parents do turn more frequently to their adult children for assistance (as adult children do to aged parents), thus creating for the children a circumstance rarely if ever experienced before. When the demand (spoken or nonverbal) for assistance is made by aging parents, and the need is misconstrued by the children with respect to its nature or extent, the result most frequently is role inversion or role reversal. The consequences of role reversal in its most blatant form are invariably inappropriate and even pernicious (Schwartz, 1979). "Parentification" on the part of the children, or the converse, "infantilizing" of the elderly, demeans and dehumanizes everyone involved (see the discussion of other aspects of infantilizing in Chapters 3 and 10), and is considered by some to be pathological (Silverstone, 1979).

The notes from a clinical case reviewed by one of the authors illustrates this not uncommon pattern of role reversal. (Again, names and identifying details have been changed to protect confidentiality.)

CASE ILLUSTRATION
Whose Guilt-Trip, Anyway?

John Broadus and his wife presented themselves to the therapist as prosperous, competent, and generous middle-aged persons. John went to great pains to explain that his eighty-year-old father and mother could no longer take care of themselves and that he had gone to some trouble to discover a high-quality medical facility for them. But, much to his chagrin, they angrily refused to give up their home and move to the facility. As he described all this it was evident that John had a very great emotional investment in his plan to move his parents. In a sense, it developed, what he was doing now compensated for the previous twenty-five years in which he had spent little time with his parents. The vehemence of their rejection of John's plan reflected a bitterness born of neglect.

John's wife took the side of the parents but revealed later that she resented the money John would spend on them, while the parents felt neglected and scorned by John and his wife. Apparently, the issue of the parents' giving up their home was only the arena in which were played out all of the resentments which had accumulated during the last twenty-five years. Because the housing move itself was a superficial aspect of this case, it was handled as family therapy and all four persons were invited to work out a totally different way of dealing with each other.

In many cases the anxiety felt by a younger person who is assuming the authority role becomes the focus of intervention. Such problems often underlie the complaints of a son or daughter about a parent residing in a nursing home. Children cannot deal openly or directly with their feelings of guilt so they attack the nursing home because it is a handy and vulnerable target. Such behavior is often a displacement of a very personal sense of failure about the past or present relationship with a parent.

Resistance to Remarriage

Another problem in the family has to do with opposition to the intended remarriage of a widowed mother or father (McLain, 1969). Typically a middle-age child registers great indignation or consternation at a parent's plan to remarry and may even try to interfere to stop it. A variety of psychological dynamics can be involved in such intrusions into parents' lives. One explanation focuses on a perceived threat to the possibility of an inheritance. The middle-aged offspring may be counting on receiving the bulk of the estate left by father or mother, and the new marriage may be seen as threatening that expectation. In such cases a premarital financial agreement is often all it takes to eliminate the opposition. In this sort of agreement both the bride and groom specify how much of their resources will be committed to the marriage and how much must be reserved to leave to the children as, perhaps, the departed mate would have wished.

In other cases, the anger or resistance toward the planned marriage of the elderly parent may stem not from monetary concerns but from complex emotional issues. It is not uncommon for some sons and daughters to believe that their surviving parent ought to dedicate the remainder of life to a ritual of single-minded devotion to the dead parent. Such stereotyped attitudes may stem from guilt associated with the child's own neglect and lack of demonstrated affection to the deceased parent. The child may now want the surviving parent to act as a stand-in fulfilling for what the child should have

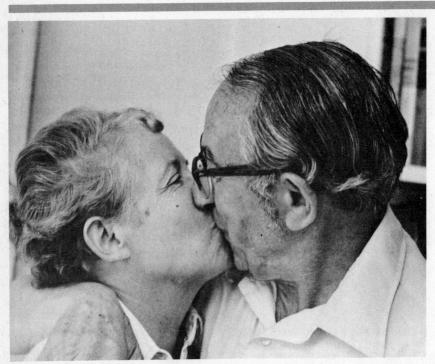

The need for and interest in closeness, affection, and intimacy can and usually does continue unabated throughout the lifespan.

fulfilled personally a long time ago. More often than not, when a daughter or son says, "Oh, mother, act your age; you are too old for that sort of thing," this may simply reflect stereotypical, myth-based attitudes about appropriate sexual behavior in the later years of life. Yet such attitudes can be a source of embarrassment and chagrin to aging parents and futher inhibit their behavior.

Whatever the particulars may be of opposition to free expression of the need for intimacy and sexuality on the part of a parent, the causes are frequently so complex that only a sensitive and experienced therapist can deal with them adequately.

A third kind of role reversal has been suggested by Neugarten as characterizing the relationship between the older husband and wife and complicating their relationship with their adult children (Neugarten & Gutmann, 1968). Neugarten tested a large sample of older persons in Kansas City on a series of Thematic Apperception cards, to try to tap their noncognitive patterns of role perception. She found that many older women seemed to have changed from expressive roles (those that have most to do with emotions) to instrumental roles (those having to do with jobs and decisions). Older men, on the other hand, often make the opposite shift. Thus as a husband and wife get older, they have to cope with a significant shift in roles. This can be most confusing to their children, who by the time they reach middle age have learned to some extent to understand and cope with father and mother. Now they begin to discover that the familiar coping strategies do not seem to apply. They must learn to listen carefully and acquire new understanding of their parents. They may resent, for example, mother's new-found independence; she begins to demand more voice in decisions, and loses some of the "softness" of her previous "mothering" role. As sociological studies established long ago, power in the family is associated with earning money, and when father and mother retire they lose a certain amount of status with each other and their children, a loss which may be reinforced by the kind of role reversal we are discussing.

Multigenerational Families

We might expect that the problems and concerns of the "sandwich generation" will be magnified and perhaps compounded by the rise of the multigenerational family in a postindustrial society. In the six-year period between 1970 and 1976, for example, the population between forty and sixty-four years of age increased by 1.9 percent, while those sixty-five years or older increased by 14.8 percent, those seventy-five or older by 16.1 percent, and those eighty-five years or older by an astounding 39.6 percent (Brody, 1979). In fact, what we are facing is a growing number of individuals in their seventies with a living parent in the nineties, part of a four- or even five-generation family. This will have profound implications for family relationships and functioning.

Widowed and Single Elderly and Their Relationships

No analysis of the older family would be complete without reference to the more than 11 million single elderly men and women. The longevity gap between men and women has yet to be bridged appreciably by modern medicine or modified life-styles. So as the older population increases in number the disproportion between the sexes also increases (Peterson & Briley, 1977). Furthermore, the salient circumstance of the rise in divorce, both for first and second marriages, promises to make a new bulge in "singleness" statistics for older persons in the next twenty years. Any examination of relationship patterns, therefore, must take these trends into consideration, if the analysis is to be at all comprehensive and meaningful (see Chapter 8).

Unless there is a radical change in marriage customs permitting some form of **polygyny**,[1] there seems to be no alternative to singlehood for the vast majority of single older women. What then are their prospects for some type of heterosexual life? There are some possible remedies.

The proliferation of retirement communities may be one answer to the segregation of single older women. In these communities single women may find opportunities for amicable associations with men (even though married) in educational classes, volunteer work, social activities, and recreational activities, and as neighbors. While an occasional swim or dance or card game with a man is not the equivalent of living with him, nevertheless this sort of relationship does provide contact and companionship. In many of these communities there are men who are perfectly willing to act as a kind of handyman and fix water sprinklers or the fence for their single female neighbors. This kind of friendship is not at all sexual, but can provide important emotional support.

A second kind of relationship, a sexual one, has developed between older single men and single women. Because the Social Security rules penalize older persons financially if they marry, many simply have long love affairs, or even live together without benefit of clergy. Certainly among the 35 percent of widows Lopata (1973) surveyed who said that they so cherished their independence that they would never remarry there are some who are not going to give up completely their emotional closeness to either men or women. And in cases where a married couple has had a long and stormy relationship, a spouse may find comfort in the arms of another person. A few have have tried communal living; some like it and some do not. Certainly there will continue to be many social experiments in which both older men and older women test new forms of intimate association. We have heard more than one middle-aged child say to an older parent, "Well, you can have relationships but you certainly are no good at marriage. Don't try that again." It seem unrealistic to assume that new cohorts of older persons will be content to be completely celibate outside marriage.

---

[1]*polygyny*—state or practice of having more than one wife at one time.

Sexual Promise of Later Years

If the sexual fires of youth are completely banked and become only cold embers in old age we may be belaboring a lost cause. But this proves not to be the case. In an earlier chapter we discussed aspects of sexuality in old age and some of the research related to it. Suffice it to repeat here that many older persons remain sexually active well into their later years and report good sexual adjustment and satisfaction. Others have given contrary reports of their perceptions of and experiences with sex in later life.

Perhaps Masters and Johnson should have placed greater emphasis on the emotional and psychological aspects of sexual adjustment in the later years. Older men and women are not merely tissues and hormones: they are individuals with long histories of unique interactions. For some these are histories of neglect, or of lack of consideration and tenderness, making it difficult for them to accept or respond to love. Perhaps that is why some long-time residents of institutions for the aged initially appear to recoil from touching and other overtures of affection. Some people are "injustice collectors," who find reward in ruminating about and reciting the faults and failings of others—conduct not conducive to sexual responsiveness. Sometimes it takes sustained intervention by an experienced therapist to help an older person surmount a traumatic past. Yet such individuals also need closeness, tenderness, and touching; sometimes it is well worth their while to spend some time in counseling.

Late Life Marital Adjustment

Much can be learned about the institution of the family from a discussion of marital adjustment, even though it is difficult to determine in specific terms how older people get along in marriage. There is considerable evidence that many marriages become boring by the middle years and never recover. There is also evidence that for many marriage does recover from the middle-aged "blahs" and is a good source of life satisfaction and morale during the remaining years together.

One longitudinal study relevant to this issue was conducted by Burgess and Wallin, who interviewed a panel of one thousand couples when they were engaged, then three years later, and again after the couples had been married up to twenty years. Peter C. Pineo, who conducted the third phase of the study, chose the word "disenchantment" to summarize the adjustment of these couples in the later years of their marriages. He found losses on most of the indices that he used to measure interaction of the couples (Pineo, 1961). Blood and Wolfe's cross-sectional sample in their classic study of 556 couples was more representative in terms of social class than was the Burgess-Wallin study, which relied on middle-class respondents, but the results were similar (Blood & Wolfe, 1960; See Figure 7–1).

A further study by Cuber and Haroff (1963) used a sample of very suc-

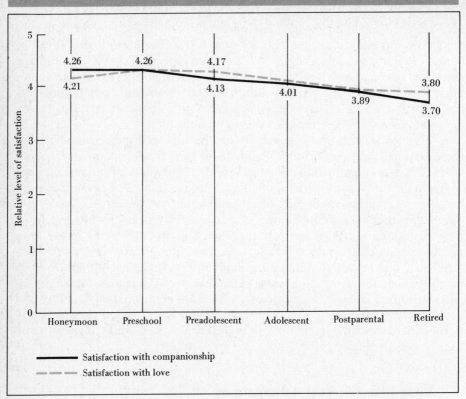

FIGURE 7–1   Wife's Satisfaction with Love and Companionship, by Stage in Family Life Cycle
Source: Blood and Wolfe (1960).

cessful upper-middle-class Americans. They categorized their findings into five classes of interaction patterns: conflict-habituated, passive-congenial, devitalized, vital, and total. Of all these types of interaction, only the vital has an aspect of "exciting sharing," and only a small group fell into this category. The largest group was that labeled "devitalized." No final statistical findings were presented, but the strong implication was that most of the respondents fall into the conflict-ridden, passive, or devitalized categories.

Lowenthal's San Francisco study (Lowenthal, Berkman, et al., 1967) embraced a stratified random sample of 280 respondents from eighteen census tracts. These respondents were interviewed three times in order to locate etiological (causal) factors in health and illness. The study concluded that "an individual who has been widowed within seven years, and who has a confidante, has even higher morale than a person who remains married but lacks a confidante." The implication is clear: in old age a marital partner does not necessarily offer profound emotional support to his or her mate. On the other hand, marrieds have a higher satisfaction rating than do widows without a confidante. There must be some couples who continue to function in vital ways with their partners, but this study also indicates some loss of communication and personal support in marriage through the erosion of time.

But not all studies show the same declining curve. Peterson's study of middle- and upper-middle-class in-movers at Leisure World in Laguna Hills, California, reported a great deal of mutual decision making, mutual dependence, and stability in the 500 couples interviewed (aged sixty-five years, on the average; Peterson, Larson, & Hadwen, 1967). He suggests that the married couples were the happiest of any group in the community, and that they had achieved a method of problem solving satisfactory to both partners. His sample, however, is limited by its middle-class bias and by being self-selected, namely, those who were moving into a retirement community.

A second mostly positive report is supplied by Feldman and Rollins (1970), who studied 240 couples in various stages of the family life cycle. In contrast to Blood and Wolfe, they found that general marital satisfaction increases after middle age and continues high during the period of retirement. But they also report that "positive companionship experiences with their spouses at least once a day or more often" decrease to a low point during retirement. The life history events used to measure these companionship experiences are "laughing together, calm discussion with each other, having a stimulating exchange of ideas with each other, and working on a project." Figure 7–2, based on this study, depicts such changes in companionship experience. While it may be that there are other sharing modes that can account for general satisfaction, marriages without laughter, discussion, sharing, or working together would seem to be dull indeed.

Peterson's findings get some confirmation from Clark and Anderson (1967), who stress the greater equality among happily married couples as contrasted to unhappy ones. These same happily married persons find marriage a source of comfort and joy when their children are grown. They support each other in illness and loneliness. On the other hand, some long-married persons blame their mates for any troubles they have and wish for termination of the marriage. Clark and Anderson found that unhappy couples cannot cope with illness. Lipman (1961) adds a further positive note in his study of the morale of couples in retirement. He believes that the retirement experience itself is instrumental in promoting the mutuality of sharing household tasks and the affective aspects of companionship, such as giving love and affection. He stresses that marriage in the later years moves away from dependence on such instrumental roles as striving for money and status, and moves toward new bonds based on mutuality of roles.

No Research Consensus

What do we make of these somewhat contradictory and incomplete studies? How can we answer our first question about the adequacy of the degree of satisfaction of marriage in the retirement years? The answer is that we cannot answer this question. All of these studies, while classic in the

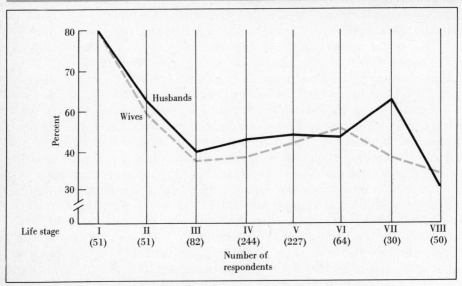

FIGURE 7–2.   Positive Companionship Experiences with Spouses
Source: Feldman and Rollins (1970).

sociological literature, are limited by class-bound and time-bound samples.
The samples are geographically limited, and the number of cases in each cell
of the life cycle is very small, too small from which to generalize. The only
safe conclusion is that we do not know much about marriage in the later
years. We are reminded that Goode (1959) described remarriage after either
divorce or widowhood as providing a better marriage, one that was certainly
"equal to good first marriages." But the last careful census study of outcomes
of second marriages, done in 1974, indicates that some 50 percent of them
will fail, and quite soon—in fact, after an average marital interval of but three
years. What we need are more comprehensive, more broadly based longitudinal studies of marriage in the later years so that we can make more depend-
able inferences from their results. In the interim we must accept the notion
that the conclusions of each of these studies are correct. Many older marriages will survive; some, as per Feldman and Rollins and Peterson, will be
happy and offer good life supports and satisfactions. In Feldman and Rollins's
study the sample is even smaller for those in the seventh stage (N = 30) than
for other stages, and in that stage there is a decided contrast of opinion as to
companionship—the *only* stage at which this occurs (see Figure 7–2)! A
great many will not be happy and, as Clark and Anderson (1967) suggest, will
not be able to bring life supports or satisfaction to their mates in marriage. It
is probable, however, that many sour marriages in late life will terminate
because the social pressures against divorce are certainly lessened both in
our laws and in the arena of public opinion.

Retirement Marriages

Remembering the hopelessly discrepant ratio of widows to widowers, it is not difficult to understand the fact that men are six times as prone to marry after age sixty-five as women. There simply are not enough men around for these women to marry. A great many of the 11.5 million older single persons in our society shun marriage, however. Lopata (1973) reports that even among her widows who described happy past marriages, some 35 percent say they would not marry again. Britton and Britton (1967) indicate that one-third of a rural sample of sixty rejected the idea of remarriage for older persons.

Another impediment to remarriage in the later years is that Social Security pays less to a married couple than to two singles, so that older lovers may have to give up part of their income in order to get a marriage license. Many instead live together without license or, if you will, in licentiousness. We have already noted earlier in this chapter the roots of some middle-aged children's opposition to their bereaved parents' marriages. This is another factor that may limit later-aged courtship. Also, loss of mobility, lessening of reserves of energy, and financial hardship may inhibit some from exploring and cultivating a possible new relationship.

All of these reasons account for the fact that there were only 60,000 marriages in 1978 among older persons. Considering the vast army of single older persons, this is minuscule. Retirement community promoters frequently boast of all the marriages that have occurred in their communities, but the aggregate is small.

If older men marry, whom do they marry? They continue the pattern initiated in their first and second marriages: they tend to marry younger women. At least 20 percent of the grooms over sixty-five married brides under forty-five. Thus, as Susan Sontag states, there is a double standard for love among older persons, in that women are labeled as "old" at a much younger age than men (see further discussion of Sontag's argument in Chapter 3).

And what happens to those who are either courageous or lucky enough to find a mate? How do these later marriages fare? McLain (1969) has provided us with a research study of 100 couples with brides over sixty and grooms over sixty-five. While these couples were married in 1960, 1961, and 1962, they were not interviewd until 1966, so that the couples had had some time for adjustment and had some perspective to their conclusions. McLain isolated six critical factors that increase the probability of successful later marriage adjustment, and we have added two more, based on our own counseling experience, for an eight-point prescription for retirement marriage success:

1. A retirement bride and groom must know each other well if their marriage is to succeed.
2. The marriage should be approved by children and friends to have a chance of success.

3. To be well adjusted in a retirement marriage, the couple must be well adjusted to retirement and other facets of aging.

4. Retirement is more successful if the couple does not try to live in a house in which one lived with another mate previously. There are "too many people" in such a house.

5. Sufficient income to underwrite the new marriage is a must.

6. Marital adjustment reflects the personal adjustment of both the wife and husband. (Most counselors would feel that this applies to marriages of any age.)

7. Couples who expect to spend their last years happily together must have a definite life plan for those years.

8. Every opportunity for premarital counseling, often involving families of the prospective bride and groom, should be explored and utilized.

Religion and Aging

The second basic social institution to be considered is that of religion. This section will take a look, as objectively as possible, at the relation between religiosity and aging. We say "as objectively as possible" because religion has received less attention by competent scientists in the field of aging (if not in all fields) than any other major social institution. One of the most recent comprehensive *Handbooks on Aging,* comprising three volumes (*The Psychology of Aging, The Biology of Aging,* and *Aging and the Social Sciences:* Van Nostrand Reinhold, 1976–77), covers almost every aspect of aging and yet makes virtually no reference to aging and religion. The same can be said of many other advanced texts on aging.

The lack of attention to this ancient social institution is puzzling. Why this neglect by psychological and sociological researchers? A partial explanation may lie in the difficulty in establishing operational definitions of religion or religious experience. Perhaps social and behavioral scientists, many without experiential background in religion, choose to ignore the subject because of its apparent complexities. Perhaps others, with a bias against the differing definitions of religious truth, conclude that the entire subject is peripheral and not worth serious scientific study. Some may perceive an increase in secularization over the past quarter-century and decide not to invest time and energy in study of an area of life that may be becoming less and less important. A further point of explanation may be the reluctance of foundations and government agencies to fund this type of investigation.

Alfred North Whitehead, in his book *Science and the Modern World* (1942), commented on the importance of science and religion in this way:

> When we consider what religion is for mankind and what science is, it is no exaggeration to say that the future course of history depends upon the decision of this generation as to the relations between them. We have here

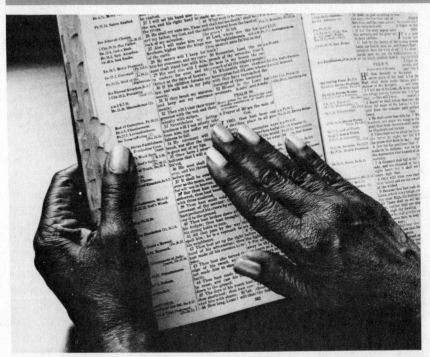

Religion continues to be a major source of satisfaction and comfort to many of the elderly.

the two strongest forces which influence men, and they seem to be set one against the other.

Has the meaning of religion changed for human beings? Is it still, as in an earlier time, a refuge from the storms of life and a symbolic affirmation of the profound meaning of life for older people? Some demographic data indicate how salient the institution of religion is in the lives of Americans. In an analysis of 35,000 households—a sizable sample—the Census Bureau discovered that *fewer* than 3 percent reported *no* religious connection or interest. About 50 percent reported attending some kind of religious gathering or ritual regularly. For the gerontologist, the pertinent question is, what about the elderly?

It is necessary to break down the general question of the relationship between religion and aging into much more definitive and specific questions if we are to throw some light on this field of inquiry:

1. What, if any, are the characteristic patterns of religious participation over the life cycle?

2. Which is more important in assessing the relationship between aging and religion, religious behavior or religious beliefs?

3. Does religious behavior or religious belief make a difference in measures of life satisfaction?

4. In what specific ways do practices and beliefs contribute to happiness, serenity, or life adjustment of older persons during their last years?

5. Does religion as an institution enable older persons to face their dying and death with greater equanimity?

6. Is it possible to differentiate the benefits to religious participants, that is, to distinguish the social aspects of religions from aspects of religious experience considered sacred?

Life Cycle Religious Participation

We are asking whether there are any characteristic patterns of religious participation that follow men and women through the life cycle. Do they attend church or synagogue more during one period of life than another? Bahr (1970) has carefully tried to answer this question by charting religious attendance by age group. He identifies several models. The one we shall refer to here is the "traditional" model. In this model, formal practice of religion is presumed to decline between ages ten and thirty, reaches its lowest point from thirty to thirty-five, and then shows a steady rise until old age. It falls off during the last years when mobility is lost. This pattern gets some support from Fichter, Mauss, and Glock (Fichter, 1954). A Gallup poll taken in the late 1970s provides additional corroborative evidence: it shows that 42 percent of adults of all faiths attend religious services in what was described as a typical week. Adults aged fifty and over had a slightly higher attendance—45 percent. This is at variance with findings over two decades earlier (Orback, 1961).

The problem with this research is that it tends to be cross-sectional for the most part. To compare religious practices of contemporary thirty-year-olds with those of contemporary sixty-five-year olds strains scientific logic. The comparison under these circumstances is between two quite different cohorts, who grew up in somewhat different cultural contexts, with differing family and community influences; the degree of secularization may have been different, too. What this really tells us is not that people become more religious in their later years, or that the old are more religious than the young. It tells us only that there is an observable or measurable difference in religious participation between generations. We do not know from this research how those persons aged sixty-five or older participated when they were thirty. Nor can we tell from these studies what the religious behavior of today's thirty-year-olds will be during *their* later years.

From studies that correlate age and religious participation we also discover very little about what religion means personally to individuals. To a thirty-year-old who has recently moved to a new community, the need for social roots and the social opportunities in church or temple involvement may be the most important aspects of religious observance. For an upwardly mobile young executive, religious and other community activities may sim-

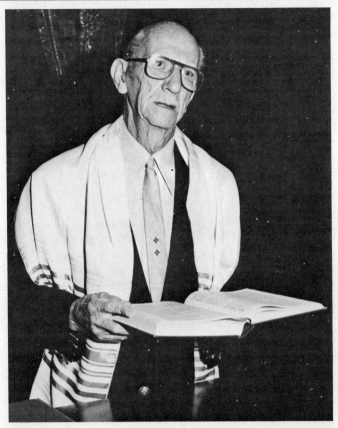

In general, people do not become religious just because they get old. The continued practice or neglect of religion appears to be more related to early training and characteristic life style.

ply be a calculated element in a long-range strategy to achieve visibility, acceptance, and, ultimately, promotion to a top executive position. For both these people, religious participation is not the same as religious belief.

In other words, simple correlations between attendance and age mean little if such investigations do not also elicit data about the motivations, attitudes, and beliefs associated with such behavior.

Religious Cognitions and Behaviors

In assessing the relation of religion and aging it is important to keep in mind that religion is a multidimensional construct. Cognitions and behaviors are two of the dimensions commonly examined in religious research. Cognitive studies of religion examine issues of commitment, faith, belief, and orthodoxy, whereas behavioral studies examine the activities, practices, and rituals associated with religion. Recent research has shown that there are two types of religious behavior, formal and informal. The distinction between formal and informal religious behaviors is especially important to our focus here, since the frequency of formal religious behaviors has been found to decline with age while informal behaviors tend to increase throughout the lifespan (Mindel & Vaughan, 1978; Moberg, 1975; Stark, 1968).

Some demographic statistics relevant to this issue are taken from data collected as part of a longitudinal, multivariate study of bereavement conducted by investigators at the Andrus Gerontology Center, University of Southern California (Thompson, Peterson, & Gallagher, 1982). This ongoing study will be discussed in greater detail in Chapter 9 because of its focus on bereavement and grief. Here we shall refer only to characteristics of the sample and to pertinent religious behaviors.

The sample included 164 older individuals, 101 widows and 63 widowers between the ages of fifty-five and eighty-nine. Table 7–5 shows demographic characteristics for two groups—those who report active religious membership and those who report a passive affiliation. As can be seen in the table, there is a difference in active versus passive religious membership

TABLE 7–5.   Demographic Characteristics: Active Membership in a Religious Group versus No Active Membership

	Reported Active Membership (N = 61)	Reported No Active Membership (N = 103)
Education		
Some school	12%	10%
High school and more	53	66
College degree and more	35	24
Age		
55 to 64	39	40
65 to 74	37	47
75 and over	24	13
Sex		
Male	38	39
Female	62	61
Employment Status		
Full-time	28	19
Part-time	16	11
Retired	56	70
Income (Yearly)		
$0 to $9,999	35	41
$10,000 to $19,999	32	27
$20,000 and over	33	31
Number of Children		
None	2	13
1 or 2	67	63
3 or more	31	24

Source: Thompson, Peterson, & Gallagher (1982).

between sexes, but virtually no difference between active versus passive membership within either sex (i.e., the percentage of active members is roughly equivalent to the percentage of passive members for men and for women). The highest percentage of passive membership appears among retired persons, a figure consonant with earlier studies, which may be explained at least in part by such factors as decreased physical mobility, lack of adequate transportation, and increase of informal religious behaviors. One interesting finding is the fact that most of those with active membership have children (98%), although the percentages are similar for those in the passive membership category.

Table 7–6 shows the frequency of religious behaviors among bereaved elderly widows and widowers. Daily prayer and meditation (presumably solitary activities) are the two most frequently reported religious behaviors. Also striking about this sample is the decided preference for talking with friends about religious matters rather than with a religious advisor (for example, clergy).

Religiosity and Life Adjustment

There have been some attempts to relate religiosity and life satisfaction, to determine whether more committed or more religious individuals evidence better adjustment in their later years than others. Havighurst and Albrecht (1953) concluded from their examination of their respondents that those who attended church were better adjusted and had better health. One might facetiously account for this as the result of better nutrition provided through church dinners. More scientifically, we might turn the equation around and speculate that healthier persons are more mobile and therefore can attend more religious affairs. Or perhaps they are better socially adjusted and thus more likely to attend social functions.

TABLE 7–6. Frequency of Religious Behaviors Among Bereaved Elderly Spouses

	Daily	Weekly	Monthly	Yearly or Less	Never
Attend Church	1%	30%	26%	9%	34%
Pray alone	65	11	7	2	15
Read sacred literature	22	17	20	9	32
Sing hymns at home	7	14	14	10	55
Meditate	34	22	12	4	29
Talk with a religious advisor	1	14	13	10	62
Talk with friends about religious matters	5	19	31	9	36
Listen to religious radio or TV programs	11	22	21	5	40

Source: Thompson, Peterson, & Gallagher (1982).

Note: Total percentages may be less than 100 due to rounding.

Barron (1958) asked an "adjustment" question, too. He wanted to know the things in life that gave older persons most satisfaction and comfort. Some 39 percent (cf. Mathieu, 1972) stated that religion and their church did so. But family and friends were cited more often than any other factor in this study.

A more recent study by Blazer and Palmore (1976) is methodologically more elegant because it is a longitudinal research effort. This study concluded that religious activity decreased over time, but that religious attitudes remained stable; that there is no relationship between religiosity and longevity, but that there is a positive relationship between religious participation and personal adjustment, and that "religion plays a significant and increasingly important role in the personal adjustment of many older persons."

A survey for the National Council on Aging conducted by Harris and associates (1975), included questions regarding religious activities. One general conclusion was that attendance at church and synagogue is slightly higher among those over than among those under sixty-five. A second finding was that the importance people ascribe to religion increases with age. Seventy-one percent of the public aged sixty-five and over feels that religion is very important in their lives, compared to only 49 percent of those under age sixty-five. However, this study recognized that two different cohorts were being compared. The Harris survey, therefore, does not suggest that in the future religion will be important to all those who live beyond sixty-five; it simply states that religion is important for the particular group that was over sixty-five in the 1970s. These conclusions come from the data set forth in Tables 7-7 and 7-8.

Religious Belief and Commitment

One of the classic studies on the impact of religion is that of sociologist Gerhard Lenski (1961), who showed the importance of religion in most people's lives. Lenski used a Detroit area sample in order to determine the effect of religious commitment on the life of individuals. His sample was one of

TABLE 7-7. The Importance of Religion in Your Life

	18–64	65 +	18–24	25–39	40–54	55–64	65–69	70–79	80+
Very important	49	71	34	45	58	65	69	71	73
Somewhat important	33	21	40	35	29	25	22	21	19
Hardly important at all	17	7	25	20	12	10	8	8	6
Not sure	1	1	1	*	1	*	1	*	2

Source: Harris and Associates (1975).

*Less than 0.5 percent.

TABLE 7-8. Attendance at a Church or Synagogue in Last Year or so

Total Public	Percent Attended Last Year	Percent within a Week or So	A Month Ago	2–3 Months Ago	More Than 3 Months Ago	Not Sure
18–64	75	71	13	7	9	*
65+	77	79	9	5	7	*
18–24	67	60	18	8	14	*
25–39	73	72	11	7	10	*
40–54	78	70	15	8	7	—
55–64	81	79	11	4	6	—
65–69	80	79	9	5	6	1
70–79	78	79	10	4	7	*
80+	68	76	10	6	8	*

Source: Harris and Associates (1975).

*Less than 0.5 percent.

the best in terms of the comprehensive way it included all elements of the population. To do this study he found it necessary to distinguish two categories of religious activity. The first had to do with involvement in a socioreligious group (i.e., the corporate type of religious activity). The second stressed private and solitary religious activities such as meditation, Bible reading, prayer, or "daily devotions." Lenski measured the influence of both types of religious behavior in the lives of the people in his sample. While he did not intend originally to examine religious behavior in any particular age group, he nonetheless discovered that in the later years religious participation in organized groups declines but the influence of religious belief does not.

Others have devoted considerable effort to specifying the dimensions of religiosity. Glock (1962) has defined five ways in which an individual can manifest religiosity: religious beliefs, religious practice, religious feeling, religious knowledge, and religious effects. Payne-Pittard (1966), using the Lenski and Glock studies as a point of departure, examined the problem from a more sociological perspective, constructing a "Commitment Scale" to measure the personal, collective, and action aspects of religion as a social institution. Eight categories of commitment measure these three elements. Table 7–9 shows the comparisons of scores by age.

This table suggests a lower level of religious commitment among youth and older persons (aged sixty-five and older) than among young and middle-aged adults. A revised scale used on a national sample of 1,000 individuals in 1968 produced results that paralleled those shown in Table 7–9.

Responsiveness of Religious Institutions

To what extent have religious organizations been responsive to an aging society? As a direct by-product of the 1971 White House Conference on

TABLE 7-9.   Comparison of Scores on the Commitment Test and the Age of Respondents

Commitment Score Frequency		AGE OF RESPONDENTS				
		15–19	20–24	25–44	45–64	65 and over
Low (N = 107)	(observed)	33	10	29	21	14
	(expected)	(24.9)	(9.0)	(29.6)	(34.1)	(9.2)
Middle (N = 180)	(observed)	46	14	45	61	14
	(expected)	(41.8)	(15.1)	(49.9)	(57.5)	(15.6)
High (N = 117)	(observed)	15	10	38	47	7
	(expected)	(27.2)	(9.8)	(32.4)	(37.3)	(10.1)
Total (N = 404)		94	34	112	129	35

Source: Payne-Pittard (1966).

Chi square is 212.8547 d.f. 8, P less than .01, V is .43.

Aging, the National Interfaith Coalition on Aging was founded. The coalition is a nonprofit corporation established in 1972 by Roman Catholic, Protestant, Jewish, and other faiths. From 1973 to 1978 the Interfaith Coalition conducted a research and demonstration project funded in part by what was then the Department of Health, Education, and Welfare. Part of its purpose was to study the education on aging offered in seminaries. The Coalition intended its survey to make some impact on the way churches and temples perceived their responsibilities to older persons. It also wanted to measure the commitment of churches and synagogues to their elderly members.

The sample of seminaries consisted of 135 schools (National Interfaith Coalition on Aging, 1976). A total of 37 seminaries of the 135 said they had at least one course in aging, and 9 had two or more courses. Some 285 courses were mentioned, but in most of them gerontology was not the main focus. Seventy-five institutions said that at least one course in gerontology was available at another nearby institution, and 54 indicated that over half of their students enroll in at least one course with substantive content related to aging. But again, how much focus there was on gerontology was not ascertained. Not a single seminary student was completing an internship in a placement setting related to aging. In view of the fact that the respondent schools collectively place about 10,000 graduates every year in positions of influence and responsibility among more than 100 million people, it is important that every effort be made to infuse the learning experience of future clergy with realistic information about the needs and characteristics of the aged people in their constituencies.

A parallel survey conducted by the American Association of Retired Persons/National Retired Teachers' Association in 1972 of 126 theological schools revealed that 24 had a special course to prepare students to minister to the aged, but in only 2 was the course required; 28 provided continuing education to programs for clergy in the area of aging; and 17 had a graduate program for special ministry to the aged (Moberg, 1975).

In spite of this rather desultory picture with respect to the training of clergy, a brighter outlook emerges from examination of the church's service activities for the aged. A great many retirement communities, nursing homes, and high-rise houses for the elderly are sponsored and operated by Methodist, Jewish, Presbyterian, Lutheran, Congregational, Baptist, Christian, Catholic, Episcopalian, and other religious groups. Some of this housing is particularly for poor elderly; for the most part, religious groups seek to serve the middle class, or the class from which the majority of their members come.

A few churches supply services that permit older persons to remain in their communities and to avoid inappropriate institutionalization. One example is the Shepherd's Center in Kansas City, Missouri. The center is the product of the charismatic leadership of Dr. Elbert Cole, a Methodist minister who rallied the cooperation of some twenty-four churches and synagogues in a geographically limited area of Kansas City to develop a center. From the beginning, the Shepherd's Center has depended on the leadership and participation of older persons themselves. The center's services and their administration are designed and overseen by a board of older persons that operates the center.

The services of the Center help to keep older persons in their homes or apartments as long as they wish to stay there. Some of the services include Meals-on-Wheels, preretirement education, transportation, repair service, telephone reassurance, friendly visitors, protective services, and health fairs.

There are other services, but these at least give some indication of how the older persons involved in the Shepherd's Center have themselves focused on the problems of aging and what programs they have initiated to help themselves, their friends and neighbors find a fulfilled life and remain in the community. Since the original Shepherd's Center was founded in Kansas City, others modeled after this program have sprung up in Atlanta, New York, and other cities. The Catholic program for the aging, HEAD, is in many ways a replication of the Shepherd's Center and its services. Many Catholic and Protestant groups in the eastern part of the country have been stimulated by HEAD to undertake much more comprehensive programs for older persons.

Most religious groups are now beginning to pay particular attention to the needs of the elderly in their neighborhoods and in their temples and congregations. Special note, for example, should be taken of the Councils on Aging of the Jewish Federations in Los Angeles, Baltimore, New York, Chicago, Dallas, and other locations.

Education and Aging

Not only are there more old people living today that ever before, but more of them are beginning to express their rising expectations regarding their adult education preferences and needs. The "baby boom" of the forties and

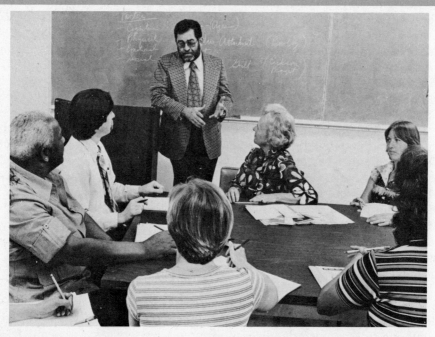

Mixed classes of young and old are a growing phenomenon in education in recent years, as more and more elderly are taking classes to seek new knowledge or to upgrade their education. Some even earn advanced degrees in late life.

fifties, which accounted for the record enrollments in high schools, colleges, and universities over the past two decades, is over. At the same time, increasing numbers of elderly persons, many of them retired, are looking to the educational system for experiences either missed or neglected in their earlier years. Surveys indicate that the aging of the American population is reflected in the age composition of those enrolled in the nation's classes. As of 1980, approximately 1,670,000 elders were involved in the school system at the college level or beyond; projections suggest that by 1990 this number will increase to well over 2,600,000 (Dean, UCLA Extension Program, personal communication, 1981). It is not surprising, therefore, that some now believe adult education for older citizens may prove to be the most challenging frontier in education in what remains of this century.

Research on Old People and Higher Education

The research on the participation of old people in late-life education is not voluminous, and tends to be more descriptive than inferential (Cowgill, 1970; Riley & Foner, 1968). Some studies had addressed themselves to determining the kinds of educational studies elders are likely to undertake, while others focus on factors that limit participation by older persons (Eklund, 1969). A large proportion of related investigations describe the expected influx of older people into the educational system (Jacobs, 1970; Seltzer, Corbett, & Atchley, 1978).

Supporting the expectation of increasing participation of older people in educational programs are the data from the most recent Harris survey. Table 7–10 shows the significant percentage rise from the 1974 to the 1981 surveys for all ages, including the old. We can clearly see the mixing of old and young students in the adult educational system.

One of the very few systematic studies available has attempted to compare selected characteristics of those older people furthering their higher education with those elderly who are not (Covey, 1980). The panel used was a random sample of 300 older people drawn from the city telephone directory. In addition, 100 questionnaires were distributed to residents of a middle-income apartment complex for older persons. Questionnaires were given to 129 older enrollees at the University of Colorado in Boulder as well, and from this list a random group of 35 students was drawn, 32 of whom participated in an interview. A total of 245 completed questionnaires were returned, providing a return rate of approximately 50 percent. Table 7–11 shows a partial tabulation of the overall results of this survey-interview study (which was reported as a preliminary investigation).

Other factors relevant to the hypotheses of the study were monthly income, occupational status, and levels of perceived social, mental, and physical activity. Additional information was elicited during interviews to ascertain whether educational objectives were being pursued for self-initiated reasons or because of perceived demands of others.

Theorizing that certain characteristics might facilitate the pursuit of academic goals, Covey found that those with a better educational background were more likely to pursue such goals. Differences between the sexes were insignificant with respect to these characteristics, as well as those related to

TABLE 7–10.   Adult Enrollment in Educational Courses at a Place of Business, School, or Community Center, 1974 and 1981
(Percentage of All Adults Surveyed)

	1981				1974			
	Total	Some High School or Less	High School Graduate/ Some College	College Graduate	Total	Some High School or Less	High School Graduate/ Some College	College Graduate
Age	*29*	7	*32*	49	*13*	*3*	*16*	*23*
18–54	38	12	38	57	18	5	18	25
55–64	11	3	14	23	5	2	8	11
65+	5	2	6	16	2	1	3	7

Source: Harris and Associates (1981).

TABLE 7–11. Level of Educational Attainment, Sex, Perceived Health Status, and Perception of Age, by Enrollment Status

		Older Students	Older Nonstudents	X² Values and Levels of Significance
Educational	Grade school	0	6 (4.4%)	
Attainment	1–3 yrs. high school	5 (5%)	22 (16.1%)	
	High school graduate	9 (8.9%)	27 (19.7%)	X² = 26.7
	1–3 yrs. college	21 (20.8%)	34 (24.8%)	P = .0001
	College graduate	22 (21.8%)	16 (11.7%)	
	Graduate work	44 (43.6%)	32 (23.4%)	
		101 (100%)	137 (100%)	
Sex	Males	38 (37.3%)	44 (31%)	X² = .78
	Females	64 (62.7%)	98 (69%)	P = .37
		102 (100%)	142 (100%)	
Perceived health	Very good	43 (42.2%)	40 (28.2%)	
status	Good	40 (39.2%)	54 (38%)	
	Average	17 (16.7%)	41 (28.9%)	X² = 8.8
	Poor	2 (2%)	6 (4.2%)	P = .06
	Very poor	0	1 (.7%)	
		102 (100%)	142 (100%)	
Age self-concept	Still young	24 (26.7%)	15 (11.4%)	
	Middle-aged	50 (55.6%)	77 (58.3%)	X² = 11.2
	Old	16 (17.8%)	38 (28.8%)	P = .01
	Very old	0	2 (1.5%)	
		90 (100%)	132 (100%)	

Source: Covey (1980).

perceived health status. Perception of one's own age, however, did make a difference; those who perceived themselves as younger (i.e., "middle-aged" or "still young") were more likely to pursue educational goals. Covey concludes that despite the youth orientation which continues to permeate the educational enterprise, older students do not accept the notion that education is only for the young. Higher incomes, white-collar status, and the perception of oneself as mentally and physically active are characteristic of the older people who are more likely to further their educations.

Diversity of Educational Roles

These data are only suggestive of the significant role that the institution of education now serves and will play in the foreseeable future. Whether they seek a credential or a degree, or would simply like the benefit of additional knowledge and skills, it is to the educational system that the elderly are turning in increasing numbers. Some of the most hallowed rituals of education (e.g., test-taking, attending every class, writing papers, etc.) may well be swept away in the process. The more older people become involved in the educational process, the more the opportunities to shape the format and content of classes to better suit their educational needs. Increasingly, curricula reflect the diverse needs and interests of these superannuated students. Classes on self-protection, money management, exercise, health care and prevention, German, Spanish, Russian, yoga, macrame, hairstyling, food preparation for good nutrition and pleasure, history of the Indians of the Northwest, knitting, needlepoint, world history, mathematics, book reviewing, art appreciation, speed-reading, folk music, chess, bridge, changing lifestyles, car care and repair, and personal growth—this is but a limited sample of the subjects being studied by older students as well as their younger counterparts.

Summary

It is clear that the American family is alive and well, and that the connectedness of elders to this long-standing institution remains intact. The majority of elderly continue to live in family settings, either as couples or with children, many in their own homes and some in the homes of others. Only a relatively small percentage live alone or in institutions. Most significant is the fact that the majority of older people prefer not to live with their adult children; nonetheless, some degree of proximity and contact with adult children and their families—"intimacy at a distance"—is a popular option.

It is also evident that religion as an institution and as a personal force continues to be important to elderly people who were raised in such traditions. But the evidence supports the conclusion that added years do not automatically increase religiosity. Rather, it appears that religious practices become less formal in the later years. Although religious organizations have lagged in training clergy specifically for work with the aged, churches and synagogues present a somewhat better picture when it comes to the sponsorship of services for the aged.

Finally, the social institution of education, long identified with a youth orientation, has begun to reflect the aging of the general population. Oldsters in increasing numbers are pursuing educational goals. The educational enterprise must make appropriate adjustments to accommodate this influx of elderly students; when older people themselves have a say in the format and content of curricula, schools and universities will truly be able to meet their needs and interests.

References

Bahr, M. H. Aging and religious disaffiliation. *Social Forces,* 1970, **49**, 59–71.

Barron, M. L. The role of religion and religious beliefs in creating the milieu of older persons. In D. Scudder (Ed.) *Organized religion and the older person.* Gainsville: University of Florida Press, 1958.

Blazer, D. B., & Palmore, E. Religion in a longitudinal panel. *Gerontologist,* 1976, **16**(1, part I), 82–85.

Blood, R. O., Jr., & Wolfe, D. W. *Husbands and wives: The dynamics of married living.* Glencoe, Ill.: Free Press, 1960.

Britton, J., & Britton., J. O. The middle aged and older rural person and his family. In E. G. Youmans (Ed.), *Older rural Americans.* Lexington: University of Kentucky Press, 1967.

Brody, E. M. Aged parents and aging children. In P. K. Ragan (Ed.), *Aging parents.* Los Angeles: University of Southern California Press, 1979. Pp. 267–287.

Clark, M., & Anderson, B. G. *Culture in aging: An anthropology of older Americans.* Springfield, Ill.: Charles C. Thomas, 1967.

Covey, H. An exploratory study of the acquisition of a college student role by older people. *Gerontologist,* 1980, **20**(2), 173–181.

Cowgill, D. O. The demography of aging. In A. M. Hoffman (Ed.), *The daily needs and interests of older people.* Springfield, Ill.: Charles C. Thomas, 1970.

Cuber, J., & Haroff, P. The more total view: Relationships among men and women of the upper middle class. *Journal of Marriage and Family Living,* 1963, **25**.

Dowd, J. J. Aging as exchange: A preface to theory. *Journal of Gerontology,* 1975, **30**, 584–594.

Dowd, J. J. Exchange rates and old people. *Journal of Gerontology,* 1980, **35**(4), 596–602.

Eklund, L. Aging and the field of education. In M. Riley & M. White (Eds.), *Aging and society.* Vol. 2. New York: Russell Sage Foundation, 1969.

Feldman, R., & Rollins, M. Marital satisfaction over the family cycle. *Journal of Marriage and Family Living,* 1970, **32**(1).

Fichter, J. *Social religion in the urban parish.* Chicago: University of Chicago Press, 1954.

Glock, C. Y. On the study of religious commitment. *Religious Education Research Supplement,* **57**, 1962.

Goode, W. J. *After divorce.* Glencoe, Ill.: Free Press, 1956.

Harris, L., & Associates. *The myth and reality of aging in America.* Washington, D. C.: National Council on the Aging, 1975.

Harris, L., & Associates. *Aging in the '80s: America in transition.* Washington, D.C.: National Council on the Aging, 1981.

Havighurst, R., & Albrecht, R. *Older people.* New York: Longmans & Green, 1953.

Jacobs, H. L. Education for aging. In A. M. Hoffman (Ed.), *The daily needs and interests of older people.* Springfield, Ill.: Charles C. Thomas, 1970.

Johnson, E., & Bursk, B. Relationships between the elderly and their adult children. *Gerontologist,* 1977, **17**(1), 90–96.

Kerckhoff, A. C. Family patterns and morale in retirement. In I. H. Simpson & J. C. McKinney (Eds.), *Social aspects of aging.* Durham, N.C.: Duke University Press, 1966.

Lenski, G. *The religious factor.* New York: Doubleday, 1961.

Lesher, R., & Peterson, J. *Religion and bereavement.* Los Angeles: University of Southern California Gerontology Center, 1981.

Lipman, A. Role concepts and morale in couples in retirement. *Journal of Gerontology,* 1961, **16**(3), 267–271.

Lopata, H. *Widowhood in an American city.* Cambridge, Mass.: Schenkman, 1973.

Lowenthal, M., Berkman, P., et al. *Aging and mental health in San Francisco:* A social psychiatric study. San Francisco: Jossey-Bass, 1967.

Mathieu, J. T. Religious aspects of death and dying. Doctoral dissertation, University of Southern California, 1972.

McLain, W. *Retirement marriages.* Monograph no. 3. Storrs, Conn.: Storrs Agricultural Experiment Station, 1969.

Mindel, C. H., & Vaughan, C. E. A multidimensionsal approach to religiosity and disengagement. *Journal of Gerontology,* 1978, **33**(1), 103–108.

Moberg, D. O. Needs felt by the clergy for ministries to the aging. *Gerontologist,* 1975, **15**(2), 170–175.

Murray, J. *Family structure in the pre-retirement years.* Retirement Study Report no. 4. Washington, D.C.: USDHEW, 1973.

National Interfaith Coalition on Aging. *The religious sector explores its mission in aging.* Athens, Ga.: National Interfaith Coalition on Aging, 1976.

Neugarten, B. L., & Gutmann, D. Age-sex roles and personality in middle age: A thematic apperception study. In B. L. Neugarten (Ed.), *Middle age and aging.* Chicago: University of Chicago Press, 1968, Pp. 58–71.

Orback, H. Aging and religion. *Geriatrics,* 1961.

Pampel. F. *Social change and the aged.* Lexington, Mass.: Lexington Books (D.C. Heath), 1981.

Payne-Pittard, B. *The meaning and measurement of commitment to the church.* Research Paper no. 13. Atlanta: Georgia State College, 1966.

Peterson, J. A. A developmental view of the aging family. In J. E. Birren (Ed.), *Contemporary gerontology: Concepts and issues.* Los Angeles: University of Southern California Gerontology Center, 1970.

Peterson, J., & Briley, M. *Widows and widowhood.* New York: Association Press, 1977.

Peterson, J., Hadwen, T., and Larson, A. *A time for work, a time for leisure: A study of in-movers.* Los Angeles: University of Southern California Press, 1967.

Peterson, J., & Payne, B. *Love in the later years.* New York: Association Press, 1975.

Pineo, P. Disenchantment in the later years of marriage. *Marriage and Family Living,* 1961, **23**, 3–11.

Piotrowski, J. Old people, bureaucracy, and the family in Poland. In E. Shanas & M. Sussman (Eds.), *Family, bureaucracy, and the elderly.* Durham, N.C.: Duke University Press, 1977. Pp. 158–171.

Riley, M., & Foner, A. *Aging and society.* Vol. 1. *An inventory of research findings.* New York: Russell Sage Foundation, 1968.

Schutz, H. G., Baird, P. C., & Hawkes, G. R. *Lifestyles and consumer behavior of older Americans.* New York: Praeger, 1979.

Schwartz, A. N. *Survival handbook for children of aging parents.* Chicago: Follett, 1977.

Schwartz, A. N. Psychological dependency: An emphasis on the later years. In P. K. Ragan (Ed.), *Aging parents.* Los Angeles: University of Southern California Press, 1979, Pp. 116–125.

Seltzer, M. M., Corbett, S. L., & Atchley, R. C. (Eds.) *Social problems of the aging: Readings.* Belmont Cal.: Wadsworth, 1978.

Shanas, E. *Old people in three industrial societies.* New York: Atherton Press, 1968.

Shanas, E., & Sussman, M. *Family, bureaucracy, and the elderly.* Durham, N.C.: Duke University Press, 1977.

Silverstone, B. Issues for the middle generation: Responsibility, adjustment, and growth. In P. K. Ragan (Ed.), *Aging parents.* Los Angeles: University of Southern California Press, 1979. Pp. 107–115.

Stark, R., & Glock, C. Y. *Religious commitment.* Berkeley: University of California Press, 1968.

Streib, G. Family patterns in retirement. *Journal of Social Issues,* 1958, 14(2), 35–45.

Streib, G. Social stratification and aging. In R. H. Binstock & E. Shanas (Eds.), *Handbook of aging and the social sciences.* New York: Van Nostrand Reinhold, 1976, Pp. 160–181.

Streib, G., & Thompson, W. The older person in a family context. In E. Shanas & G. Streib (Eds.), *Social structure and family: Intergenerational relations.* Englewood Cliffs, N.J.: Prentice-Hall, 1965.

Sussman, M. The family life of old people. In R. H. Binstock & E. Shanas (Eds.), *Handbook of aging and the social sciences.* New York: Van Nostrand Reinhold, 1976. Pp. 218–239.

Thompson, L., Peterson, J., & Gallagher, D. Multiple factors in coping with grief in the elderly (ongoing investigation, unpublished). Los Angeles: University of Southern California Gerontology Center, 1982.

Treas, J. Aging in the family. In D. Woodruff & J. Birren (Eds.), *Aging: Scientific perspectives and social issues.* New York: Van Nostrand, 1975. Pp. 92–108.

Whitehead, A. N. *Science and the modern world.* New York: Macmillan (Mentor Books), 1942.

For Further Reading

Clements, W. M. *Ministry with the aging.* San Francisco: Harper & Row, 1981.

Cross, K. P. *Adults as learners: Increasing participation and facilitating learning.* San Francisco: Jossey-Bass, 1981.

Frankfather, D., Smith, M., & Caro, F. *Family care of the elderly.* Lexington, Mass.: Lexington Books (D. C. Heath), 1981.

Marshall, V. W. *Last chapters: A sociology of aging and dying.* Monterey, Cal.: Brooks/Cole, 1980.

Payne, B. Religious life of the elderly: Myth or reality? In J. Thorson & T. Coole (Eds.), *Spiritual well-being of the elderly.* Springfield, Ill.: Charles C. Thomas, 1980.

Aging and Minority Status: The Castes of Thousands

Chapter 8

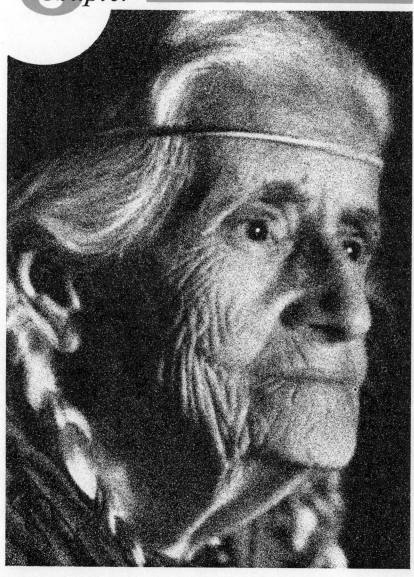

Prescription for eternal youth:
  Avoid fried fods which angry up the blood.
  If your stomach disputes you, lie down and pacify it with cool thoughts.
  Keeep the jucies flowing by jangling gentle as you move.
  Go very lightly in the vices, such as carrying on in society—the society
    ramble ain't restful.
  Avoid running at all times.
  And don't look back.
    Something may be gaining on you!
  Leroy "Satchel" Paige

The elderly in America constitute a relatively small but growing seg-ment of our national population. Today, one of approximately every nine people is sixty-five or older—roughly triple the proportion of elderly in this country in 1900, but about half the projected proportion of elderly in the United States just fifty years from now.

In contrast to the stereotypic view of the elderly as a homogeneous sub-population, old people in fact are as diverse as the rest of the population, with respect to geographic location, habitat, life-style, physical features, adaptive capacities and capabilities, motivation, socioeconomic status, social activities and contacts, family background, occupational history, educational preparation, and countless other characteristics. While a number of common experiences do provide the basis for group identity and serve to distinguish older from younger cohorts, the distinctiveness and individuality of elderly persons seem, at times, to defy attempts at meaningful description of the group as a whole.

Are the Aged a Minority Group?

Older people are a minority in our society, statistically speaking. The term "minority," however, has taken on a special significance in recent years, and is more often used to label a group of persons that differs with respect to one or more identifiable physical, social, or economic characteristics from the normative and generally more powerful "majority" group. Are older people a "minority" in the special sense of the word?

As it turns out, this is a rather controversial question. Barron (1953) is credited with having been the first to suggest that the aging process confers minority status on the elderly, a position that was later championed by Rose (1968) in his description of the "subculture of aging." According to Rose, aging individuals tend gradually to limit their realm of social interaction to their age peers, in part because of the "pull" or social attractiveness of such persons, but more commonly because of the "push" of disengagement, which serves to isolate older people from other segments of society.

Yet "the extent of isolation from the larger society . . . varies from one older person to the next. Thus, different older people have different degrees of involvement in the aging subculture" (Rose, 1968, p. 30). This differential involvement makes minority group identification more difficult to establish for older persons; age *qua* age may not be a very salient or meaningful dimension for ascription of minority status (Streib, 1968). Nonetheless, Rose argued, those elderly who do become dissociated from the mainstream of social activity share "the signs of group identity that previous sociological studies have found in ethnic minority groups. . . . evidence of the growing group identification among older people in the United States today is available to even the casual observer" (1968, p. 34).

The case for identifying the elderly as a unique and distinctive subculture or minority seems to depend largely on the phenomenon of disengagement, through which the older individual and society itself go through a process of mutual withdrawal (commonly exemplified by retirement from a job or occupation). The tendency of the older person to become uncoupled from the structures and functions of society is thus reinforced as society pushes the old aside to make room for more youthful replacements. Although disengagement does occur in some contexts and among some older persons, it is but one style of adjustment to later life, and can hardly be described as the typical response to aging. Indeed, Lemon, Bengston, and Peterson (1972), Maddox (1968), Neugarten, Havighurst, and Tobin (1968), and a host of others have pointed to the continued activity of many older persons as an equally valid response pattern. The widespread variability of the frequency and intensity with which the elderly pursue different behavioral options seems to suggest that, although the elderly may share certain needs and concerns as a group, their diversity precludes describing them as a distinct subculture or a "minority" in the special sense of the word.

In large measure this diversity is explained by the fact that "cultural [and] other minorities account for much of the heterogeneity within the elderly population" (Smith et al., 1978, p. 59). About 10 percent of the population sixty-five or older is either black, Hispanic, Asian-American, or native American, or belongs to another ethnic group of color (Harris, 1981). Furthermore, perhaps 35 percent or more of the remainder of elderly persons in the United States are immigrants (15 percent) or the children of immigrants (20 percent) who identify with a particular European ethnic heritage (Meyers, 1980). There exist more or less identifiable differences among (and within) these groups in terms of the respective levels of cultural distinctiveness, cultural identification, and degree of assimilation or incorporation into the mainstream of American society (cf. Gordon, 1964; Trela & Sokolovsky,

1979). While "ethnic differences, like any other obvious divergence from the norm, are viewed by the majority society as undesirable deviations" (Markson, 1979, p. 343), the recent renaissance of ethnicity (cf. Novak, 1973) has afforded legitimacy to participation in culturally distinct life-styles and patterns of behavior. It should not be surprising to find that, although

> the onset of physical and social changes that accompany the aging process produce some similarities among all elderly individuals [t]here does not appear any evidence . . . that the ethnic group member's "roots" become merely a part of the remembered past when the individual becomes older [Gelfand, 1981, p. 104].

Despite the fact that nearly half of the elderly population identifies with an ethnic minority group, relatively little is known about the contributions of ethnicity and ethnic distinctiveness to patterns of aging (and vice versa). Moreover, much of what has been reported in this area to date must be viewed with caution. While many studies of minority aging were triggered by the growth of interest in minorities in general in the 1960s and 1970s, relatively few were conducted by investigators who were themselves members of ethnic minority groups. The possibility that the assumptions, interpretations, and conclusions made by nonminority investigators may reflect an ethnocentric "middle-majority" bias in the study of ethnic minority aging cannot be overlooked. More than simply posing a threat to the ecological validity of research findings reported in some of these earlier studies, this bias may have had a pervasive influence on the formulation, conduct, and analysis of subsequent studies. As a result, a number of negative myths and stereotypes may have inadvertently been perpetuated to account for the phenomena of ethnic aging.

No doubt one of the more pervasive of these myths is that membership in an ethnic minority group precludes "successful aging;" that for the aging individual little if anything is gained and a great deal is lost by virtue of belonging to an ethnic minority group. While it may be true that greater risks to financial security, health maintenance, and longevity are associated with aging in some ethnic groups (primarily those of color) in comparison to the white majority, it does not necessarily follow that ethnic group members are less satisfied with their lives or that they cope less effectively with life change in later years than their white majority counterparts. This myth, among others regarding the minority aged, has clouded our understanding of the role of ethnicity in the lives of the elderly for too long (Hendricks & Hendricks, 1977). The remedy for this situation lies in the adoption of a more balanced perspective—one which recognizes that gains and losses are characteristic of the lives of *all* peoples across the entire lifespan (cf. Chapter 9), and which further accounts for the perception of gains and losses as such within an ecologically valid cultural context.

In any discussion of minority issues and aging there is another important group to be reckoned with. While women generally outnumber and outlive men and thus are not proportionally a minority of the general population at any point during the lifespan, they do share a number of problems and concerns which derive from their historically less-than-equitable treatment as psychosocial and economic entities. Although, once again, the variability among women with respect to many characteristics and patterns of behavior may be great, the common life experience of female socialization has been described by Lopata (1971) and others (e.g., Kuhn, 1980; Wolleat, 1980) as sufficiently pervasive to permit the legitimate ascription of minority status to women in general, and older women in particular (cf. Beauvoir, 1974; Sontag, 1972).

With these thoughts in mind, we shall turn to the central issues under consideration in this chapter:

1. What are some of the contributions (positive and negative)of ethnicity to the behavioral patterns and adaptive responses of minority members in their later years of life? How do these differ (if, in fact, they do) from those of the aging majority?

2. What are some of the contributions (positive and negative) of the process of female socialization to the behavioral patterns and adaptive responses of women in later life? How does the experience of aging differ for men and women? How does it differ among women with respect to marital status and **parity**?[1]

3. Does the aging process accentuate or attenuate the problems of minority status for women and ethnic groups?

4. What are the advantages and disadvantages of membership in more than one minority group over the lifespan (e.g., being a female member of an ethnic group)? Do these advantages and disadvantages change in frequency or intensity with increasing age?

5. What are the prospects for society's treatment of aging minority members in the future?

Ethnic Minorities

As mentioned earlier, ethnic minorities currently comprise nearly half the population of Americans aged sixty-five or older. Approximately 78 percent of these ethnic elders are members of first-generation descendants of white European families who arrived in America either before World War II ("old immigrants") or afterward ("new immigrants"). The remaining 22 percent includes ethnic groups of color whose ancestors lived in America before the advent of white settlers or were transported from other parts of the world to work as slaves or servants, or who are members or descendants of groups that, like many white ethnics, migrated to the United States to escape oppression

[1] *Parity:* number of children born

in their homelands and to seek opportunities for improved quality of life in this country. Figure 8–1 depicts the reported country of birth of immigrants arriving in the United States between 1951 and 1980.

White Ethnic Minorities

The proportion of white ethnic elders is substantial, due to the massive influx of immigrants from Europe over the past century. Their representation within the ranks of older minority members will likely decrease in the future, however, as the result of (1) the declining flow of persons emigrating from Europe to the United States in recent years; (2) the "generational shift in ethnic saturation" (Kastenbaum, 1979) through which successive generations of foreign-born persons who live and grow old in America identify

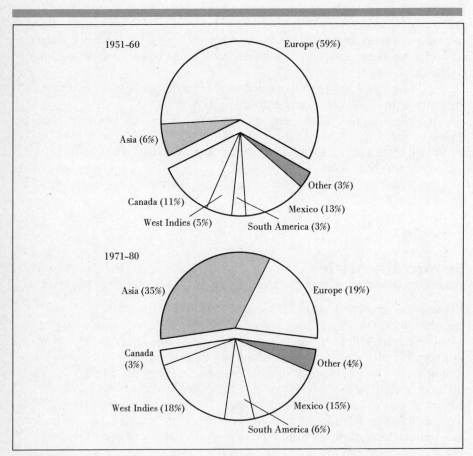

FIGURE 8–1. Reported Country of Birth of Immigrants to the United States, 1951–80.
Source: Statistical Abstract of the United States, 1980.

themselves (and are identified) less in terms of their ethnic roots and more as "Americans"; (3) the expected rise in the numbers of aged Hispanics, Asian-Americans, and other minorities of color over the next several decades.

White ethnics represent a wide variety of national origins and cultures—Greeks, Hungarians, Poles, Latvians, Lithuanians, Estonians, Italians, Yugoslavians, Irish, Germans, Russians, and many others. As might be expected, group and individual differences distinguish elderly white ethnics with respect to the length of time they have resided in the United States (old versus new immigrant status), the physical, social, emotional, and economic environments in which they live, and the degree to which they have become assimilated and incorporated into the mainstream of American life. Quite obviously, those older minority individuals who live within their own ethnic enclaves are more likely to find support and reinforcement for the preservation of their culture than are elders who live in more culturally or ethnically heterogeneous locales. In addition, those living in essentially ethnic communities may have more opportunities for passing along the artifacts and history of their ethnic group to future generations.

In contrast to the notion of the "melting pot," according to which all ethnic groups are subsumed without distinction into one large, happy American family, it appears that the model which better describes the behavior patterns of many white ethnic elders is that of "integrated pluralism" (Trela & Sokolovsky, 1979). This model suggests that the ethnic identity of minority members is reinforced by social ties and activities that exist against the backdrop of American life. The response of white ethnic elders to the pressures of social conformity in this country has been tolerant and compliant to a degree. Yet these individuals are still dedicated to the preservation of their unique cultural identity, often becoming more involved and immersed in ethnic group activities in their later years.

In her study of "emotional needs of elderly Americans of Central and Eastern European background," Mostwin (1979) attempted to identify the ethnic contributions to the needs for love, survival, and creativity—and how these needs were fulfilled—among elderly Americans of Estonian, Latvian, Lithuanian, Hungarian, and Polish descent. Not unlike elderly from the majority, the respondents surveyed in this investigation preferred to express their love for family members in the context of "intimacy at a distance" (see Chapter 7). While few ethnic elders were found to live with their adult children, many enjoyed frequent contact with their children and grandchildren and often eschewed government or other support in favor of maintaining ties of dependency with these family members. Their needs for survival were expressed in the strong desire to preserve their cultural heritage through the continued use of their native languages, the display and enjoyment of art and music, and observance of national and religious customs. Finally, their needs for creativity were satisfied through individual or social activities which often included an ethnic or religious component.

Gutmann (1979) analyzed the kinds of ethnic support systems which best met the needs of white ethnic elderly from eight different groups

(Estonians, Greeks, Hungarians, Italians, Jews, Latvians, Lithuanians, and Poles) living in the Washington, D.C., and Baltimore area. Despite the availability to these individuals of a variety of formal support services, Gutmann discovered that roughly three-fourths of the ethnic elders sampled generally did not take advantage of such services—probably because their needs were being met in other informal ways, often by family members. However, results also suggested the existence of barriers to formal support services. Such barriers were often linguistic, but adherence to traditional values also reduced the appropriateness of such services in the eyes of many of these older individuals. Those elders born in the United States as well as those who had migrated to this country following World War II tended to rely on formal support services to a greater extent than those who came to America before the war. This finding was perhaps due to the fact that the "new immigrant" groups were better educated and more aware of the existence and nature of such services than the latter, or possibly it is the result of differences in levels of incorporation into American society and willingness to participate in social institutions. Elders in Gutmann's sample generally expressed greater confidence in members of their families and ethnic friendship networks for

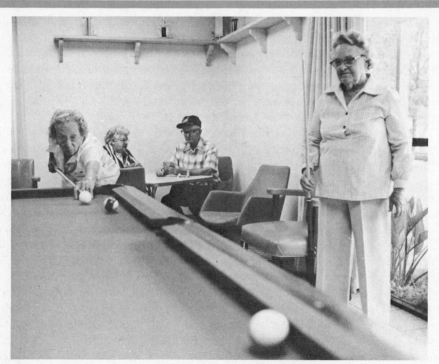

New friends and activities help counteract the loss of morale of many elderly women as their social roles become attenuated and their economic base becomes more precarious.

social support, and indicated relatively high rates of participation in ethnic organizations and activities in their later years.

Another study of white ethnic elders was conducted by Cohler and Lieberman (1979) to determine the nature of personality changes among male and female members of Irish, Italian, and Polish ethnic groups living in Chicago. Data used to analyze personality change in this study were collected by means of questionnaires, speech samples, and personality tests administered to members of these three ethnic groups ranging in age from forty to eighty years. The results of this investigation suggested that while Polish- and Italian-American men and women experienced complementary shifts in personality similar to those described by Neugarten et al. (1964)—that is, women became more assertive and achievement-oriented in their later years while men became less so—Irish-American men and women both continued to operate in a more assertive, active mode, at least through age eighty. Cohler and Lieberman concluded that "personality change across the second half of life is not independent of cultural context and . . . aging may accentuate differences in modal or ethnic personality" (p. 242). However, their findings may have been confounded by significant differences in status-related characteristics between the higher-income Irish and the lower-income Italians and Poles they sampled. Social class rather than ethnic membership differences may have produced their results. In addition, this study was based on a cross-sectional analysis of personality differences, which may have confounded cohort-related historical variability in personality factors with personality change over time. While it may indeed be the case that ethnic differences such as those described by Cohler and Lieberman exist, it is not possible to draw this conclusion from these results alone.

Quite obviously, these studies offer only a rather cursory glance at the wide range of behavior exhibited by white ethnic elders. Nonetheless, they do suggest the continuing importance of ethnicity in the lives of older persons, and may serve to stimulate additional research along similar or related lines in the future.

Nonwhite Ethnic Minorities

The history of nonwhite ethnic minorities in the United States is rather different from that of their white ethnic counterparts. While white ethnics are generally rated "low" in terms of ethnic distinctiveness, nonwhite minority members usually range from moderately to highly distinctive in comparison to majority groups (no doubt reflecting differences in racial as well as cultural distinctiveness). Nonwhite ethnic groups have been described as members of "quasicastes" (Blau, 1974) and "caste-like minorities" (Ogbu, 1978) due to the pervasive limitations upon their social and economic mobility perpetuated by majority members (i.e., "invidious pluralism"; Trela & Sokolovsky, 1979). Whereas many white ethnic groups have managed to do quite well in their adoptive society from the standpoint of economic status, nonwhite eth-

nic minorities have experienced a greater incidence and degree of economic
hardship in this country. For example, in 1972 the median family incomes of
foreign-born Russians, Poles, and Italians living in the United States were
$13,929, $12,182, and $11,646, respectively—better than the average Ameri-
can family, given the fact that the national median income independent of
ethnic heritage that year was $11,000 (Gans, 1974, and Thurow, 1976, cited
in Markson, 1979). The median family income of American blacks that year,
however, was only about 60 percent of the national median income of
whites—roughly $6,600. Ten years later, the situation for black families
appeared to be worse relative to their white counterparts, as Figure 8–2 suggests. The annual median income of Hispanics and other nonwhite ethnic
groups is little better—with the exception of those individuals of Japanese
descent who seem to have been more successful in breaking through the
economic barriers erected against people of color in the United States.
Unfortunately, these patterns appear to be characteristic of the economic
welfare of many nonwhite ethnic minorities throughout the lifespan, as the
comparative data for elderly whites, blacks, and Hispanics shown in Table 8–
1 implies (see also Critical Discussion, Chapter 5).

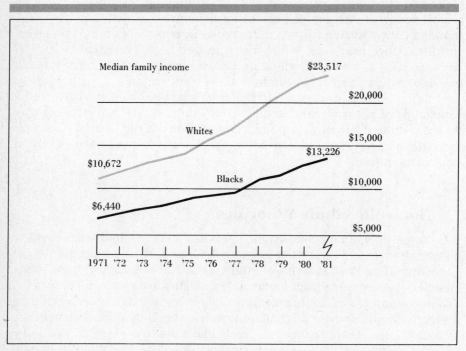

**FIGURE 8–2.   Relative Median Family Income of White and Black American
Families, 1971–81.**
Source: U.S. News and World Report, Aug. 2, 1982, 95(8), 8.

TABLE 8–1.   Income and Income Sources of Black, Hispanic, and White Aged in the United States

	Black	**Hispanic**	**White**
Median individual income			
female, 65–69 years	$1,170	$1,270	$1,608
70–74 years	1,098	1,248	1,525
75+ years	974	1,189	1,362
male, 65–69 years	1,956	2,659	3,817
70–74 years	1,711	2,101	2,892
75+ years	1,503	1,735	2,229
Percent persons with income under $2,000			
female	83.4	77.3	67.5
male	59.8	47.4	34.0
Percent persons without income			
female	14.0	21.0	13.0
male	5.9	5.8	2.9
Median family income by family type			
husband (65+ years old)–wife	$3,250	$4,373	$5,050
female (65+ years old)–head	2,904	3,897	5,772
Percent of all aged families living in poverty	38.8	25.4	15.6
Percent of all aged unrelated individuals in poverty	71.7	58.1	48.8

Source: U.S. Bureau of the Census, *Census of Population, 1970: Detailed Characteristics,* Final Report PC(1)-D1, United States Summary (Washington, D.C.: Government Printing Office, 1973).

Double Jeopardy?

In 1964, the National Urban League published a report indicating that the economic problems inherent in the black experience in America are compounded by the problems of growing older. "Double jeopardy," the descriptive label applied to the plight of aging blacks, has since come to be applied to the status of many other nonwhite minority group members in their later years as well, and now has given rise to the notion of "multiple jeopardy," the problematic situation of minority persons who are aging and female. While the concept of double jeopardy suggests that older minority members suffer the combined negative effects of racism and agism, two more recent hypotheses propose that minority membership may help to offset some of the problems encountered in the aging process (the "ethnic compensation" model; Trela & Sokolovsky, 1979), or that the aging process may ultimately level or reduce the gaps between minority and majority status (the "age-as-leveler" hypothesis; Bengston, 1979; Dowd & Bengston, 1978; Kent, 1971). As is often the case, none of these three descriptions of the interaction of minority membership and aging is sufficient alone to account for the evi-

dence presented to date. Rather, each one appears to have some limited utility in explaining specific components of the minority aging experience.

For example, Dowd and Bengston (1978) designed an investigation in
which differences in age and ethnicity with respect to status, life satisfaction,
and social interaction patterns were studied in more than 1,200 individuals.
A stratified sample of black, Mexican-American, and white Los Angeles residents ranging in age from forty-five to seventy-four was surveyed in an
attempt to test the double jeopardy hypothesis. Following an analysis of their
results, Dowd and Bengston discovered that with respect to economic status
and self-perceived health status, differences in age were accentuated by differences in ethnicity. Economic status and health status declined with
increasing age and increasing ethnic distinctiveness, thus offering some support for the notion of double jeopardy. In contrast, however, black and Mexican-American respondents indicated a greater frequency of social interaction with family members as a function of age when compared to white
respondents, a finding which is consistent with the ethnic compensation
hypothesis. (Whites were not classified with respect to ethnicity in this
study.) Finally, measures of life satisfaction were found to decrease in variability among the three ethnic groups with increasing age, providing confirmation of the age-as-leveler position. What is important to note about this
study in particular is the fact that three different explanations, based on very
different assumptions about the interactive effects of ethnicity and aging,
were required to account fully for the results obtained. Had this investigation
been limited to a study of economic and health status exclusively, or of life
satisfaction, or of patterns of social interaction, for example, only one of the
three hypotheses would have received support. Thus, depending on the
nature and number of variables chosen to study the interactions of ethnicity
and aging, it might be possible to gather evidence in support of only one
hypothetical formulation when in fact others might be more relevant and
more valid explanations of the data or of related phenomena. In sum, given
the relative paucity of information concerning the interactions of ethnicity
and aging, it is better to look at as much of the picture as possible, rather
than restricting one's focus too much, in order to maintain the balanced perspective described earlier in this chapter.

Interaction of Ethnicity and Aging

Another caution is in order at this point. Varghese and Medinger (1979)
have proposed that "poverty is the situational deficit most salient to the status
of the minority aged" (p. 99). While economic status is certainly influential
in determining the extent to which cultural and ethnic expression may be
possible over the lifespan, and may be a very powerful contributing factor to
the life-style and "life chances" (cf. Trela & Sokolovsky, 1979) of a particular
ethnic group, it seems that many discussions of ethnicity and aging confound
the notion of an ethnic minority group with that of an "ethclass" (Gordon,
1964)—that is, a social group defined by ethnic background or heritage *and*

socioeconomic status or class membership. Failure to control for economic class membership may lead to erroneous and invalid conclusions about the role of ethnicity per se in the lives of aging individuals, thus fueling the fires of negative myths about the dynamics of minority aging (cf. Bell, Kasschau, & Zellman, 1976). The question is, independent of economic status, how do ethnicity and aging interact?

Speaking to this issue, Trela and Sokolovsky (1979) write:

> When social class is controlled, very little evidence exists suggesting that various ethnic groups have specific needs, although there may continue to be life expectancy differences [from group to group] . . . and other life chances may be somewhat differently distributed. Rather, . . . the needs of the elderly appear to be essentially similar regardless of economic background. *What does vary is the way ethnic groups respond to these needs* [p. 133; italics added].

These comments suggest a possible answer to our question. It appears that if we examine the interaction of "ethclass" and aging, the double jeopardy hypothesis best describes the treatment of elderly members of minority groups. But when we remove variability due to class membership and examine the interaction of ethnicity and aging independent of economic status, we find that the needs of various ethnic groups are similar in their later years. In this instance, the aging process reduces group differences—consistent with the "age-as-leveler" hypothesis. Yet even though "the needs of the elderly appear to be essentially similar," the role ethnic groups play in fulfilling these needs suggests that ethnicity does indeed contribute to the lives of elderly persons, providing various levels of support in the later years—thus validating the hypothesis of ethnic compensation.

Ethnic Compensation

Given this background and orientation, we now turn to a brief discussion of the ways in which the responses of four nonwhite ethnic minority groups provide compensatory support for their elderly members. Our discussion will focus on blacks, Hispanics, Asian-Americans, and native Americans—the groups represented in the special sessions of the 1971 White House Conference on Aging that led to the formulation of specific resolutions for support for minority elderly. Four points to keep in mind in this consideration of ethnic compensation are: (1) there are major differences *between* minority groups and their responses to elderly members; (2) there are major differences *within* minority groups and their responses to elderly members; (3) minority groups and their elderly members are distributed in geographically unique ways or patterns in the United States; (4) historic and political factors have contributed to the uniqueness of each cohort of minority elderly (adapted from the Federal Council on Aging, 1978, as cited in Fujii, 1980).

Black Americans and Aging

Although there is little information concerning the aging black population that is not linked to variables describing economic status and welfare, some clues as to the role of the black subculture in the experience of aging are apparent. About 8 percent of the black population in the United States is sixty-five or older—a somewhat smaller proportion than reported for the white population in this country (Fujii, 1980). Roughly three-fourths of elderly black persons live in urban areas, often in moderately close proximity to family members. Elderly blacks lead lives that may be described as "stable" with respect to at least two major characteristics: residential mobility and role transition. Most elderly blacks change their residential location very infrequently, and most continue to play very important, focal roles in patterns of family interaction. The relatively high status afforded these elderly individuals as a result is consistent with the findings of Cowgill and Holmes (1972) in various reports of cross-cultural ethnicity and aging.

Jackson (1972) has concluded that older black Americans live in a modified extended family context for the most part. That elderly blacks generally report seeing their children about once a week on the average suggests that, not unlike white majority and white ethnic elderly, older black individuals prefer parent-child relationships characterized by intimacy at a distance. Nonetheless, Billingsley (1968) has reported that among families headed by older women, the probability of "adopting" children under the age of eighteen from elsewhere within the extended family network is five times greater for blacks than for whites. This informal "adoption" procedure provides family continuity, reinforcing the roles and status of elderly black women in the family and providing opportunities for the transmission of values and customs to "adoptive" children. In addition to building important cross-linkages between primary family components within the extended network, this custom often adds to the income of elderly black women charged with the responsibility of raising another's child. It should be noted that this informal transfer of child-raising responsibilities among family units described by Billingsley has at least one other counterpart: in Puerto Rico, a distinction is commonly made between one's *hijos* (children one has raised) and one's *hijos de crianza* (literally, children one has "created"; one's biological offspring). As has been noted for white ethnic groups, family solidarity against the larger backdrop of American life helps to preserve group norms and customs for black Americans, although for blacks ethnic pluralism has a large negative component (Trela & Sokolovsky, 1979).

Evidence for the latter point is provided by the fact that public and private service organizations and institutions seem somewhat insensitive to the needs of older blacks. While the very infrequent institutionalization of black elderly has been cited by some as indicative of the strengths of the black American family, for example, a more relevant explanation appears to be that very few long-term care institutions in this country have made provisions for or would consider welcoming elderly blacks as part of their clientele. As a result, the members of an older black individual's family network assume greater responsibility for the delivery of services. Whether such patterns of interdependency among black family members contribute to the greater optimism and higher morale of older blacks (as observed by Dowd & Bengston, 1978), compared to older whites, remains to be seen.

While these generalizations point up the contributions of the black family to the experience of aging family members, it must be recognized that there may be important regional and local differences which contradict such observations. Additional research is required to determine the extent to which this is a representative picture of ethnicity and aging for black Americans.

Hispanic Americans and Aging

If little is known about the interaction of ethnicity and aging for the black population, even less information exists to describe the relationship of Hispanic culture and heritage to life in the later years. Fewer than 5 percent of the Hispanic population living in the United States is sixty-five years old or older; however, there are differences in the various subgroups of that population. For example, about 4.2 percent of Mexican-Americans, 2.4 percent of Puerto Ricans, and 6.4 percent of Cubans are counted among the ranks of elderly Hispanics, in addition to an indeterminate number of older persons from Central and South America and other countries. The majority of older Hispanics live in urban areas (86.3 percent; Fujii, 1980); Mexican-Americans tend to live in metropolitan sections of cities in the western and southwestern part of the United States, Puerto Ricans live primarily in the environs of New York City, and Cubans tend to be concentrated in Miami. These major differences in geographic location, coupled with the uniqueness of each ethnic subgroup, complicate the situation as we attempt to determine the role of ethnicity in the lives of Hispanic elderly in general.

Although there is some question as to the extent to which the extended family figures in the lives of older Hispanics who reside in the United States, it appears that older Hispanic persons seem to prefer interactions with family and friends which permit communication in their national language to those beyond the bounds of the family-friendship network which require communication in English. Older family members are afforded relatively high status in the family setting, not unlike the situation of older blacks. The common emphasis on childbearing and the production of large families provides women with many children an especially privileged position in the family unit—a position which often carries the additional responsibility of child care for grandchildren and other family or friendship-network offspring.

While relatively little else can be reported at present with respect to the interaction of ethnicity and aging for Hispanics living in this country, the Critical Discussion included in this chapter describes a recent study of "100+ over 100," an investigation of more than 100 Caribbean centenarians living in Puerto Rico (Snyder & Schwartz, 1981), which provides additional information about the contributions of ethnicity to longevity and survivorship in a Hispanic subgroup.

Asian-Americans and Aging

Like Hispanic Americans, Asian-Americans are members of more than one ethnic subgroup. Although the composition of the group at large may vary as a function of classification schema employed, the most liberal grouping includes individuals of Japanese, Chinese, Korean, Vietnamese, Thai, Burmese, Pilipino, Cambodian, and Hawaiian descent, as well as those ancestors (or who themselves) came from any of the Pacific islands. It goes without saying that very little of a meaningful nature can be concluded about the role of ethnicity in the lives of aging Asian-Americans in general, given the great diversity of these various subgroups. Undoubtedly, the linguistic problems faced by many elderly members of these subgroups have led to some measure of group cohesiveness and isolation from the mainstream of American society, perhaps resulting in networking among older persons. The rapid push of many younger Asian-Americans to become acculturated and assimilated may eventually pose some threats to the traditionally high status of elderly family members who find security and comfort in more traditional ways and customs.

For subgroup-specific information about the contributions of ethnicity to aging among Asian-Americans, Meyers (1980) has suggested several volumes of the Campanile Press's series, *Cross-cultural Study of Aging Minority Elders in San Diego,* as excellent reference sources. Among the volumes available in this series are those addressing ethnicity and aging among Chinese, Guamian, Japanese, Pilipino, and Samoan elders (see "For Further Reading" at the end of this chapter).

CRITICAL DISCUSSION ▬▬▬

"100+ over 100"—the Old-Old of Puerto Rico

One of the statistics often quoted in discussions of the minority elderly is that at no time in our nation's history has life expectancy at birth for such persons either matched or exceeded that of their white majority counterparts. Nonetheless, a number of relatively recent studies suggest that there may be a "cross-over" in life expectancy rates for minorities and whites in later life. Some (e.g., Jackson, 1972) have interpreted this phenomenon to mean that the greater hazards and hardships of minority relative to majority life produce a selective effect on survivorship. Those who are successful in mastering their fates develop a special "immunity" that helps insure their survival through the young-old, middle-old, and old-old years.

As all aging individuals continue to survive for longer periods of time, interest has grown among research scientists and investigators in identifying and studying those factors associated with extension of the lifespan. Two of the authors of this text are among those who have attempted to investigate the factors related to longevity in a group of ethnic minority elders, the centenarians of Puerto Rico (Snyder & Schwartz, 1981).

Puerto Rico is a tiny island of approximately 3,000 square miles, located east of Cuba, Haiti, and the Dominican Republic in the center of the Caribbean basin. Like the continental United States, about 10.5 percent of its population of 3.5 million people are at least sixty years old. Unlike the United States, the island seems to have produced an unusually sizable proportion of very, very old persons; in 1981, the number of centenarians living in Puerto Rico was estimated at approximately 2,200. A 1977 study undertaken by the island's agency on aging, La Comissión de la Gericultura, was one of the first to reveal information about the status of these superannuated survivors. Based on the findings of this study, Snyder and Schwartz decided to conduct a more detailed and extensive descriptive analysis of survival patterns of the centenarian elderly in Puerto Rico.

Working together with a number of their students, Snyder and Schwartz developed and administered an extensive questionnaire to 101 centenarians living in Puerto Rico and its neighboring island, Vieques, during 1980–81. The "100+ over 100" individuals sampled ranged in age from 100 to 118 years of age, and included forty-three men (average age 105) and fifty-eight women (average age 103).

Because period and cohort effects are so influential in determining the status of elderly persons, it is important to provide some background information about the life context of the individuals who participated in this study. When this centenarian cohort was born, the Spanish government had been in exclusive control of the island for more than 350 years; Spanish remains the dominant language of the island, particularly for social, family, religious, and political functions. These respondents were already young adults at the time of the Spanish-American War, following which Puerto Rico was ceded to the United States in 1898. The society in which the centenarians lived was largely agrarian for most of their lives. Opportunities for formal education were limited to the elite, and the impact of technology introduced by American business and commerce was not felt to any degree until this cohort was well into its seventh decade of life.

Given the general finding that variability among the elderly tends to increase with increasing age, Snyder and Schwartz hypothesized that individual differences would likely be great enough to obscure most major trends in behavior or demographic characteristics in this sample. Surprisingly enough, they found relatively little individual variability among the 101 individuals they studied. Indeed, a number of their findings have been replicated in studies of centenarians in Southern California (personal communication, Committee for an Extended Lifespan, 1982) and in Russia (Benet, 1974), among other diverse locations. The range of variables studied by Snyder and Schwartz was extensive; only the more general behavioral and demographic trends observed in the sample of centenarians from Puerto Rico will be reported here. First, centenarians were the progeny of relatively long-living parents, who themselves had exceeded the normal expectations of about forty years of life a century ago by an average of forty years for the parents of male centenarians and twenty to thirty years for the parents of centenarian women. Centenarians were born into large families and themselves produced families averaging about eight children. Extended families provided much social support for their members, including the centenarian elderly. Approximately 64 percent of centenarians lived with younger family members at the time of the study, and fully one-third were the eldest members of five-generation extended family networks. In addition, close friends were observed to have been adopted into the family through the *compadrazco* or the "godfather" system, thus extending the realm and influence of the family (and the centenarian family member) beyond strict kinship ties and strengthening intergenerational bonds throughout a larger community of people.

Physical health and well-being are, of course, matters of great interest with respect to the survival of the old-old. Much like the sample of centenarians from Soviet Abkhasia described by Benet (1974), these survivors appeared to have been a remarkably healthy cohort. While approximately 65 percent reported that their health at the time of the study was worse than it had been in the past, the remaining respondents indicated that their current health status was just as good, if not better, than in previous years. Three-fourths of men and women had been hospitalized at least once in their lives, but not until after they had passed their ninetieth birthdays in the majority of instances. Hospitalization was most frequently related to cardiovascular complaints, osteoporosis, diabetes, and other problems associated with chronic ailments.

What about the use of tobacco and alcohol? Fifty percent of the women and seventy-eight percent of the men used the former, including cigarettes, cigars, pipes, and tobacco-chewing in roughly equal proportions. One-third of women used alcohol, as did almost six of every ten men.

Patterns of eating, sleeping, and sexual activity were all moderate in terms of both frequency and duration. Most centenarians slept an average of seven to nine hours nightly, as they had done most of their lives. Most also consumed food on a routine basis three times daily; consumption patterns had changed little over the lifespan, and generally included less beef and animal fat and more grains, legumes, fruits, and vegetables than the "typical" American—and Puerto Rican—diet of today.

Other frequently reported characteristics of this elderly sample included a strong tendency toward fatalism and religious belief, decreasing levels of activity over time in their later years, increasing amounts of solitary activity, and widespread reports of economic insufficiency (despite the fact that the level of home ownership was high). When asked about their own perceptions of what had contributed to their extended years, however, responses became considerably more variable. Some reported that good food, eating well, drinking, and having a good time are essential ingredients to a good, long life. Others stated just as emphatically that hard work, faith, abstention from vice (including tobacco and alcohol), and piety are prerequisites for achieving centenarian status. Most concurred, however, that faith in the Deity, consumption of fresh rather than preserved foodstuffs, plenty of rest and tranquillity, and passive compliance have been the most important contributors to their advanced years. Although responses to Snyder and Schwartz's queries about advice that centenarians might give to younger persons so that they, too, might live to be at least 100 were also rather variable, in general respondents counseled passivity, faith in the Deity, tranquility, and maintaining a proper appearance before the world. Compliance, eating well, sleeping long hours, and avoiding vices were also common recommendations to younger cohorts.

These results, describing centenarians in an ethnic minority population, are strikingly similar to those reported in a recent newspaper article from a study of 1,000 American centenarians by the Committee for an Extended Lifespan (*Los Angeles Times,* Feb. 12, 1982). Remarkably, the findings from this tremendous sample of old-old persons in the United States is parallel a large number of items from the study of ethnic minority elderly in Puerto Rico. *All* of the following findings reported by the Committee on Extended Lifespan replicate those of Snyder and Schwartz:

—They [the sample of 1,000 centenarians] do nothing in excess. If they drink, it's in moderation. Tobacco users indulge in cigars, pipes, or chewing. The few that smoke cigarettes do not inhale. Few are fat. They are not given to binges of any kind.

—They're early risers. Usually, this also involves the habit of early retiring [to bed].

—A high proportion are devout believers. They have led what they consider a spiritual life, accepting all experiences as "God's will."

—They've kept busy all their lives. Few are dreamers or loungers. A large number have been self-employed. The majority attribute their survival to hard work.

—They are self-protective. Commonly used phrases were "taking care of myself," and "never letting anything bother me." And they've been self-sufficient as much as possible.

Perhaps more than any other set of phenomena, the parallel findings of these and other recent studies of centenarian status lend credence to the "age-as-leveler" hypothesis. While ethnicity may play a significant role in the lives of the elderly in at least some ways, it appears that the achievement of centenarian status deemphasizes the variability of ethnicity and underscores the commonality of adaptiveness over time.

Native Americans and Aging

Unlike black and Hispanic elders, older native Americans live less frequently in cities and more often in rural locations, nearly three-fourths of which are in the southern and western parts of the United States. Of the 5.7 percent of native Americans aged sixty-five years or older, slightly better than one-fourth continue to live on reservations, while the majority reside in farm and nonfarm communities (Fujii, 1980).

Again, unlike black and Hispanic elders, older native Americans are members of an ethnic group whose ancestors predated other settlers in this country. Pursuant to some of the difficulties involved in negotiations for rights to land and natural resources between the United States government and the descendants of the original native American residents of these disputed areas, several attempts have been made by the government to promote more rapid acculturation and assimilation of segments of the native American population into American society. As a result of some of these efforts, the contributions of ethnicity to aging for native Americans may have become less significant in more recent years. With the increasing modernization of the United States, many customs and practices associated with the native American nomadic-hunter heritage became largely a matter of written or spoken record. The fact that approximately 45 percent of elderly native Americans live in urban areas suggests the decreasing importance of ethnicity and the trappings of reservation life for older members of this group. To reiterate, the great variability in tribal groups and their distribution throughout the country precludes a more thorough treatment of unique patterns of interaction between ethnicity and aging for each of these groups. For additional information on this topic, the reader is referred to *The Elder American Indian* (Dukepoo, 1980), in the list "For Further Reading" at the end of this chapter.

Working with Nonwhite Minority Elderly

The diversity of nonwhite ethnic minority elderly within and beyond the boundaries of group membership provides a unique challenge to the helping professions as they attempt to identify culture-relevant strategies and approaches to meeting the service needs of these individuals. Katz and Libbee (1980) have developed a workshop-based training program for nonprofessional (i.e., volunteer and paraprofessional) service providers geared specifically to consciousness-raising and the development of appropriate avenues for learning and attitude change in response to this challenge. While it is important to recognize that the effectiveness of service provision outcomes may vary from situation to situation, even within what might appear to be a relatively homogeneous community of nonwhite elders, Katz and Libbee offer some helpful advice about the impact of service provider attitudes on service program effectiveness, shown in Table 8-2. To these comments should be added the observations of Kuypers and Bengston (1973), who

TABLE 8-2. Working with Minority Elderly

Attitudes That May Not Be Helpful in Working with Minority Elderly	Possible Effects of That Attitude on Effectiveness	Attitudes That are More Likely To Be Effective in Working with Minority Elderly
Color is unimportant—we're all the same under the skin.	Disregards the important part of a person's identity and experiences.	Recognize and appreciate differences in culture and race.
A member of one ethnic group can understand what it means to be a member of another ethnic group. (Learning from schoolbooks, courses, television, religious teachings, etc. may be helpful in better understanding others but does not teach everything.)	Blinds people from seeing areas that they need to learn about other racial and ethnic groups.	Recognize that no matter what level of awareness you may have, there is still more to learn. Be open to learning. Don't wait to be told—ask!
Minority elderly have the same needs and preferences as white elderly (e.g., they like the same music, read the same magazines, are interested in the same activities).	Minority elderly would be reluctant to come to Senior Citizen Center.	Recognize that the needs of minority elderly may be different from those of white elderly. Solicit input from minority elderly in developing programs.
All people of an ethnic or racial group are alike in their attitudes and concerns.	Generalizes, stereotypes, and boxes minority elderly. Ignores individual differences.	Minority members are human—with individual needs, feelings, aspirations, and attitudes.
I know what is best for the elderly, including minority elderly (e.g., telling a black woman that it is not good for her to stay home and watch soap operas).	Makes minority elderly defensive and alienated. May induce anger. No one will accept help when told it is for their "own good" or decided upon by someone else.	Be a resource person to minority elderly persons—not a savior. Help serve the person's needs. Mutually define what those needs are.
I'm perfectly trustworthy, sincere, and committed to my job. Minority elderly should recognize that.	This attitude has no effect on dissolving the distrust that may exist because of cultural conditioning. Puts distrust on a personal level rather than on a cultural level.	Awareness that distrust may not be personally directed. Recognize that distrust may be legitimate. Take risks to confront distrust and be committed to working on it with the other person.

Source: Katz & Libbee (1980).

265

point out that only when the elderly have a voice in the planning of policies and programs intended for their benefit can these policies and programs be truly responsive to their needs. With the expected growth in numbers of non-white elderly in our society over the coming years, it is essential that the "critical link between talking about the problem[s] . . . and moving toward action" (Katz & Libbee, 1980, p. 329) be developed by group members in order to insure maximally effective outcomes.

Women

Though American women hardly constitute a minority in the statistical sense at any point in the lifespan, numbers alone do not a minority or majority make, as Kobata, Lockery, and Moriwaki (1980) so cogently point out. Rather, "it is clear that the salient variables defining minority status refer to patterns of relationship, the distribution of power and assumed differences in character traits" (p. 449).

These remarks were made with reference to ethnic minority groups, but they are equally applicable to women, whose roles and status have been circumscribed throughout their collective lifespans in our society. As Rohrbaugh (1979) argues, this is not to say that "all women are alike" (or even that "all older women are alike," if we choose to focus on the later years alone). The tremendous diversity of women with respect to many characteristics and functions—ethnic background, marital status, parity (i.e., number of children), residential location and circumstance, mobility, educational attainment, employment history, financial status, self-sufficiency, future expectations, and others (not to mention age) underscores the undeniable heterogeneity of this population. Nonetheless, the processes of "growing up female" and "growing old female" in a society which implicitly sanctions the differential treatment of women in accord with a double standard of behavior at *every* age cannot but have a pervasive, universal effect on the life-styles, belief systems, self-perception, and personal adjustment of these individuals over time. Rohrbaugh (1979) asserts, "Although the importance of gender varies from one area of life to another, from one setting to another, and from one group of women to another, gender is inescapable. It is probably the most important determinant of any individual's life experience" (p. 3).

Perhaps it comes as no surprise to find that the "vulnerabilities and the strengths resulting from the shared experience [of women] have led to negative and positive consequences for the . . . well-being of [this minority group]. . . ." (Kobata, Lockery, & Moriwaki, 1980, p. 449). Just as we observed in the case of ethnic minorities earlier in this chapter, however, one of the negative consequences of the female experience is the set of myths and stereotypes about the behavior of women that colors their treatment across the lifespan. The fact that even the strengths of women are often evaluated in negative, preconceived terms has contributed to the "no win" situation of many women, and does them a gross disservice. A more balanced view that recognizes positive as well as negative outcomes of the female experience is required to achieve an understanding and appreciation of women as they approach and live out their later years.

One obvious advantage of being female (in contrast to belonging to an an ethnic minority group) is revealed in statistics concerning life expectancy. While ethnic minority groups tend to have shorter life expectancies than their white majority counterparts, on the average, women generally live seven years longer than men. Today, in fact, American women may expect to live to an average of eighty-one years, significantly longer than the seventy-four years expected by their brothers. These figures may vary somewhat as a function of ethnic group membership (as suggested above), of socioeconomic status, or of a number of other apparently longevity-linked variables, of course, but the relative advantage of women with respect to survivorship is a constant. Or is it? Does the bonus of a longer life for women guarantee them an additional few years of comfortable, satisfying, and enriching experience, or does the extra time add an additional burden to an already overburdened life? What, exactly, are the pros and cons of relatively greater survivorship for women today?

Aging as a Women's Issue

With the simultaneous progress in consciousness-raising about the experience of being female and the process of aging has come the recognition that aging is, in a very real sense, a women's issue. One of the results of differential longevity between the sexes is that for every 72 men in this country sixty-five or older, there are approximately 100 elderly women. Put another way, this formula translates to 1.4 elderly women for every older man—wonderful for aging men, but deplorable for aging women interested in an exclusive relationship with a peer of the opposite sex. According to the most recent Harris poll (1981), approximately one-fourth of elderly women are married and living with their spouses, while slightly better than three-fourths of elderly men find themselves in similar circumstances. If we recalculate our formula to determine the relative proportions of *unmarried* men and women sixty-five or older, however, we find that there are only 23 unmarried elderly men for every 100 unmarried elderly women in this country. Why the drastic reduction in the relative numbers of unmarried men in the later years and the disproportionate increase in unmarried women?

The answer lies in the double standard, a behavior code that rewards the actions of one group while punishing similar actions of another. Sontag (1972) has written a particularly biting essay about "the double standard of aging" which addresses the disproportionate availability of unmarried men and women later in life. In her essay, Sontag points to the fact that women are defined (and confined) by the perceived need to preserve physical appearance, while men define themselves in terms of actions, activities, and the power these afford. As women grow older, the battles to preserve their beauty become more difficult to win; presumably by the time "old age" has arrived, the war is lost for good. While women are struggling with their appearance in the later years, men in contrast are reaping the benefits of earlier labors. During the middle adult years, power continues to accumulate so that by the time "old age" arrives, most men have achieved considerable status. According to the double standard, young women are attractive because they are beautiful (relative to older women) and older men are attractive because they are powerful (relative to younger men). Thus, the argument goes, older men will limit their choices for companionship to younger women. Unfortunately, younger men also tend to limit their choices for companionship to younger women—the sanctions against older woman–younger man dyads are sufficiently punitive to reduce their frequency to a minimum. For the woman who has defined herself by her appearance, the war has been lost before the first battle ever began. What little consolation may be afforded by the fact that women usually marry men who are older than they are—a situation which essentially maximizes the advantages of their relative attractiveness—is of little value as they grow older, given the data on life expectancy. If women can be expected to outlive men of the same age by seven years, then a younger woman who marries an older man can expect to survive him by even longer. When she becomes a widow, she will be entering her late forties, perhaps, or her fifties or sixties—allegedly the age of waning physical beauty—with a third to a half of life yet to live and the prospects for another relationship dimming fast. In Simone de Beauvoir's words, "She has been taught only to devote herself to someone, and nobody wants her devotion anymore" (1974, p. 649). How did this state of affairs develop—and how can it be changed?

Being/Female and Doing/Male: Will the Force Be with You?

Chodorow (1971) has observed that the powerful-powerless dichotomy that seems to characterize the relative positions of men and women across the lifespan in our society is not a necessary condition. Anatomy is *not* destiny, to contradict Freud. Rather, general cross-cultural patterns of socialization provide role continuity for female children—but for male children, the extent to which role continuity versus discontinuity is provided is a culture-specific phenomenon. In less developed societies, both male and female children experience greater role continuity as they grow up—the kinds of activities in which they engage as children are highly similar to those in which they engage as adults. In more developed societies, however, only female children are socialized through role continuity; male children are exposed with increasing frequency to situations which demand novel, discontinuous behavior compared to those of early childhood. In this latter case, the resulting distinction between the female and male experience may be described as "being versus doing" (Horney, 1932).

While the condition of being is that of a steady state, a passive, constant existence, the experience of doing is active, changing, a dynamic flux. According to this perspective, once female children have matured into adulthood, the steady state period has begun. Any future change is not occasioned by activity, but by *entropy*—the inevitable, progressive disorganization which leads to the collapse of the steady state system (cf. Rifkin, 1980). On the contrary, maturing male children continue to engage in activities that repeatedly provide them with a sense of masculine identity and seemingly offset or mask the inevitable process of entropy, at least for a while.

Just as a steady state is best maintained by little conflict and much compliance and cooperativeness, a dynamic flux is best promoted by achievement and competition. Women *are* cooperative, while men *act* competitive. By virtue of their cumulative achievements, men become powerful relative to women; this power is translated into authority and the establishment of behavioral norms for society. Rohrbaugh (1979) elaborates,

> The male bias has created a "Catch 22" for women. A woman cannot win when she is defined and evaluated totally in male terms. . . . Why has the female always been defined in male terms? The answer can be expressed in one word: *power.* Since males are viewed as more powerful, females are automatically viewed as passive, dependent, and even somewhat helpless [p. 463]. . . . The essential ingredient . . . is power: power as access to money, prestige, and advancement; power as the ability and the right to control the behavior of others; power as the expression of dominance and ownership. And in all these areas the male comes out on top. He has the power, and the woman has none [p. 7].

So it is that women, socialized into role continuity, are ultimately devalued by the physical changes that accompany the aging process—the changes that alter their outward appearance and threaten the steady state of their "being." And so it is that men who have experienced role discontinuity from childhood accumulate greater power and value as the reward of continued activity over time. Although female being may sometimes be differentiated into doing—a transformation that in at least some instances may provide women the opportunity to accumulate power and status—male doing must not be dedifferentiated into being, at the risk of powerlessness and the diffusion of self. While larger numbers of younger women are being socialized according to the model of role discontinuity, the negative sanctions against male socialization by means of role continuity in our culture preclude any complementary crossover in learned patterns of behavior. The ultimate outcome of this female trend away from "being" may, to a certain extent, reduce the social inequities of men and women in the future. But what about women who have been socialized according to more traditional norms and standards? In particular, what are the implications, advantages, and consequences for women sixty-five and older today of earlier training histories?

For the most part, today's cohorts of elderly women whose lives have been patterned after the role continuity model have been oriented toward the maintenance and care of their families. In this context, traditional role fulfillment has been provided by the challenging and demanding tasks of minimizing conflict, satisfying needs, and promoting harmony among family members. Women who have succeeded at these early-through-midlife tasks seldom have been commended for their invisible, self-sacrificing efforts to maintain the expected steady state of the status quo. But when the equilibrium of life has been disrupted, invisible efforts have often been transformed into visible deficiencies.

Nevertheless, the majority of life situations for continuity-trained women have probably been manageable from within the realm of their circumscribed life experience. Patience, compliance, passive manipulation, and perseverance are employed resolutely to assuage minor life crises. Whenever these qualities of being prove ineffective in solving a problem and achieving a return to homeostatic equilibrium, the "helpless" strategy of "capitulate and delegate" provides an easy escape: The woman admits her lack of experience and competence in responding to the critical discontinuity and delegates the responsibility for its resolution to her husband. But dealing with the original problem has not been the only outcome of this transfer. Through this avenue the husband's "will to power" has been reaffirmed and validated in strategic action, while his wife has demonstrated her mediocrity through inaction.

Emancipation of Later Life

For women who have lived by the rules of compliant continuity, defining themselves as their husbands' subordinates, authentic self-expression of needs, wants, and desires has often been postponed or surrendered until later life. Dependent upon their husbands for psychological, social, and economic definition and support, nevertheless at least *some* women socialized in this manner have come to realize the anger that frustrated self-expression can create. For those who have devoted their lives to the socialization and nurture of their children, the "empty nest" years may provide the first real opportunity for the assertion of personhood. With the exodus of adult children from the family home, many women have returned to the classroom and the labor force, have turned avocations into life-styles and programs for action, and have sought discontinuities in their lives from which to learn and grow. For others, however, dependence upon a husband may supersede self-expression. This group of women has been so well socialized, so successfully trained, that only one life event may be jarring enough to shake them from their mold.

The single life event that a man, no matter how powerful, cannot manage for his wife is his last. For the older woman who has built her entire life around that of her husband, his death is perhaps the first occurrence of discontinuity with which she has had to deal since the beginning of their lives together. The death of her husband, occurring on the average about seven years before her own death, may be a terrifying experience for the woman whose coping strategies have been limited to passivity and compliance throughout her adult life. The action demanded in response to this over-whelming discontinuity can no longer be initiated by her spouse—she must assume final responsibility for her own life. Chances are great that her spouse will have handled their financial affairs, property, legal documents, commer-cial arrangements, and other "man's business" for the duration of their shared existence, and that she will have been entirely ignorant (by mutual consent) about that important facet of their relationship. "All too often a woman without a man is a socially isolated, invisible individual with no money, no clear social roles, and few emotional supports" (Rohrbaugh, 1979, p. 464).

Certainly the death of a husband is a stressful event. For women who have begun to seek self-fulfillment during the later years with their husbands, the grief and bereavement they experience is just as real and as painful as it is for women who have invested their being exclusively in the lives of their mates. Yet, as Peterson and Briley (1977) have noted, becoming a widow not only symbolizes the end of a relationship with a husband, but the beginning of a new or renewed appreciation of the woman's self as a valid person. That the death of a husband can result in both loss *and* gain in this fashion is shown in the following case illustration.

CASE ILLUSTRATION
Something for Myself, Too

Mr. Z., eighty-one years old and dying of cancer, requested an appoint-ment at the Adult Counseling Center in order to resolve some of his con-cerns about his condition. While he was receiving counseling from one of the peer counselors there, Mrs. Z., his seventy-six-year old wife, who accompanied him on his visit, was invited to participate in an interview with one of the authors.

During the early part of the session, Mrs. Z. was preoccupied with her concerns about her dying husband's morale. She was also attempting to clarify her role for herself as wife, companion, nurse, etc., with respect to her husband. It was evident from the many questions she asked that her anxieties about her husband's welfare and the pressures she felt to "do the right thing" by him were profound and authentic. She left no doubt that her concern for this man around whom her life had revolved for some forty-seven years of married life was sincere.

It was also apparent to the interviewer that Mrs. Z. was struggling with a hidden agenda. When the dialogue began to focus on her expec-tations for her own life following the imminent death of her husband, she became more agitated, even tearful. At that point she began to ver-balize the expected apprehensions about her future. But suddenly Mrs. Z. looked directly at the interviewer, paused a moment, and then remarked thoughtfully, "I want to do what I can to care for my husband and help him during the weeks or months left to him. That's only part of it, though. I want to do something for *myself* too. I want to invest some of my energies into myself, my own life and future."

> And from those succinct words, the interviewer realized that Mrs. Z., socialized though she had been as a "helpmate" for her husband, was beginning a profound and necessary struggle to rediscover herself as a person.

As Peterson and Briley (1977) have concluded, "The need for the widowed to achieve emotional independence from their deceased mates recognizes that they now are new individuals with new status and that there are still many chances for a creative life" (p. 125; (8)-28 cf. Welch, 1982).

Fortunately, women are not alone in their struggle for self-identity—they have each other. Contrary to the notion advanced by some sociobiologically oriented investigators (e.g., Lionel Tiger and Robin Fox) that only males are capable of peer bonding, women are beginning to benefit from the bonds developed through group experience. Rohrbaugh (1979) provides the following insight into the bases and varieties of bonding for women:

> ... each and every woman can begin to reexamine her assumptions about what it means to be female, and how she wants to live her own life. She can begin to search for solutions that reflect her own experience and the experiences of the women around her.

> Millions of women have already begun [this process]. . . . They have turned to other women to share, to give support, to define themselves in female rather than in male terms. They gather in each others' homes, at schools and churches, in Women's Movement offices. . . . In talking with each other these women are doing more than reevaluating their own feelings and life styles; they are creating a female solidarity and activism that reflects a positive view of the female experience. Women are not simply dependent, passive, and weak; they are also independent, assertive, and strong.

> Female solidarity has a tremendous social impact; it gets things done. . . . In female solidarity lies not only a woman's personal strength, but also her social force [p. 468].

This is true for women at every age, but the solidarity of women in later life can be an especially rewarding, stimulating, comforting, and strength-giving resource, regardless of marital status, parity, or other variables or characteristics (cf. Wolleat, 1980). With increasing numbers of older women forecast for our society in the coming decades, bonding and the discovery of personhood may make the later years of their lives "the best yet to be."

Summary

This chapter began by examining the thorny question of whether the aged can rightfully be described as a minority group in the political sense of the term. The chief argument in favor of such a designation derived from the relative isolation or segregation of the aged from the larger society, but this is a notion which has received less than universal support. Another dimension considered is the interaction of minority status, ethnicity, and aging, conclusions about which may be contaminated by an ethnocentric "majority" bias on the part of investigators unfamiliar with the unique characteristics of interrelationships of these factors.

The initial analysis of ethnicity and aging examines the needs of white ethnic minorities and how those needs are met. Nonwhite ethnic minorities are discussed as well, with particular reference to the disparity between their economic status and well-being and that of the Caucasian majority in this country. The concept of "double jeopardy" in this connection suggests that elderly minority members may suffer the combined negative effects of racism and agism. It is suggested that poverty is the situational deficit most salient to the status of minority aged.

Within the context of "ethnic compensation" for the problems of minority aging, an analysis of four nonwhite ethnic minority groups is presented. These groups, identified by the 1971 White House Conference on Aging as the major ethnic minority groups of interest and concern in the establishment of meaningful, culturally relevant social policy, are aged black Americans, aged Hispanic Americans, aged Asian-Americans, and aged native Americans. The unique challenge to individuals in helping professions in working with nonwhite minority elderly is described.

The final section of the chapter is devoted to an examination of women as a minority group—not in the statistical sense, but as a group differing from the more powerful normative group, men. From this perspective, aging is characterized as a women's issue, and discussed in terms of the double standard that dictates the ways in which males and females are socialized into adulthood and aging. The emancipation of women in the later decades of life is described and discussed in terms of the potential for reawakened motivation of older women to achieve a greater sense of selfhood and their opportunity in the later years for self-actualization.

References

Barron, M. L. Minority group characteristics of the aged in American society. *Journal of Gerontology,* 1953, **8**, 477–482.

Beauvoir, S. de. *The second sex.* New York: Vintage Books, 1974.

Bell, D., Kasschau, P., & Zellman, G. *Delivery services to elderly members of minority groups: a critical review of the literature.* Santa Monica, Cal.: Rand Corporation, 1976.

Bengston, V. Ethnicity and aging: Problems and issues in current social science inquiry. In D. Gelfand & A. Kutzik (Eds.), *Ethnicity and aging: Theory, research, and policy.* New York: Springer, 1979. Pp. 9–31.

Billingsley, A. *Black families in white America.* Englewood Cliffs, N.J.: Prentice-Hall, 1968.

Benet, S. *Abkhasians: The long-living people of the Caucasus.* New York: Holt, Rinehart and Winston, 1974.

Baul, P. M. Parameters of social structure. *American Sociological Review,* 1974, **39**, 615–635.

Committee for An Extended Lifespan, San Marcos, Cal.: 1982. Personal Communication.

Chodorow, N. Being and doing: A cross-cultural examination of the socialization of males and females. In V. Gornick & B. K. Moran (Eds.), *Women in sexist society: Studies in power and powerlessness.* New York: Basic Books, 1971. Pp. 259–291.

Cohler, B. J., & Lieberman, M. A. Personality change across the second half of life: Findings from a study of Irish, Italian, and Polish-American men and women. In D. Gelfand & A. Kutzik (Eds.), *Ethnicity and aging: Theory, research, and policy.* New York: Springer, 1979. Pp. 227–245.

Cowgill, D. O., & Holmes, L. (Eds.). *Aging and modernization.* New York: Appleton-Century-Crofts, 1972.

Dowd, J. J., & Bengston, V. L. Aging in minority populations: An examination of the double jeopardy hypothesis. *Journal of Gerontology,* 1978, **33**(3), 427–436.

Federal Council on Aging. *Policy issues concerning the minority elderly—executive summary report and final report.* San Francisco; Human Resources Corporation, 1978.

Fujii, S. M. Minority group elderly: Demographic characteristics and implications for public policy. In C. Eisdorfer (Ed.), *Annual review of gerontology and geriatrics.* Vol. 1. New York: Springer, 1980. Pp. 261–284.

Gans, H. More equality: income and taxes. *trans-action,* 1974 (Jan.–Feb.), **11**(2), 62–66.

Gelfand, D. E. Ethnicity and aging. In C. Eisdorfer (Ed.), *Annual review of gerontology and geriatrics.* Vol. 2. New York: Springer, 1981. Pp. 91–117.

Gelfand, D., & Kutzik, A. (Eds.) *Ethnicity and aging: Theory, research, and policy.* New York: Springer, 1979.

Gordon, M. *Assimilation in American life.* New York: Oxford University Press, 1964.

Gutmann, D. Use of informal and formal supports by the ethnic aged. In D. Gelfand & A. Kutzik (Eds.), *Ethnicity and aging: Theory, research, and policy.* New York: Springer, 1979. Pp. 246–262.

Harris, L., & Associates. *Aging in the '80s: America in transition.* Washington, D.C.: National Council on the Aging, 1981.

Hendricks, J., & Hendricks, C. D. *Aging in mass society: Myths and realities.* Cambridge, Mass.: Winthrop Publishers, 1977.

Horney, K. The dread of women. *International Journal of Psychoanalysis,* 1932, **13**, 359.

Jackson, J. J. Black aged: In quest of the phoenix. In *Triple jeopardy—myth or reality?* Washington D.C.: National Council on Aging, 1972. Pp. 27–40.

Kastenbaum, R. Reflections on old age, ethnicity, and death. In D. Gelfand & A. Kutzik (Eds.), *Ethnicity and aging: Theory, research, and policy.* New York: Springer, 1979. Pp. 81–95.

Katz, J. H., & Libbee, K. S. Working with minority elderly: A training program. In C. J. Pulvino & N. Colangelo (Eds.), *Counseling for the growing years.* Minneapolis: Educational Media Corporation, 1980. Pp. 323–331.

Kent, D. P. The elderly in minority groups: Variant patterns of aging. *Gerontologist,* 1971, **11**(part 2), 26–29.

Kobata, F. S., Lockery, S. A., & Moriwaki, S. Y. Minority issues in mental health and aging. In J. E. Birren & R. B. Sloane (Eds.), *Handbook of mental health and aging.* Englewood Cliffs, N.J.: Prentice-Hall, 1980. Pp. 448–467.

Kuhn, M. Grass-roots gray power consciousness raising. In M. M. Fuller & C. M. Martin (Eds.), *The older woman: Lavender rose or gray panther?* Springfield, Ill.: Charles C. Thomas, 1980. Pp. 223–227.

Kuypers, J. A., & Bengston, V. L. Social breakdown and competence: A model of normal aging. *Human Development,* 1973, 16(3), 181–201.

Lemon, B. W., Bengston, V. L., & Peterson, J. A. An exploration of the activity theory of aging: Activity types and life satisfaction among in-movers to a retirement community. *Journal of Gerontology,* 1972, 27(4), 511–523.

Lopata, H. Z. Widows as a minority group. *Gerontologist,* 1971, 11(part 2), 67–77.

Maddox, G. L. Persistence of life style among the elderly: A longitudinal study of patterns of social activity in relation to life satisfaction. In B. L. Neugarten (Ed.), *Middle age and aging.* Chicago: University of Chicago Press, 1968. Pp. 181–183.

Markson, E. W. Ethnicity as a factor in the institutionalization of the ethnic elderly. In D. Gelfand & A. Kutzik (Eds.), *Ethnicity and aging: Theory, research, and policy.* New York: Springer, 1979. Pp. 341–356.

Maxwell, R. J., & Silverman, P. Information and esteem: Cultural considerations in the treatment of the aged. *International Journal of Aging and Human Development,* 1970, 1, 361–392.

Meyers, A. R. Ethnicity and aging: Public policy and ethnic differences in aging and old age. In E. W. Markson & G. R. Batra (Eds.), *Public policies for an aging population.* Lexington, Mass.: D. C. Heath, 1980. Pp. 61–79.

Moore, J. W. Situational factors affecting minority aging. *Gerontologist,* 1971, 11(part 2), 88–93.

Mostwin, D. Emotional needs of elderly Americans of Central and Eastern European background. In D. Gelfand & A. Kutzik (Eds.), *Ethnicity and aging: Theory, research, and policy.* New York: Springer, 1979. Pp. 263–276.

National Urban League. *Double jeopardy: The older Negro in America today.* Washington, D.C.: Author, 1964.

Neugarten, B. L., & Associates. *Personality in middle and late life.* New York: Atherton, 1964.

Neugarten, B. L., Havighurst, R. J., & Tobin, S. S. Personality and patterns of aging. In B. L. Neugarten (Ed.), *Middle age and aging.* Chicago: University of Chicago Press, 1968. Pp. 173–177.

Novak, M. *The rise of the unmeltable ethnics.* New York: Macmillan, 1973.

Ogbu, J. U. *Minority education and caste: The American system in cross-cultural perspective.* New York: Academic Press, 1978.

Peterson, J. A., & Briley, M. L. *Widows and widowhood: A creative approach to being alone.* Chicago: Association Press/Follett, 1977.

Rifkin, J. (with T. Howard). *Entropy: A new world view.* New York: Bantam, 1980.

Rohrbaugh, J. B. *Women: Psychology's puzzle.* New York: Basic Books, 1979.

Rose, A. M. The subculture of the aging: A topic for sociological research. In B. L. Neugarten (Ed.), *Middle age and aging.* Chicago: University of Chicago Press, 1968. Pp. 29–34.

Smith, W. D., Burlew, A. K., Mosley, M. H., & Whitney, W. M. *Minority issues in mental health.* Reading, Mass.: Addison-Wesley, 1978.

Snyder, C. L., & Schwartz, A. N. Physiological, psychological, and social characteristics of 101 Caribbean centenarians. Paper presented at the 12th international Congress of Gerontology, Hamburg, West Germany, 1981.

Sontag, S. The double standard of aging. *Saturday Review,* Sept. 23, 1972, 29–38.

Streib, G. Are the aged a minority group? In B. L. Neugarten (Ed.), *Middle age and aging.* Chicago: University of Chicago Press, 1968. Pp. 35–46.

Thurlow, L. C. Not making it in America: The economic progress of minority groups. *Social Policy,* 1976, **6**(5), 5–11.

Trela, J. E., & Sokolovsky, J. H. Culture, ethnicity, and policy for the aged. In D. Gelfand & A. Kutzik (Eds.), *Ethnicity and aging: Theory, research, and policy.* New York: Springer, 1979. Pp. 117–136.

Varghese, R., & Medinger, F. Fatalism in response to stress among the minority aged. In D. Gelfand & A. Kutzik (Eds.), *Ethnicity and aging: Theory, research, and policy.* New York: Springer, 1979. Pp. 96–116.

Welch, M. A widow finds new life. *Modern Maturity,* Aug.–Sept. 1982, **25**(4); 79–82.

Wolleat, P. L. Counseling the elderly woman: A sex-role perspective. In C. Pulvino & N. Colangelo (Eds.), *Counseling for the growing years.* Minneapolis: Educational Media Corporation, 1980. Pp. 185–196.

For Further Reading

Cheng, E. *The elder Chinese.* San Diego: Campanile Press, 1978.

Dukepoo, F. *The elder American Indian.* San Diego: Campanile Press, 1980.

Federal Council on the Aging. *National policy concerns for older women: Commitment to a better life.* DHEW Publication No. (OHD) 76-20956. Washington, D.C.: USDHEW, 1976.

Fuller, M. M., & Martin, C. M. (Eds.) *The older woman: Lavender rose or gray panther?* Springfield, Ill.: Charles C. Thomas, 1980.

Gutmann, D. Observations on culture and mental health in later life. In J. E. Birren & R. B. Sloane (Eds.), *Handbook of mental health and aging.* Englewood Cliffs, New Jersey: Prentice-Hall, Inc., 1980. Pp. 429–447.

Havighurst, R. J., Neugarten, B. L., & Tobin, S. S. Disengagement and patterns of aging. In B. L. Neugarten (Ed.), *Middle age and aging.* Chicago: University of Chicago Press, 1968. Pp. 161–172.

Hsieh, T., Shybut, J., & Lotsof, E. Internal vs. external control and ethnic group membership. *Journal of Consulting and Clincial Psychology,* 1969, **33**, 122–124.

Ishikaza, W. H. *The elder Guamian.* San Diego: Campanile Press, 1978.

Ishikaza, W. H. *The elder Samoan.* San Diego: Campanile Press, 1978.

Ishizuka, K. C. *The elder Japanese.* San Diego: Campanile Press, 1978.

Jacobs, R. H. A typology of older American women. *Social Policy,* 1976, 7, 34–39.

Lopata, H. Z. *Occupation: Housewife.* New York: Oxford University Press, 1971.

Lowy, L. *Social policies and programs on aging.* Lexington, Mass.: D. C. Heath, 1980.

Pampel, F. *Social change and the aged.* Lexington, Mass.: D. C. Heath Company, 1981.

Peterson, R. *The elderly Pilipino.* San Diego: Campanile Press, 1978.

Reiter, R. R. (Ed.) *Toward an anthropology of women.* New York: Monthly Review Press, 1975.

Stanford, E. P. *The elder black.* San Diego: Campanile Press, 1978.

Tiger, L. *Men in groups.* New York: Vintage Books, 1970.

Valle, R., & Mendoza, L. *The elder Latino.* San Diego: Campanile Press, 1978.

Zola, I. K. "Oh where, oh where has ethnicity gone?" In D. Gelfand & A. Kutzik (Eds.), *Ethnicity and aging: Theory, research, and policy.* New York: Springer, 1979. Pp. 66–80.

The Later Years: Gains and Losses

9 *Chapter*

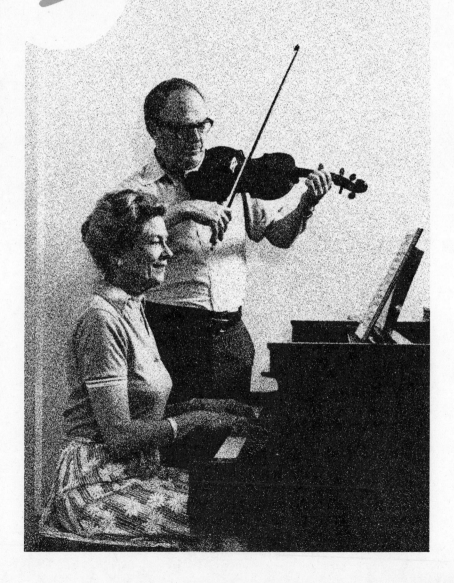

Being 70 is no crime . . . but it's no joke, either.
  Golda Meier

Multiple loss is the concept most frequently associated with aging. Loss continues to be the pervasive theme and dominant tone of professional articles and texts and scientific meetings on aging. This is true despite the fact that the word "loss" rarely appears in indices of books on aging.

Any review of the literature on aging makes it abundantly clear that clinicians and researchers alike have so thoroughly documented the losses of old age that they have contributed substantially even if inadvertently to old age's negative image and at times to feelings of thwarted hope and even to despair.

A more balanced perspective of the lifespan, however, suggests the premise of this chapter, namely that *both* gains and losses are characteristic of *every* chronological period of life. There are, for example, both advantages and disadvantages to being an adolescent. The manifest equation is that the asset of high levels of adolescent energy is balanced by the deficit of lack of life experience. The same principle applies to the sixth, seventh, eighth, and ninth decades of life and beyond. Diminished levels of energy in later life may impose unwanted limits, but the richness of accumulated experience potentiates a wide choice of coping strategies. In other words, the oldster has learned that it is not necessary to reinvent the wheel, which the youngster has not yet learned.

The literature on aging has also managed to counterbalance the negative image of old age by exposing many supposed losses of aging for the myths they are. For instance, the stereotypes about the inevitability of loss of intelligence (I.Q.) in the later years (Baltes & Schaie, 1974; Schaie, 1974), loss of capability for work (Jacobson, 1980), loss of capacity to enjoy sexual activity (Runciman, 1975), loss of adaptive capacity (Bengston, 1973; Langer & Rodin, 1976), loss of touch, smell, and even taste sensitivity (Engen, 1977; Kenshalo, 1977) have been demonstrated to be negative distortions of the more balanced view. We shall in this chapter examine specific instances of gains and losses in later life, beginning with consideration of some major loss factors and the issues associated with them.

Losses

Losses are daily facts of living, encompassing an extremely wide and varied range of possibilities. A short list of significant losses could conceivably include the loss of vital capacity, loss of a breast through mastectomy, loss of a leg or fingers, loss of a job, total loss of vision or loss of an eye, loss of a significant sum of money or of regular income, loss of status, loss of an important object (a wedding ring or treasured heirloom), loss of "face." Given the uniquely personal nature of the perception of and response to loss, the list could be expanded ad infinitum. Figure 9–1 provides a model for conceptualizing the circular nature of the loss cycle. The model indicates how the biopsychological factors implicated in the cycle feed upon themselves, with negative consequences, when appropriate modifications in perceptions or attitudes fail to interrupt or intervene in the cycle (Cousins, 1980).

Suicidologists are sometimes called upon for etiological explanations of why a seemingly innocuous or minor loss provokes the final act of self-destruction. The explanatory paradigm involves the understanding that each experience of loss, if not effectively resolved, tends to be cumulative (cf. the discussion of stress in Chapter 2). In one sense, each loss may add some degree of demoralization. The "small" loss brings into play all the other prior negative feelings associated with previous deprivations, and the most recent incident tips the balance in favor of suicide: a case of the straw that broke the camel's back.

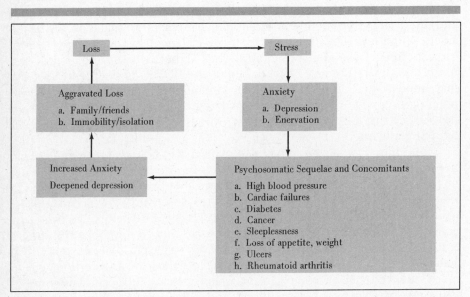

FIGURE 9–1.   The Loss Cycle Process
Source: Peterson (1982).

Even within this context gains and losses can be seen to coexist. For some well-motivated individuals with a high degree of ego strength each loss becomes an occasion for gain. Aged individuals of this sort have learned how to marshal internal as well as external resources to adapt to change and loss. For such persons each loss does not translate into demoralization and dysfunction; rather, the occasion of loss satisfactorily resolved provides the basis for anticipating and meeting the next challenge. Peterson and Briley (1977) have suggested that even the loss of a mate can direct attention to new horizons and reveal opportunities for new achievements and satisfactions.

Death and Dying

Discussion of death and dying ought to begin with a simple definition of death, quite apart from its many connotative meanings. Such a definition, however, no longer appears to be easy to produce. In an earlier time death was signaled when the heart stopped beating and breathing ceased. These were unequivocal signs then. They are not necessarily so now. Because of legal and medical implications, the question of when death actually occurs has become a controversial one.

Clinical signs of death are straightforward and fairly standard. Among these are cessation of respiration and heartbeat, changes in pupillary reflex, lack of sensitivity to electrical stimulation, pallor, hypostasis, rigor mortis, and relaxation of the sphincter (Cassell et al., 1972; Mant, 1976).

At another level of complexity is cellular death. Successful transplantation depends upon removing organs from donors before cellular death occurs. As Mant (1976) phrases the question, " ... when is the person from whom the organ is to be removed in a state which is incompatible with the persistence of life?" The more rapidly the organs are removed, the greater the chances for the grafted organ to survive.

A third aspect of the contemporary debate about when the actual onset of death occurs involves "brain death." This event is marked by a flat EEG (electroencephalogram) pattern, indicating a lack of electrochemical activity and therefore a lack of brain function.

Some vital brain cells, if deprived of oxygen for even a relatively short time, will die and cannot be restored or replaced. Other parts of the brain appear to be hardier and may survive temporary trauma. In the process, the individual may lose "personality," thought processes, and voluntary movement, and yet maintain a heartbeat (Mant, 1976).

In the Western world a final judgment regarding death is recorded on a death certificate that specifies time and cause of death. Schneidman (1976) estimates that 10 to 15 percent of all coroners' cases are "equivocal" as to cause of death. Schneidman thinks that the death certificate is anachronistic because it is based on the premise that a person is only a "biological machine" to which "things happen." He would introduce the dimension of intentionality under a new category on the death certificate: "imputed lethality," with four designations—"high," "medium," "low," and "absent." He describes each of these dimensions carefully. For instance, the low imputed lethality "would indicate that the decedent played some small but insignificant role in effecting or hastening his own demise" (Schneidman, 1976). Adding this dimension would provide basic research data about the mental status of any individual and give a much fairer summary of the death episode.

How It Is To Die

It is generally accepted that the loss of a significant other (spouse, intimate friend, child) affords the most traumatic stress to the bereaved, second only to the loss of self (i.e., self-esteem). The seminal work of Holmes and

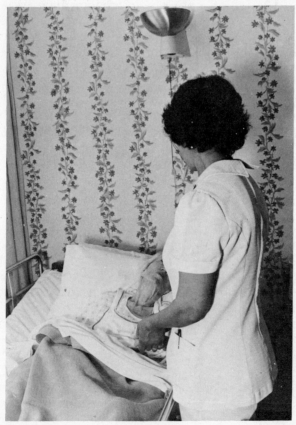

The introduction of the hospice in the United States from England humanizes the dying process and enables the old to share their feelings, to be with family and understanding staff, and to die with dignity.

Rahe (1967; cf. Chapter 2) places such loss at the top of life stresses. Dying and death therefore affect two populations: those who are experiencing the event and those who are closest to them.

No one has returned to describe what it is like to be dead—not to think, laugh, or love. But we do know something about the feelings and reactions of persons regarding death. Kalish (1976) lists three reasons why the meaning of death is different for older persons:

1. The anticipated lifespan is normally foreshortened. . . .
2. Older persons . . . often perceive themselves as not having sufficient futurity to deserve a major investment of the resources of others. . . .
3. Older persons receive more reminders of impending death from within their bodies. . . .

Kalish reasons that these factors encourage disengagement pyschologically and socially, to provide a detachment that would make the last days meaningful. One can then "turn inward, contemplate the meaning of the past in reminiscence, concern for the past and future, and pull back from the emotional pain that occurs when attachments are lost or broken" (Kalish, 1976).

The same writer suggests three meanings of death for older persons. The first has to do with the way a sense of finitude organizes our time. Table 9–1 shows the answers of 434 Los Angeles County residents to the question "What would you do if you knew you were to die in thirty days?"

The second meaning is *death as loss.* There is a devastating sense of loss of self, with all the self's meaningful relationships. Schneidman's book (1976) ends with a poem written by a very sensitive young man when he was dying. The last lines are:

> Step lightly, we're walking home now.
> The clouds take every shape.
> We climb up the boulders, there is no plateau.
> We cross the stream and walk up the slope.
> See, the hawk is diving.
> The plain stretches out ahead.
> Then the hills, the valleys, the meadows.
> Keep moving, people. How could I not be among you?

TABLE 9–1.   Role Choices with Limited Life Expectancy, by Age
(In Percentages)

	20–39	40–59	60+
Marked change in life-style, self-related (travel, sex, experiences, etc.)	24	15	9
Inner-life centered (read, contemplate, pray)	14	14	37
Focus concern on others, be with loved ones	29	25	12
Attempt to complete projects, tie up loose ends	11	10	3
No change in life-style	17	29	31
Other	5	6	8

Source: Kalish (1976).

"How could I not be among you?" is an anguished cry of loss that poignantly reflects all of our own abhorrence at losing the clouds, the stream, the birds, the people—life. There are other losses.

A third reaction is that death is punishment for sin. Kalish tested this in his study and found this attitude in force more in the case of the death of a young person than of an older one. As a matter of fact, if an older person has suffered a long and painful illness, death may be viewed as a blessing.

Conspiracy of Silence

Gerontologists also have recognized that the study of dying and death is not done without some reluctance. Humans cherish life so highly that they find it difficult to contemplate its end. While the harvesting hand of time cannot be stayed, the reality of death is often denied in many subtle ways: by the elaborate cosmetic artfulness of the undertaker, by the vocabulary of the mourners, by the conspiracy of silence on the part of the family and even of professional helpers. In his early investigations of attitudes toward death, Feifel (1959) found that many physicians were not able to deal realistically with death. Physicians' distorted notions about the awareness of either patients or their families regarding impending death made it difficult, if not impossible, for them to help patients cope with the reality of death. In doing interviews for his study of death and death role expectations, Matthieu (1972) found in interview after interview that older persons said, "I'm glad to talk with you about death. My doctor and my minister won't discuss it and I'm tired of talking with my undertaker." Not only physicians but also nurses, clergy, and psychiatrists deny death by shunning both the topic and the dying person. Feifel had reported much the same experience.

Such denial forecloses opportunities for those approaching death to cope psychologically or spiritually with all of the emotions that contemplation of their end might arouse, and with the opportunity to complete the unfinished business of their personal histories. Intimates are thus denied honest and meaningful interactions with the dying person. The attention which gerontology has given to this last significant experience of life has proved to be a useful stimulus to improving the situation. A number of colleges and universities now are giving students the opportunity to face the reality of death, to study research about dying, and thus to modify their attitudes toward the dying process. Some of the issues that need to be investigated in terms of the process of dying and death are raised by these questions:

1. Is there some consistent process in the dying trajectory?
2. What valid kinds of supports during this process prevent loneliness and pain?

3. What are the current rituals with which we cope with death? Are they changing?
4. How do we constructively cope with bereavement, grief, and mourning?

The Process of Dying

Elizabeth Kübler-Ross has given us the most explicit and detailed analyses of the psychological stages of dying, which she called "coping mechanisms at the time of terminal illness" (Kübler-Ross, 1969). The stages she has proposed are:

1. *Denial and isolation* ("No, not me, it can't be true"). First reactions include shock, horror, disbelief. Many think the diagnosis was in error, a mistake. Some insist on a second opinion, then begin a desperate search for a "miracle cure."

2. *Anger, rage, envy, resentment* ("Why me?"). In this phase, the patient vacillates between rage and anger, directed indiscriminately toward the physician, toward God, toward the hospital, toward family members, etc., and self-pity. The patient suffers an increased sense of inner chaos and disorganization, and inability to make or carry out any plans.

3. *Bargaining* ("If you'll let me . . . then I'll . . ."). The press at this stage is for a way out of the horrible predicament at whatever price, so the patient begins to bargain with God, with the hospital staff, etc. The patient promises to be a better person, a better spouse, to begin religious practice, to do good works. Kübler-Ross points out that these bargains are rarely kept.

4. *Depression* ("What's the use?"). This is the "bottoming out" stage, characterized by guilt, shame, grieving over one's "sinfulness," deep sadness. It is here, Kübler-Ross believes, that the patient especially needs permission and encouragement to express depression and grief to others.

5. *Acceptance.* At this stage the terminally ill patient, having worked through the earlier reactions, begins to develop some sense of detachment from the things and people of his or her world. According to Kübler-Ross, this is not despair or resignation. It is coming to terms with the reality of the situation, which is why Kübler-Ross has termed it "acceptance." This stage is quiet, a peaceful waiting for the impending end to life.

These steps in the dying process were first identified in a seminar at the University of Chicago in which dying patients were interviewed about their feelings. One pervasive theme important to Kübler-Ross is the observation that *hope* persists through all of these stages.

Some have questioned the inevitability and universality of these stages of dying by noting that not all persons progress through each stage, nor always in the sequence proposed. Schneidman, an experienced investigator of the phenomenon of suicide, is one who has questioned these stages of dying:

> My own limited work has not led me to conclusions identical with those of Kübler-Ross. Indeed, while I have seen in dying persons isolation, envy,

bargaining, depression, and acceptance, I do not believe that these are necessarily "stages" of the dying process, and I am not at all convinced that they are lived through in that order, or for that matter, in any universal order. What I see is a complicated clustering of intellectual and affective states, some fleeting, lasting for a moment, a day, a week, set, not unexpectedly, against the backdrop of that person's total personality, his "philosophy of life" (Schneidman, 1973).

Schneidman rejects the notion of a unidimensional pathway to death, feeling that there is a constant alternation between acceptance and denial. Likewise, he detects among his interviewees many who exhibit on one level of consciousness a need to be aware of death and on another a need not to know. In spite of the valid questions Schneidman and others have raised about stages of dying, however, Kübler-Ross deserves the credit given her for being one of the very first to have studied and described systematically and in detail the affective and psychological aspects of the dying process.

In contrast to this approach, Weisman, a Harvard psychiatrist, has studied the myths that preclude physicians in particular from having effective interactions with the dying (Weisman, 1972). Some of these myths about dying are:

1. Only suicidal and psychotic people are willing to die. Even when death is inevitable, no one wants to die.
2. Fear of death is the most natural and basic fear of humans. The closer they come to death, the more intense the fear becomes.
3. Reconciliation with death and preparation for death are impossible. Therefore, say as little as possible to dying people, turn their questions aside, and use any means to deny, dissimulate, and avoid open confrontation.
4. Dying people do not really want to know what the future holds. Otherwise, they would ask more questions. To force a discussion or to insist upon unwelcome information is risky. The patient might lose all hope. S/he might commit suicide, become very depressed, or even die more quickly.
5. After speaking with family members, the doctor should treat the patient as long as possible. Then, when further benefit seems unlikely, the patient should be left alone, except for relieving pain. He will then withdraw, die in peace, without further disturbance and anguish.
6. It is reckless, if not downright cruel, to inflict unnecessary suffering upon the patient or his family. The patient is doomed; nothing can really make any difference. Survivors should accept the futility, but realize that they will get over the loss.
7. Physicians can deal with all phases of the dying process because of their scientific training and clinical experience. The emotional and psychological sides of dying are vastly overemphasized. Consultation with psychiatrists and social workers is unnecessary. The clergy might be called upon, but only because death is near. The doctor has no further obligation after the patient's death.

A further observation that should be added to this list is the common fallacy that the old are most likely to fear death. Virtually all surveys support the notion that the old are most fearful not of death itself, but of the anticipated pain, disfigurement, inconvenience, helplessness, and other indignities associated with the dying process.

Weisman goes on to point out that these fallacies do all kinds of mischief. For example they lead physicians into inconsistencies and justify physicians' penchant for avoiding death issues themselves. They help physicians feel somewhat easier about their own withdrawal from dying patients. The fourth fallacy, which says the patient "doesn't want to know," absolves the physician from talking about it. Weisman asserts that the most dangerous fallacy of all is oversimplification through stereotyping patients, when each person ought to be treated as a special case.

Social Death

An extended illness and the resulting protracted process of dying has been observed to lead to the phenomenon called "social death." For example, in cases where an individual goes into a coma and remains comatose over a long period and shows only clinical signs of life, the survivors often will exhibit all the usual signs of bereavement and grief, as if the dying person were already deceased. Nor is it unusual for nurses, physicians, and others attendant on those caught up in this drawn-out process to tend to give less attention to or even ignore the dying individual, who is responded to as if already dead. Physicians and nurses are trained to save lives and to fight death. Dying therefore represents for many so trained a professional failure and personal defeat. They find themselves frustrated and angry over the condition of the dying person in spite of their best efforts, at times to the point of developing physical symptoms themselves (Benoliel, 1971).

Equally poignant is the very same reaction by family members to elderly kin with severe multiple disabilities who are viewed as already having lost contact with reality. Such an old person has lost touch with society, no longer participates or is in any fashion involved with family relationships or family affairs, has lost that subtle but vital interface with daily life that distinguishes the socially alive from the socially dead. For the kin, instrumental, cultural, and social processes have ostensibly terminated. Social communication has long since ceased. The family regards the aged individual, isolated and withdrawn, as if already dead. And their bereavement may be just as real and their grief just as painful as if physical death had already occurred, a fact not always fully appreciated by observers (Fulton & Fulton, 1971).

The When of Dying

It would appear on the face of it that *when* people die is a matter quite beyond individual control, the exigencies of disease and human frailty being what they are. Some want to live to an older age than they expect to live (Reynolds & Kalish, 1974). Others do not expect to live as long as they in fact do (Snyder & Schwartz, 1981).

One factor that complicates the issue of when people die is the phenomenon of those individuals who continue to survive, for longer or shorter periods, in the face of contraindicating evidence, signs, and conditions. There is a considerable amount of anecdotal evidence about persons in a terminal state for whom medicine has given up all hope and for whom death seems imminent, who manage to "hang on" for days or even weeks until a beloved son or daughter finally reaches the deathbed. Then following the reunion, death occurs. Some anecdotal evidence suggests that the dying individual manages to survive until some anticipated event—a birthday, an anniversary—has arrived; almost immediately afterwards, death ensues.

So far as the authors can determine, only one systematic study (a statistical assessment) of the connections between deathday and birthday has been reported. The purpose of the analysis was to see how dying people react to one special event, their birthdays, to learn whether some people postpone their death until *after* their birthdays. The study (Phillips, 1972) examined only the deaths of famous people. One reason for this was that the birthdays of famous people were assumed to be especially rewarding and celebrated. A second reason was that it is easier to examine the deaths of famous than of ordinary people.

Figure 9–2 depicts the results, which support the conclusion that some people do, in fact, time their deaths to coincide or follow an anticipated special event. For example, many have noted that both Thomas Jefferson and John Adams died on July 4, 1826, exactly fifty years after the signing of the

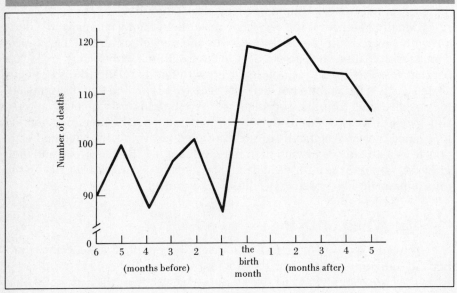

FIGURE 9–2.   Deaths Before, During, and After Birth Month
Source: Phillips (1972).

Declaration of Independence. It may be easier to believe that this was not coincidence if we read Jefferson's last words, quoted by his physician (Peterson, 1970):

> About seven o'clock of the evening of that day he [Jefferson] awoke, and seeing my staying at his bedside, exclaimed, "Oh, Doctor, are you still there?" in a voice, however, that was husky and indistinct. He then asked, "Is it the Fourth?" to which I replied, "It soon will be." These were the last words I heard him utter.

A second factor that complicates the issue of when people die can be identified with the technology of modern medicine which can maintain clinical signs of life mechanically in a comatose person almost indefinitely. In such cases the timing of death would appear to be largely at the discretion of those who control the machinery.

We may conclude from these studies and observations that although we are learning more about the process of dying, the research is still in its early state. Service providers who work with dying persons, however, will achieve additional understanding from Kübler-Ross, Schneidman, Weisman, Feifel, Matthieu, and others whose work has given us additional insights into the dying process.

Supports for the Dying Person

Moving from the question of what constitutes the dying process to an analysis of what supports are available for the dying person, there are some concrete examples of help and some research studies that offer specific insights.

In his study of rural Montana, suburban Pasadena, and retirement home (Laguna Hills) samples, Matthieu (1972) asked about supports when "thinking about death." Table 9–2 summarizes his findings. Several observations of this study are significant. There is, first of all, a rather remarkable consistency of response from these three diverse samples. Second, even in the rural sample only about one-third of the respondents say they depend upon religion as their support in thinking about death. On the other hand, "remembrance

TABLE 9–2. Religion as a Comfort when Thinking of Death

Which of the Following Comforts You Most As You Think of Death?	PASADENA (N = 189)		LAGUNA HILLS (N = 183)		MONTANA (N = 115)	
	N	%	N	%	N	%
My religion	62	32.8	58	31.7	43	37.4
Love from those around me	49	25.9	51	27.9	29	25.2
Memories of a full life	78	41.3	74	40.4	43	37.4

Source: Matthieu (1972).

of things past" (the life review) turns out to have much power in giving support.

All of our research sources speak of the value of allowing dying persons to talk about their death trajectory. Weisman (1972), in particular, emphasizes the need for a most sensitive response pattern on the part of the helper. While sensitivity is essential, the positive effect that openness and responsiveness can have is well illustrated in case studies presented by all the researchers. Accessibility for intimate sharing is obviously the opposite of the withdrawal tendencies implicit in the fallacies about the dying that Weisman believes are typical of physicians.

Because of the history of denial of death by Western society generally and because of the rejecting and withdrawing tendencies of doctors, nurses, clergy, and other service providers, it became apparent that some new form of institutional caring would be required to overcome these inhibitions. One place where changes were made was the University of Chicago Medical Hospital, which introduced new ways of helping the dying as the result of the experience and teaching of Kübler-Ross, referred to earlier. In many other cities as well her influence has encouraged medical staffs to modify their approaches to the dying.

A second and even more unique response to this need has been made at the innovative St. Christopher's Hospice in London. Dr. Cicely Saunders is the medical director there and most of the reports on this creative approach to death came from her (Saunders, 1980). St. Christopher's is modeled after the hospices located in medieval towns to care "for the sick and poor." The basic aim of St. Christopher's is to build a new type of institutional community, involving doctors, nurses, staff, patients, and their families, where the last weeks of life can be humanized, full of joy, and relatively painless. Analgesics are given freely, but no heroic, technological methods for prolonging life are ever used. All staff and members of families are trained to have a new attitude toward death so that the dying person is surrounded by positive supports during the course of the terminal illness. Thus, compassion, a good deal of training, and continuing contact with family and friends help patients have a decent and "appropriate" death.

St. Christopher's also has a research and teaching function. It does research on aspects of care for terminally ill patients to try to help those in charge better understand conditions for ultimate help to patients, and it trains other doctors and nurses in its techniques. Saunders has visited America many times. A number of institutions similar to the original hospice in England have now opened in the United States. A critical issue is whether it is sound public policy to try to build hospices all over the United States or whether it might not be possible to educate our medical and nursing staffs and nursing home and hospital administrators in such a way that the spirit, attitudes, and processes that are responsible for St. Christopher's effectiveness could be adopted by existing hospitals and nursing homes in the United States.

The Value of Ritual

The funeral ceremony, cemetery rituals, black clothing, armbands, the eulogy, the wake, sitting shiva, funeral processions and parades are only a few of the many ceremonies and rituals that symbolize the passage of the dead and serve the grief needs of the living. The commemorative process begins when a person dies. If the individual has died in a nursing home or a hospital, the physician remains the chief actor. Although usually they act as "symbols of life rather than death," physicians must shift from that role to one in which they act, if only temporarily, as the ones who tell the family about the death and circumstances surrounding it, and offer what comfort they can (Kalish, 1976; Warner, 1965). In doing so, physicians still must protect their essential identity as healers, as well as their own self-images, and convince themselves that their skills were used appropriately to do everything possible to prevent that death.

The family must now call in a second professional to handle the body, prepare it for burial, and make arrangements for burial and, perhaps, for the funeral itself. This is the undertaker, who plays several roles. In one sense, the undertaker stands beside the minister as a counselor to help the family through its crisis of grief. The undertaker's preparation of the corpse so that the dead person looks good or at least peaceful during final viewing is given prominence. Warner (1965) observes that the undertaker must "take the ritually unclean, usually diseased, corpse with its unpleasant appearance and

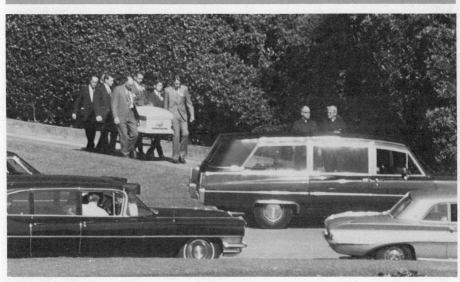

Bereavement and grief are as difficult for the elderly as they are for the middle-aged. The elderly are especially vulnerable to the effects of the loss incurred at the death of a spouse, a relative, or a life-long friend.

transform it from a lifeless object to the sculptured image of a living human being who is resting in sleep." Our society's social and psychological defense mechanisms are nowhere better displayed than in this mandate to make the dead look as if still alive and "only sleeping."

The undertaker has also assumed the role of manager of the commemorative ritual, and arranges the casket, flowers, family, friends of the family, and other mourners. Warner says:

> In one sense [the undertaker] is the producer who fashions the whole enterprise so that other performers, including the minister, the eulogist, the organist, the vocalist, family, and mourners can act becomingly and get the approval and praise for the funeral's success and receive the sensuous satisfaction that the funeral's symbolism evokes.

Undertakers have developed a series of public relations maneuvers aimed to add to the alacrity with which mourning family members will pay for all of this. It is widely claimed by mortuaries that viewing the body in the "slumber room" is a significant form of grief therapy. To see the person who was devastated by illness "transfigured with peace and happiness" is the justification for the great amount of energy expended by morticians (Baird, 1972). Jessica Mitford, however, examined this ritual in great detail and found it wanting as grief therapy (Mitford, 1978).

A second contention of funeral directors is that embalming and a tightly sealed casket help prevent decomposition. In one famous case, *Chelini* v. *Silvio Nieri,* Chelini sued Nieri, the undertaker, because upon disinterment he found his mother's body in an advanced state of decomposition. Out of the trial emerged the fact that embalming in no way slows down decomposition and a "seal-type" casket only hastens decay. Chelini won the case (Baird, 1972).

A common myth is that cemeteries are nonprofit. Cemetery land is tax-free, based on the supposition that the operation is nonprofit, which probably stems from the days when a church or city maintained the plots. But more recently cemetery promoters charge a large fee, as well as levying additional charges for "perpetual care" (Baird, 1972). The mausoleum in which crypts are piled on top of each other simply saves land and maintenance for the cemetery proprietor.

Some action has been taken in response to the high cost of dying. In almost every large city, funeral societies have sprung up. One pays a very modest fee to belong to one of these organizations. The society contracts with a funeral director who agrees to provide its members with funeral services at minimum cost, depending on the type of casket and funeral that are selected. These funeral societies are really cooperatives, run by elected boards of directors (Nora, 1962).

Another option that is increasingly popular is cremation. The general practice is to cremate the body, scatter the ashes, and hold a memorial service later. Usually no coffin or urn is present at the memorial service. The urn or other container of the ashes, sometimes a miniature casket, may then be placed in a mausoleum, which can then be visited by family and friends. The cost of cremation is a fraction of what it costs to embalm a body, purchase a casket, and inter it. Moreover, some environmentalists are making strong pleas for cremation, arguing that urban land is becoming too scarce to use for cemeteries.

A congressional committee held hearings on the funeral industry across the country during the summer and fall of 1976. Included in the testimony were many examples of price gouging and other unfair business practices. On the other hand, a great many morticians have served their communities well for a great many years, and have earned the respect of those communities. It is probable that the pressure of funeral societies, crematoria, and public opinion may force the funeral industry to moderate many of its policies and become more realistic in its claims. Yet the vast majority of Americans still choose an old-fashioned funeral complete with casket and burial rituals. This is traditional in America, and these customs will not soon be abandoned.

Bereavement and Grief

Much of the data about dying reminds us that psychological factors have a profound effect upon even healthy people. For years it has been known that widows and widowers have a higher mortality rate than married men and women of the same age. In addition, a peaking of mortality rate in widowers during the first year of bereavement has been observed. Young and his colleagues (Young, Benjamin, & Wallis, 1963) found an increase in the death rate among 4,486 widowers over the age of fifty-four of almost 40 percent during the first six months of bereavement. Granger Westberg, author of *Good Grief* and trainer of therapists in psychosomatic healing at the Illinois Psychiatric Institute, has reported research which showed that at least half of all admissions to hospitals followed a significant loss (Westberg, 1982, personal communication). What remains to be added to the equation is the psychological impact of bereavement. Holmes and Rahe's (1967) schedule of life change events permits rank-ordering of significant events on the basis of increasing impact. Such recent life changes are good predictors of physical breakdown and illness. At the top of the rank-ordered list—that is, the recent life change with the greatest psychological impact and attendant risk—stands "death of a spouse." This may account substantially for the findings of Young and Westberg.

Parkes (1972) has done a systematic review of the literature on grief, as well as research of his own directed toward the development of what he calls a "biological theory of grief." This theory views grief as a stressor that elicits the sympathetic part of the autonomic nervous system while inhibiting the parasympathetic system. Thus bereavement incites an alarm reaction, much akin to fear or stress. He reports that the data do not provide consistent support for this view.

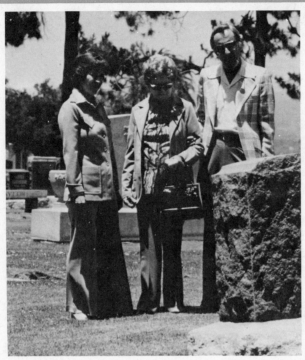

Loss of kin or friends is particularly difficult for the elderly whose support network tends to shrink.

Acute and episodic pangs of grief are expressed, according to Parkes, through a series of phases of behavior. These include:

1. Searching ("I can't help looking for him everywhere"; "I walk around searching for her.")
2. Illusions ("I keep thinking I see him in a crowd"; "I imagine I hear her moving about in another room.")
3. Withdrawal (avoidance of close friends or familiar places; disbelief that the loss has really occurred; developing emotional numbness; attempts to rationalize the loss or "make sense of it")
4. Guilt and anger (self-reproach over some act or omission that might have harmed the dying person; anger or protest over the pain and grief caused by the "desertion" of the dead one)
5. Attempts to gain a new identity (developing new expectations about one's life or self and new roles)

The classical study of grief reactions is that of Eric Lindemann (1944), who studied the responses of 101 persons who lost close relatives in the nightclub fire in Boston. He gives a somewhat different series of responses than Parkes:

1. *The syndrome of physical distress.* The survivor experiences sighing, choking, shortness of breath, digestive troubles, and exhaustion.
2. *Preoccupation with the image of the deceased.* Other persons fade away while the survivor is obsessed by rememberances of the lost person.
3. *Feelings of guilt.* The bereft feel responsible for the death.
4. *Hostile reactions.* The survivor feels irritability, anger, and some concern that the present state of instability may lead to insanity.
5. *Loss of pattern.* Old roles are disrupted, life is out of joint.

A third study is significant. Schoenberg, Carp, Peretz, and Kutscher (1970) asked 133 professional consultants (ministers, psychologists, and psychiatrists) to list significant aspects of grief. Their findings indicated that:

1. Ninety-nine percent of the respondents thought that the death of a mate would result in depression, loss of weight, sleeplessness, and despair.
2. Ninety percent thought that the bereaved would have dreams about the deceased.
3. Seventy-five percent thought that a widower would experience impotence and diminished sexual desires.
4. Seventy-four percent expected the bereaved to fantasize or have illusions about the presence of the dead person (compare Lindemann's findings on "images")
5. Seventy-three percent thought the bereaved would seek advice.

Schoenberg et al. also asked their respondents for a suggestion regarding coping behaviors that would be helpful. Ninety-one percent thought that talking with someone who had the same experience would be very useful. Ninety percent thought that continuation of a work role was helpful, and 85 percent recommended remarriage in the future. The idea of sharing with others who have been in the same loss situation has been actualized by the CRUSE widow-to-widow groups in England and by the spontaneous growth of innovative experimental groups of a similar sort in this country.

Self-Help and Widow's Groups

In looking at ways in which groups can be used to facilitate the grief process, Barrett (1974) organized groups of three different kinds of widows. Half of her sample said they had never thought about the death of their husband before it occurred, and two-thirds of them had never considered what it would be like to be a widow. Their average income, even though half of them worked, was about one-half of what it had been at the time of their husband's death.

The first group Barrett organized was called a *self-help group* because the leader was only a facilitator and not a teacher. She helped members of the group help each other. This type conformed to what is generally referred to as a widow-to-widow group in England and in some locales in this country. The second group was called the *confidante group*. Barrett used interpersonal discussion techniques and group activities where individuals were paired and participated as couples. In this group the leader tried to facilitate a "helping relationship" for each pair.

The third group was labeled a *woman's consciousness-raising group*. In discussions, the focus was on ways in which sex roles were viewed by the widows in the group, with such topics as "Sexuality among Widows: Are You Still a Wife?" Each of the groups gathered for two hours a week for some eight weeks. These three groups were then matched with a control group.

Several measures were used to determine whether the groups had any impact on the attitudes and values of the participants. One measure was "predicted future health." This is a measure of the sense of well-being and optimism. Subjects in all groups showed growth in self-esteem and all were appreciative of being women. Those who participated in the experimental groups showed higher hopes for future health in contrast to the control group. All groups were less depressed as the result of their participation, but the control group stressed health problems and loneliness more than the other three. The confidante group became more active in social roles and showed greater positive change in self-esteem than the others. Significantly, all three treatment groups decided to continue meeting even when the experiment was over. Barrett concluded that each of these groups had much to offer in assisting widows toward adjustment and in growth of emotional well-being. In England almost all communities now have a chapter of the CRUSE widow-to-widow program. There are few such programs in the United States, although the American Association of Retired Persons is actively engaged in promoting such a program now.

Gains versus Losses

The supportive network around an individual plays an important role in the balanced perspective of later life. More central to the concept of late life gains (versus losses) is the notion of coping with loss. The answer to the question implied in this concept lies in the relative strength of those factors perceived as positive (gains) or negative (losses). Two recent studies provide pertinent data.

One of these studies reports a detailed analysis of life histories obtained from nationally representative samples of 500 seventy-year-old men and 500 seventy-year-old women. The findings of the report were based on an assessment (i.e., clinical judgments) of the dynamics of the lives of these individuals. The study focused on identifying the critical factors determining both an individual's current quality of life and the same individual's quality of life over the lifespan.

The major findings include confirmations of the importance of health and material well-being. It was concluded that these factors are especially critical if they are negative, that is, when they represent losses. Health was a major negative (loss) factor, by a big margin (Flanagan, 1982).

Figure 9–3 shows the single dominant factors in determining current quality of life and Figure 9–4 indicates the parallel response as judged over the lifespan.

From Figure 9–3 we can see that having a spouse is judged a positive factor by far more older men (53%) than older women (17%) as far as current quality of life is concerned. This is in sharp contrast to the lifespan responses depicted in Figure 9–4; there 55 percent of the men judged "spouse" to be the single positive dominant factor, and 43 percent of the women make the same response. No doubt the greater survivorship of women in the past accounts for the difference in their response to current and lifespan interpretations of quality of life. Additionally, one may speculate that elderly women are at this point reflecting a lower degree of dependence upon their spousal relationship than would be true of the men, and also that women are able to find satisfactions in alternative relationships more readily than men seem to be able to do.

The latter interpretation tends to be supported by the respondents' perceptions of children as a dominant positive factor both in current quality of life and over the lifespan. From Figures 9–3 and 9–4 we note that 27 percent and 28 percent, respectively, of the women (and only 8 percent of the men) indicate that children are a dominant positive contributor to quality of life (i.e., as an adjunct to successful coping with loss).

Two remarkable shifts are seen to occur in the later years with respect to health and material well-being as negative (loss) factors. As a current negative factor, loss of health is endorsed by 40 percent of the women and 33 percent of the men, whereas loss of material well-being (money, possessions) is endorsed by 21 percent and 18 percent of women and men, respectively. This contrasts sharply with the overall lifespan picture. In Figures 9–3 and 9–4 we see loss of health endorsed as a negative factor by only 11 percent of women and 7 percent of men, and loss of income or money endorsed by 27 percent of women and 23 percent of men. When one compares the findings on health in this study with the findings of a 1974 Harris poll (cf. Table 2–3 in Chapter 2), according to which 21 percent of a national sample of older people stated that "health was a top priority concern," and with the results of a 1981 Harris poll, which indicated that over 70 percent of adults sixty-five or older feel that health status has improved for older Americans, it is obvious that some discrepancy exists. This may be due to the fact that different kinds of questions were asked in each survey. In addition, even though 21 percent cited health as a top priority concern in the 1974 Harris study, other older persons (i.e., the remaining 79 percent) may regard health as an important, but not necessarily the most important, factor. In any case, it is clear that in a number of instances the views of the aged are not in harmony

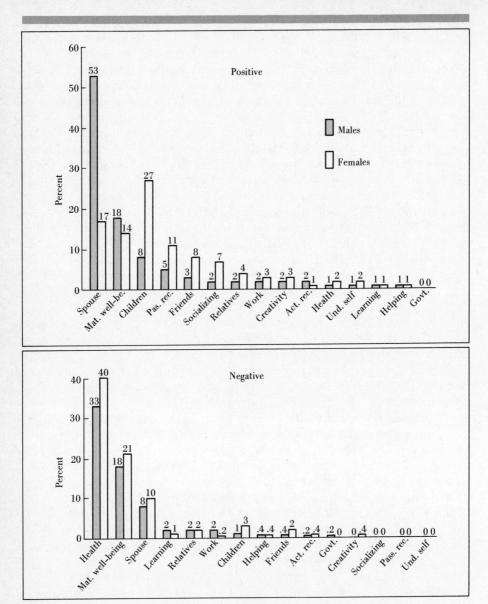

FIGURE 9–3.   The Single Dominant Factor in Determining Current Quality of Life
Source: Flanagan (1982).

with the views of younger people about them. It is also evident that health and money, while important, are by no means the exclusive or even the over-whelming concern of older people, as younger generations have been led to believe.

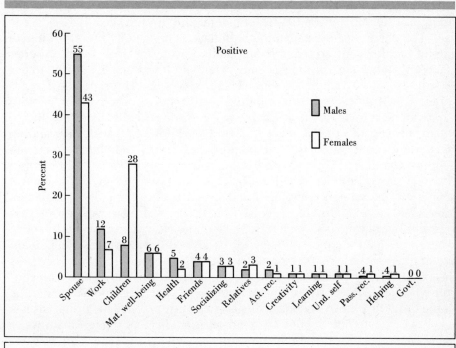

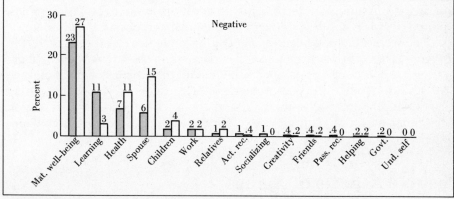

FIGURE 9–4. The Single Dominant Factor in Determining Quality of Life Over the Lifespan
Source: Flanagan (1982).

Coping with Bereavement

Preliminary analyses of new data from a study of grief by Thompson, Peterson, and Gallagher at the University of Southern California's Andrus Gerontology Center lend credence to the foregoing. The general hypothesis of this study of bereavement proposes that "cumulative loss when related to an adequate or inadequate support system and to greater or lesser coping strength results in a given degree of mental and physical health."

This theoretical formulation could have been tested in terms of loss of gainful employment, in terms of amputation, in terms of abortion, in terms of a criminal indictment such as embezzlement; it was finally decided to test its validity with a sample of widows and widowers. The rationale for this choice was Holmes and Rahe's finding that loss of spouse had the greatest impact upon individuals (see Chapter 2). A three-year study was conducted which investigated the "grief work" of 230 widows and widowers and an equal number of controls who did not lose their mates. Individuals from both samples were interviewed six weeks after the loss, six months after the onset of bereavement, and one year after the loss. The last interview of the control sample has now been completed and initial results have been tabulated. Early analyses of the findings support this theoretical framework as relevant to certain significant aspects of loss. Some of the early statistical results show, for example, that the mortality rate for widows and widowers is 300 percent higher than for those in the control (nonloss) group, and that morbidity rates (hospitalizations) are twice as high for the bereaved in comparison with controls whose relationships are intact. In terms of severe reactions, the ratio is on the order of 10 to 1, bereaved versus controls. Final statistical analysis has not yet been completed, but to date all of the indicators suggest that loss of mate constitutes a significant determining factor with respect to both psychological and physiological decrements. In addition, as Granger Westberg has reported, loss is a significant clue to both mental and physical adjustment.

The patterning of percentages of coping strategies employed, as shown in Figure 9–5, very clearly demonstrates once again the strength of the family-friend support network as a positive element in the gains of late maturity. Most striking of all is the use of memories (in excess of 90 percent of the respondents employed this strategy), a much more frequently used means of coping than affiliation with groups (other than religious organizations) and the seeking of specific information.

Positive Aspects of Aging

It is as important, if not more so, to our understanding of the aging process to appreciate the gains inherent in these later years as it is to focus myopically on senescent pathologies and decrements. Nevertheless, one does not negate the existence of the other.

The simple fact remains that there are now well over 23 million persons in the United States over sixty-five years of age, the great majority of whom are able to function reasonably well. The question asked by Butler (1975) is merely an echo of the question asked by many: "Why survive?" The answers inevitably will first and foremost be individual and personal. Some more general responses offered here need to be considered for our own understanding of aging.

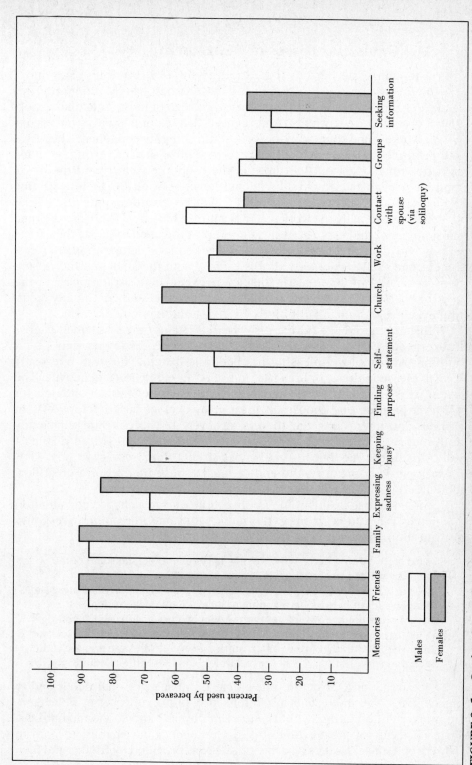

FIGURE 9–5. Coping Strategies Used by Caucasian Respondents in Response to Spouse's Death

Source: Thompson, Peterson, & Gallagher (in progress)

The Gains and Losses of Retirement

Although some persons regard retirement as a severe loss and find it difficult to envision new horizons and to develop new uses for their time, this is certainly not true of all older persons—not even of most. The relative popularity of so-called early retirement suggests that in our postindustrial society not all workers find their work or work settings highly congenial. The visual and print media have enabled many to recognize the interesting, enticing activities which exist outside those of the shop, the factory, and the office. Retirement enables many to shed the burden of a boring job, thereby gaining the freedom to expend the same energy in more rewarding pursuits.

For a great many the work world is a mixed blessing. There are the time constraints and the responsibilities imposed by the need to satisfy the expectations and demands of superiors, the marketplace competition, the customers, one's fellow workers; all this is laced with the anxieties and frustrations generated by internal dissonance between high aspirations and the need to "perform" on the one hand and, on the other, the continually recurring evidence of human fallibility, perplexity, and ignorance.

In contrast, old age (along with "retired" status) would seem to offer as little else does, the freedom to be oneself. Once the pressing need for career building and employer-pleasing has been dissipated, who does one really have to please in dress, in life-style, in use of time, in choice of activity? The senior years usher in the welcome freedom to structure energies and time for whatever purpose one chooses. A great many persons have untapped latent abilities and interests which they were never able to cultivate sufficiently until they were freed from day-to-day job requirements. It is true that most work structures time, but it usually does so in a rigid, restrictive way. Thus for many in later maturity, the end of regular work life means a great deal more freedom.

Some remarks made by an elderly couple during a chance encounter in a mountain campsite with one of the authors illustrates the point. In response to a question, they said:

> What are we doing here? Why, we now have time to pursue some of the interests we had to curtail when we ran a store. Now we can get away. We're here to watch birds; there are some interesting species up here in these pines. When we leave here we're planning to join a couple dozen friends at a neighboring college. We're going to sit in a two-day seminar on "shelling." After that most of us will be going on up to the beach with our snorkels and hunt shells. After that, we're off up north for several weeks with our children and grandchildren. . . . We never had time to do these things before.

The freedom to structure one's time to pursue personal needs and to pursue one's own interests is also a reflection of the relief from the responsibilities of child rearing, with its attendant physical and economic burdens. The availability of greater blocks of discretionary time enables the old to rediscover themselves, to savor the satisfactions provided by friends and family, and allows older couples to rediscover each other. There is "permission," appropriateness, as well as opportunity for older persons to try new and different things, and to explore the bittersweet rewards of the life review as fully as one might explore new and enticing activities. In essence, the opportunity to indulge oneself in ways and to an extent that earlier family and career demands inhibited is one of the major gains associated with growing old.

As indicated earlier (see Table 2–3 in Chapter 2), health and economic well-being are perceived by younger persons to be top priority issues of old age. These are important to the old, too. But it may well be that the gains of later life described here can provide the necessary balance weighing against increasingly limited economic means and the accrual of physical disabilities to make extended longevity worthwhile.

Wisdom of Old Age

Significant shifts in cognitive and intellectual appraisals in later life, at times labeled a deficiency when measured in the context of an experimental laboratory, may in fact represent another significant gain inherent in old age. A sample of older male research participants were observed to think "in blocks" (Birren, 1959). That is, rather than sort through a variety of impressions elicited by presented stimuli, these elderly individuals tended to "solve the problem" by arriving at a gestalt, an integrated cognitive configuration of the whole. The tendency was to ignore minor details and to perceive whole patterns.

Under certain circumstances this tendency might prove to be disadvantageous. For most circumstances, however, it can prove to be very practical. It enables older persons to "see life and see it whole." It is a capacity that derives from the rich experience of years: to have observed the growth and fading of fads and fancies, the repeating patterns of time and history's ebb and flow. By some it is called perspective, the knowledge that there is really nothing new under the sun in the domain of human knowledge and experience. It is the essence of wisdom.

Nothing could summarize the gains of later life as well as the following excerpt from *The Delights of Growing Old:*

> I cannot tell how I shall behave when aches and decrepitude come or that illness which will thrust me, roughly or not so roughly, out of this world. . . . it does not seem to me sensible to dwell upon unpleasant things before they even happen. I only beg that I may, without weakening, remain true to the oaths that I have inwardly sworn: honor the life dwelling within me to its very last, and even if only a spark remains to me, treat it still as a holy flame. (Doudeket, 1966).

Summary

In spite of the persistent association of unremitting loss with aging, a more balanced view is suggested: namely, that both gains and losses are associated with *every* period of life. Loss does occur across time, and death is one such major loss, both to the dying person and to those most closely associated with him or her. When death actually occurs is still a controversial issue.

Death has many different meanings to different people. Many, including a number of professional helpers, deal with dying by means of a conspiracy of silence, to the detriment of all concerned. Kübler-Ross, one of the very first to study the emotional and psychological aspects of the dying process, has formulated a series of stages through which dying persons are likely to progress, although the universality of these stages has been questioned. Social death is a very special case wherein the individual, though physically alive, is perceived to be and is even treated as if already deceased—and the pain of bereavement is just as real. Allied to this notion is the not altogether rare phenomenon of individuals who appear to "time" their own demise to coincide with or follow an important anticipated event.

Religion serves as one component of support for the dying person, as does the hospice program originated in England. Death rituals are important psychological supports for the bereaved. At the same time, considerable empirical evidence supports the view that spouses (especially for men) and children contribute greatly to life satisfaction and thus balance loss. Health factors and economic well-being also contribute, but not to the extent usually assumed by younger persons.

The effects of retirement are mixed. They represent both loss and gain. For many older individuals it opens the door to a new sense of freedom to indulge themselves in the pursuit of long-deferred interests and activities.

References

Baird, J. The funeral industry in Boston. In E. Schneidman (Ed.), *Death and the college student.* New York: Behavioral Publications, 1972.

Baltes, P., & Schaie, K. W. Aging and I.Q.: The myth of the twilight years. *Psychology Today,* 1974, 7, 35–40.

Barrett, C. J. The development and evaluation of three-group therapeutic intervention for widows. Doctoral dissertation, University of Southern California, 1974.

Bengston, V. L. Self-determination: A social-psychologic perspective on helping the aged. *Geriatrics,* 1973, **28**(12), 118–130.

Benoliel, J. Q. The practitioner's dilemma: Problems and priorities. In R. Davis (Ed.), *Confrontation with dying.* Los Angeles: University of Southern California, Andrus Gerontology Center, 1971. Pp. 31–41.

Birren, J. *The psychology of aging.* Englewood Cliffs, N.J.: Prentice-Hall, 1959.

Butler, R. *Why survive? Growing old in America.* New York: Harper & Row, 1975.

Cousins, N. *The anatomy of an illness.* New York: Bantam Books, 1980.

Cassell, E., Kass, L., et al. Refinements in criteria for determination of death: An appraisal. *Journal of the American Medical Association,* 1972, **221**: 48–54.

Cousins, N. *The anatomy of an illness.* New York: Bantam Books, 1980.

Engen, T. Taste and smell. In J. Birren & K. W. Schaie (Eds.), *Handbook of the psychology of aging.* New York: Van Nostrand Reinhold, 1977. Pp. 554–561.

Feifel, H. (Ed.) *The meaning of death.* New York: McGraw-Hill, 1959.

Flanagan, J. C. *New insights to improve the quality of life at age 70.* (Prepared for NIA, NIH, and DHHS, Bethesda, Md.; Grant No. 1, RO1, AGO 2453-01.) Palo Alto, Cal.: American Institutes for Research in the Behavioral Sciences, 1982.

Fulton, R., & Fulton, J. A psycho-social aspect of terminal care: Anticipatory grief. *Omega,* 1971, **2**, 91–100.

Holmes, R., & Rahe, R. The social readjustment rating scale. *Journal of Psychosomatic Research,* 1967, **11**, 219–225.

Jacobson, B. *Young programs for older workers.* New York: Van Nostrand Reinhold, 1980.

Kalish, R. Death and dying in a social context. In R. Binstock & E. Shanas (Eds.), *Handbook of aging and the social sciences.* New York: Van Nostrand Reinhold, 1976. Pp. 483–507.

Kenshalo, D. Age changes in touch, vibration, temperature, kinesthesis, and pain sensitivity. In J. Birren & K. W. Schaie (Eds.), *Handbook of the psychology of aging.* New York: Van Nostrand Reinhold, 1977. Pp. 562–579.

Kübler-Ross, E. *On death and dying.* New York: Macmillan Company, 1969.

Langer, E. J., & Rodin, J. The effects of choice and enhanced personal responsibility for the aged: A field experiment in an institutional setting. *Journal of Personality and Social Psychology,* 1976, **34**(2), 191–198.

Lindemann, E. Symptomatology and management of acute grief. *American Journal of Psychiatry,* 1944, **101**, 141–148.

Mant, A. K. The medical definition of death. In E. Schneidman (Ed.) *Death: Current Perspectives,* Mayfield, N.Y. 1976.

Matthieu, J. Dying and death role-expectation: A comparative analysis. Doctoral dissertation, Department of Sociology, University of Southern California, 1972.

Mitford, J. *The American way of death.* New York: Fawcett/Crest, 1978.

Nora, F. *Memorial associations: What they are—how they are organized.* New York: Cooperative League of America, 1962.

Parkes, C. M. *Bereavement: Studies of grief in adult life.* New York: International Universities Press. 1972.

Peterson, J., & Briley, M. *Widows and widowhood: A creative approach to being alone.* New York: Association Press, 1977.

Peterson, M. *Thomas Jefferson and the new nation.* New York: Oxford University Press, 1970.

Phillips, D. Deathday and birthday: An unexpected connection. In I. Tamer, F. Mosteller, et al. (Eds.), *Statistics: A guide to the unknown.* San Francisco: Holden-Day, 1972.

Reynolds, D., & Kalish, R. Anticipation of futurity as a function of ethnicity and age. *Journal of Gerontology,* 1974, **29**, 224–231.

Runciman, A. Problems older clients present in counseling about sexuality. In I. Burnside (Ed.), *Sexuality and aging.* Los Angeles: University of Southern California Press, 1975.

Saunders, C. St. Christopher's Hospice (excerpted from *St. Christopher's Hospice Annual Report, 1971–72*). In E. S. Shneidman (Ed.), *Death: Current perspectives.* 2nd ed. New York: Mayfield, 1980.

Schaie, K. W. Translations in gerontology. From lab to life: intellectual functioning. *American Psychologist,* 1974, **29**, 802–807.

Schneidman, E. *Deaths of man.* New York: Quadrangle, 1973.

Schneidman, E. The death certificate. In E. Schneidman (Ed.), *Death: Current perspectives.* New York: Mayfield, 1976.

Schoenberg, B., Carp, A., Peretz, D., & Kutscher, A. (Eds.). *Loss and grief: Psychological management of medical practice.* New York: Columbia University Press, 1970.

Snyder, C. L., & Schwartz, A. N. Physiological, psychological, and social characteristics of 101 Caribbean centenarians. Paper presented at the 12th International Congress of Gerontology, Hamburg, Germany, 1981.

Warner, W. The city of the dead. In R. Fulton (Ed.), *Death and identity.* New York: Wiley, 1965.

Weisman, A. *On death and dying: A psychiatric study of terminality.* New York: Behavioral Publications, 1972.

Young, M., Benjamin, B., & Wallis, C. Mortality of widowers. *Lancet,* 1963 (2),454.

For Further Reading

Becker, E. *The denial of death.* New York: Free Press, 1973.

Cohen, K. P. *Hospice: Prescription for terminal care.* Germantown, Md.: Aspen Systems Corporation, 1979.

DuBois, P. M. *The hospice way of death.* New York: Human Sciences Press, 1980.

Freese, A. *Help for your grief.* New York: Schocken Books, 1977.

Hamilton, M., & Reid, H. F. *A hospice handbook: A new way to care for the dying.* Grand Rapids, Mich.: W. B. Eerdmans, 1980.

Jury, M., & Jury, D. *Gramp.* New York: Grossman, 1976.

Kastenbaum, R., & Aisenberg, R. *The psychology of death.* New York: Springer, 1978.

Kleyman, P. *Senior power: Growing old rebelliously.* San Francisco: Glide Publications, 1974.

Lack, S., & Buckingham, R. W. *First American hospice: Three years of home care.* New Haven, Conn.: Hospice, 1978.

Moss, B. B. Hospice and terminal care. *Seminars in Family Medicine,* 1982, 3(1), 51–56.

Rossman, P. *Hospice: Creating new models of care for the terminally ill.* New York: Association Press, 1977.

Schneidman, E. *Death: Current perspectives.* 2nd ed. New York: Mayfield, 1980.

Stoddard, S. *The hospice movement: A better way of caring for the dying.* Briarcliff Manor, N.Y.: Stein & Day, 1978.

Watson, W., & Maxwell, R. *Human aging and dying: A study in cultural gerontology.* New York: St. Martin's Press, 1977.

Wheeler, H. Goodbye to mandatory retirement. *Modern Maturity,* 1978, 21, 9–11.

Environment as the Context for Aging

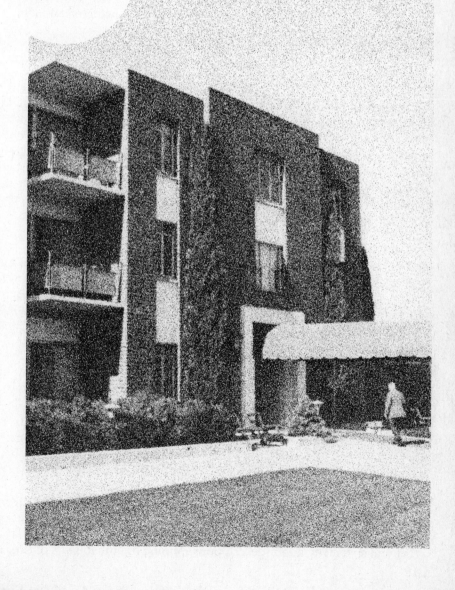

If life is a matter of getting older then it is bound to be a sad and mournful
business, because you are leaving in the dust behind you life's glories
dead. On the other hand, if life is a matter of growing older,
deepening your affection, extending your field of knowledge,
heightening your sense of beauty, expanding your areas of service,
bearing your suffering more nobly, sensitizing your awareness of
God's presence, then it is a joyful, and not a mournful, business.
Dr. Melvin Sheatley, Jr.
Los Angeles Times, *August 6, 1967*

The notion of environmental impact upon the health, psychological well-being, and behavior of the human organism is neither new nor novel. It enjoys a long, well-entrenched, and respected history in the study of human behavior. A substantial and growing body of theoretical knowledge and empirical data (Altman, 1975; Hall & Lindzey, 1970; Hawley, 1950; Lawton, 1970, 1974; Lewin, 1936; Moos, 1976; Murray, 1938; Proshansky, Ittelson, & Rivlin, 1970; Sommer, 1969) has made it clear that the interface of humans and their environments is characterized by an active, dynamic process of exchange.

Most of us readily assume the environment to be a relatively stable "given," a static backdrop to the human drama played out upon life's stage. From a more scientific viewpoint, individuals are seen to interact continuously with their environments, modifying and being modified in complementary fashion by the elements of their surroundings (Bevan, 1968; Sells, 1963). Humans, in fact, are the only members of the animal kingdom capable of substantially creating and refurbishing their environments to serve survival needs and to provide satisfaction and comfort.

Egon Brunswik, one of the first psychologists to adopt an ecological perspective, and Roger Barker, another pioneer in ecological psychology, were early exponents of the necessity for study of the human organism in its natural ecological environment in order to understand how it functions. Recognizing the dynamic, symbiotic relationship between person and environment multiplies the difficulties in attempting to define environmental impacts. The interrelationships among biological factors, psychological and social influences, and the physical environment are especially complex with respect to a population as variegated and diverse as the elderly. On what basis do we define the boundaries of the environment? Does it make sense to describe the environment in general terms, or are we bound to individual or cultural specificity in our descriptions? Among the inhabitants of Chicago,

Houston, and Athens are babies, dogs, elderly persons, college students, and rats. Do they all share the same environment?

Moos (1976) has followed a number of historical trends that underlie the recent stimulation of interest in human surroundings. The past two decades have been witness to two trends in particular that will serve as the focus of this chapter. The first trend is the growing attention directed toward the person-environmental transactional perspective (cf. discussion in Chapters 1 and 4). The second trend, especially notable within the past ten years, is the generation of new and systematic efforts to measure the environments of older people and to identify ecological features which affect and contribute to their perceived "quality of life." Both trends are important to the field of gerontology as we come to the realization that our understanding of the aging process will remain seriously deficient without additional knowledge of the context in which behavior occurs.

Classification of Environments

Broadly defined, the environment of the elderly has been divided into the *macroenvironment* and the *microenvironment* with respect to physical considerations. The environment may be described in more than purely physical or design-related terms, however. For example, the *group environment* pertains to the behavior of individuals acting as groups in some structural relationship to a given person (Altman & Lett, 1970); the *personal environment* consists of interactions with significant others; the *suprapersonal environment* refers to "the characteristics of the aggregate of individuals in physical proximity usually expressed as the average or the mode" (Lawton, 1980); and the *social environment* represents such phenomena as sociopolitical movements and institutions, cultural values, legal traditions, and economic cycles (cf. Chapter 4). Classifying the older person's environment with respect to all of these dimensions becomes an important task in understanding the context of behavior.

Rudolph Moos and associates (e.g., Kiritz & Moos, 1974) have additionally identified three environmental dimensions based on the social impact of personality characteristics which may be helpful in describing the functional surroundings of the elderly:

1. *Relationship dimensions,* which assess the extent to which individuals are involved in the environment and the extent to which they help and support each other. Examples include involvement, affiliation, peer cohesion, and expressiveness.

2. *Personal development dimensions,* which assess the basic directions toward which self-enhancement activities tend to progress in a particular environment. These dimensions are exemplified by autonomy, independence, and responsibility

3. *System maintenance and system change dimensions,* reflected in degrees of order, organization, clarity, control, and innovation.

Lawton (1980) has further discussed the salience of such environmental dimensions as simple versus complex, quiet versus noisy, and beautiful versus ugly. The following case illustrations will illuminate the importance of these environmental dimensions to the lives of three elderly people.

Case Illustration
Mrs. S., a Widow

Mrs. S., an eighty-three-year-old widow, is a first-generation American who has spent virtually all of her adult life in middle-class apartments near the central city sections of a large metropolitan community. She has been widowed about eight years; her three children are now grown. One daughter lives with her family in another large city 300 miles away; her son and his wife, city dwellers as well, live even farther from her. Contacts with these children range from occasional to rare. A third daughter lives within a few minutes' driving distance and has almost daily contact with her mother.

  For many years Mrs. S., who never learned to drive a car, was able to shop and devote herself to a variety of interests, including extensive volunteer work. These activities were made possible by virtue of the proximity of shopping centers, well within walking distance of her home, and the availability of accessible, affordable public transportation. Following the death of her husband, Mrs. S. moved into a private room in a congregate-living retirement setting. From this base she is able to maintain her shopping and volunteer activities, although these are now limited by her reduced energy level and by her apprehensions about going out late in the day or at night. She experiences some frustration now that her major activities are confined to and focused within her present institutional setting. Many of her friends and acquaintances are scattered throughout the metropolitan area, and her social contacts are reduced to occasional phone calls and even less frequent excursions by public transportation or when a ride by car is offered by friends. Her acceptance of the status quo in no way eliminates her sense of constraint about her relative lack of mobility.

CASE ILLUSTRATION
Mr. and Mrs. B., an Inner-City Couple

Mr. B. is in his late sixties and Mrs. B. is in her mid-seventies. They live in a small "kitchenette apartment," consisting of a bedroom, a bathroom, a living-dining area, a tiny kitchen, and a small service porch, in a large run-down tenement building in an inner-city complex of similarly run-down apartment buildings. This is the latest in a series of low-cost apartments which the B.'s have called home over a period of years.

They have one child, an adult son, who lives far away and who maintains periodic contact with his parents by letter. Mr. B. still leaves the apartment almost daily to make his contacts as a salesman, although he expresses growing concern over his wife's failing memory and increasing loss of energy and physical strength. A concerned neighbor once requested the attention of the Visiting Nurses Association for Mrs. B., who appears to have great difficulty in preparing her own meals while Mr. B. is gone. That visit revealed that Mrs. B. is underweight and quite frail, has low blood pressure, and finds that meal preparation has become an almost impossible task—her old-fashioned cast iron pots and pans are too heavy and are mostly stored in inconvenient shelves close to the floor. Living in a third-story apartment with no elevator, about six blocks from the nearest market, discourages Mrs. B. from attempts to leave her home for even minimum shopping. Mr. and Mrs. B. cannot afford a TV but do have a small, battered table radio which she plays constantly. Mr. B. worries much about his wife, who seems for the most part spiritless, apathetic, discouraged, and sad. She spends most of her day idly leafing through the newspaper and old magazines which neighbors provide, or sitting on an unmade bed listening to the radio, which she says she enjoys immensely.

These case studies and other accounts of the lives of older people raise questions important to gerontologists with respect to environmental effects upon the behavior of the elderly:

1. To what extent is the environment a source of stress and ill health when an older person attempts to function within a setting which is incompatible with his or her needs and preferred life-style?

2. Should we accept as "ideal" the perspective that older people are expected to adjust to their environments, or should we adopt the view that efforts be directed toward the design of appropriate environments which "fit" the older person?

3. What factors in the social and designed environment affect the health and well-being of elderly individuals?

4. Are there "ideal" environments for the elderly? What constitutes the optimal fit between the older person and the environment?

5. How are the various aspects of environment assessed, operationalized, and measured so as to make them amenable to systematic and meaningful modification?

Selected Theoretical Perspectives

Most theories of personality and human behavior of necessity have incorporated references to environmental variables with varying degrees of focus, emphasis, and detail. Rather than providing a comprehensive review, we have chosen to highlight several theoretical formulations which are most congruent with the person-environment transactional approach (cf. Schwartz, 1974), the major thesis of this text.

In certain respects, behavioral ecology grew from the seeds planted by Gestalt psychologist Kurt Lewin. Lewin's field theory, like Koffka's ideas about the "behavioral environment," was an outgrowth of the older sciences of physics and chemistry. In Gestalt psychology, the "way in which an object is perceived is determined by the total context or configuration in which the object is embedded" (Hall & Lindzey, 1970). Thus behavior will vary in part as a function of differing environmental contexts. Henry Murray (1938) broadened earlier concepts by including in his personality theory not only the familiar concept of individual needs but also the less well-known concept of environmental press.

Environment and Competence

Within this general framework, and drawing heavily on Murray's concepts, Lawton (1980; Lawton & Nahemow, 1973) has proposed a succinct yet elegant formulation. The "ecological model of adaptation and aging" is schematized in Figure 10–1, in which the vertical axis represents competence of the individual (ranging from low to high) and the horizontal axis represents environmental press (from weak to strong).

According to Lawton and Nahemow:

> The essential contribution of the model is to indicate that adaptive behavior and/or positive affect may result from a wide variety of combinations of individual competence and environmental press. The shaded areas on both sides of the central diagonal thus represent areas of positive outcome; at any point in these areas one might say that the level of demand (environmental) is in balance with the person's ability to respond to that demand. . . . The central line labeled "adaptation level" (AL) represents points where environmental press is "average" for whatever level of competence the person in question has [1973, pp. 11–12].

The Lawton-Nahemow model very nicely schematizes the subtle variations that occur continuously in individuals and environments and the give-and-take, push-pull exchange between the two. Their model has much heuristic value and achieves considerable predictive as well as explanatory power with respect to the behavior of older people when variations in capacity to respond (adaptation or competence value) and the variability of environmental press (demands of the environment) are considered.

Mrs. B.'s situation, described in our second case study, exemplifies the relationship between competence, environmental press, and negative affect. As environmental press increases in strength for Mrs. B. as the result of loneliness and the presence of physical obstacles and impediments to activity, Mrs. B.'s diminished competence (reflected in her low blood pressure, spotty memory, and muscular weakness) will most likely decrease her adaptive level and thereby lead to an increase in negative affect.

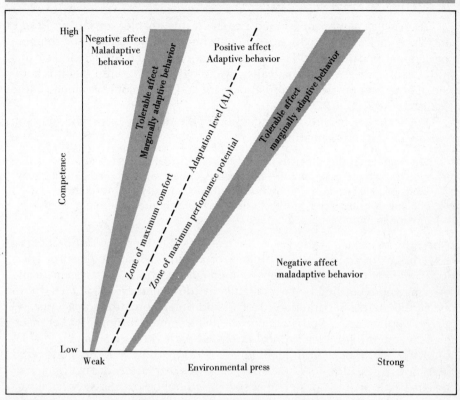

FIGURE 10–1.   Ecological Model of Adaptation and Aging
Source: Lawton & Nahemow (1973).

Environment and Health

Sargent (1972) has suggested that health is a process of person-environment interaction within a specific ecological context. Person and environment are thus viewed as one system. From this perspective, health may be defined in terms of the adaptive capacity of a person in relation to his or her environmental circumstances. When adaptation succeeds, the person can be considered healthy; when it fails, the person is ill. Health may therefore be construed as

the ability of the organism to function effectively within a given environment. . . . since the environment keeps changing, good health is a process of continuous adaptation to the myriad of microbes, irritants, pressures, and problems which daily challenge man [Dubos, 1968; cf. Carlson, 1975].

Other Ecological Approaches

Brunswik's views, mentioned earlier in this chapter, deserve a prominent place among those which have contributed to the person-environment transactional perspective of aging. Brunswik drew attention to the fact that "both historically and systematically psychology has forgotten that it is a science of organism-environment relationships and has become a science of the organism" (1957, p. 6).

Roger Barker is a notable exception to the majority of psychologists in this respect. Barker commented,

> Who can doubt that changes in our environment ranging from new levels of
> radiation, to increased numbers of people, to new kinds of medicine, and new
> kinds of social organization, schools and governments are inexorably
> changing our behavior, and that our behavior is, in turn, altering our
> environment [1963a, p. 19].

He and his associates at the Psychological Field Station (Kansas) pioneered the technique of "behavior mapping," a procedure devised to discover operational elements of person-environment transactions by systematically observing and recording behavioral and environmental events *in vivo* within specific time frames (Barker, 1963b). In addition to providing concepts and theories applicable to a broad range of environmental milieus, Barker made significant methodological contributions as well. Robert Sommer (1969), employing methodological techniques developed by Barker, conducted extensive investigations of behavioral responses in a variety of environmental contexts in his analysis of personal space. Although Sommer's research was not age-specific, his intriguing studies may readily be adapted to the study of aging and environment.

Designed Environment Variables

Basing his experimental work on the postulate that human behavior is the outcome of a functional relationship between the individual and a specific social or mechanical environment, O. R. Lindsley (1964) has cogently argued the utility of developing geriatric **prosthetic**[1] environments as a free operant conditioning mode. His approach reflects a strong Skinnerian influence. He describes ways in which manipulation or modification of the physical environment can compensate for sensory deficits and also produce positive reinforcements (rewards) necessary to improve nonproductive or maladaptive behaviors in later life. Lindsley was one of the first investigators to point out that we have not begun to exhaust the vast possibilities for developing prosthetic devices for the aged that will prevent their being penalized as a consequence of multiple physical losses.

---

[1]*prosthetic:* compensating; providing appropriate support to permit normal functioning in the presence of disability or dysfunction

Working from the same general perspective, Kermit Schooler (1969, 1975, 1981) has addressed the ever-recurring question: Does the nature of the social environment make a difference to the elderly and, if so, in what ways? His investigation of the relation of social interaction to morale of older persons illuminates the complex nature of these variables and the necessity of assessing them with reference to environmental configurations.

The Macroenvironment: States, Communities, Neighborhoods

As noted previously, the terms "macro-" and "microenvironments" refer to the dimension of scale. In this section, we will focus on larger-scale environments, including states, communities, and neighborhood settings.

Where do older people live? The assumption that the southwestern "sunbelt" states have the highest concentration of older people is a popular, yet inaccurate, stereotype. In 1977, as Table 10–1 shows, Florida had the highest concentration of persons aged sixty-five or older. This no doubt reflects the inclination of many older people to seek a warm climate. Although there has been generally heavy migration from northeastern and north central states to southern and southwestern states, California, Arizona,

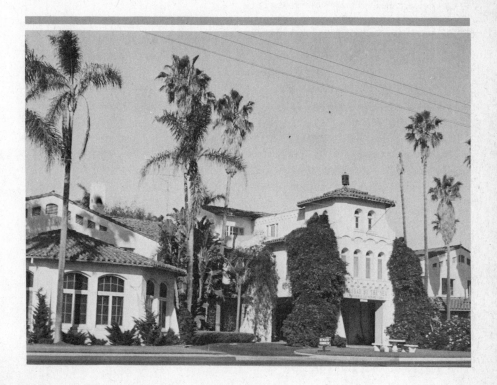

TABLE 10–1. High and Low State Values of Selected Characteristics of the Older Population, United States, 1970

Population Characteristic	High Value	Low Value
1. % of state population aged 65+	14.8 (Fla)	6.4 (Nev)
2. %of elderly living in urban areas	90.5 (RI)	35.4 (Vt)
3. % of elderly living in rural farm areas	16.8 (ND)	0.3 (RI)
4. % of elderly living alone or with non-relatives ("Primary Individuals")	31.1 (Ark)	21.4 (NC)
5. % of elderly married and living with spouse	61.0 (Fla)	33.3 (Ala)
6. % of elderly living dependently in child's household	18.1 (NY)	3.9 (Ore)
7. % of elderly in institutions of all types	8.0 (ND)	2.3 (Fla, WVa)
8. % of elderly who are native to state	82.7 (Ky)	9.1 (Ariz)
9. % of elderly who are foreign born	35.2 (NY)	0.7 (Miss)
10. % of elderly who are non-white	35.9 (Miss)	0.3 (Vt, NH)
11. % of elderly who moved to state between 1965 and 1970 (in-migrants)	20.8 (Ariz)	1.2 (NY)
12. % of elderly who left state between 1965 and 1970 (out-migrants)	10.9 (Nev)	1.9 (Ark, Tex
13. % of elderly who received any income in 1969	98.8 (Kan)	86.1 (Wash)
14. % of elderly receiving income with income below $3,000	85.8 (Miss)	45.1 (Conn)
15. % of elderly males in labor force	36.4 (Wis)	17.6 (Conn)
16. % of elderly employed males in white-collar occupations	51.8 (NY, NJ)	26.2 (SD)
17. % of elderly-headed households living in owned homes	81.0 (Kan)	45.9 (NY)
18. Median years of school completed by women aged 70–74	10.5 (Ariz, Nev)	7.6 (La)
19. Number of elderly males per 100 elderly females (sex ratio)	100.1 (Mo)	64.3 (Mass)
20. Average number of children ever born to elderly women who ever married	3.6 (Utah, ND)	1.5 (Wyo)

Source: Kart & Manard (1976).

Nevada, New Mexico, Idaho, and Hawaii (as of 1977) were still underrepresented in terms of percent population of older persons relative to the national norm. This may mirror significant migration patterns of younger families in pursuit of jobs and better housing opportunities over the past decade. It may also reflect migratory patterns of rural to urban relocation, although these trends are only speculation based on data available at the present time.

In a study of the residential status of older Americans, Kart and Manard (1976) investigated selected population characteristics, a list of which appears in Table 10–1. Their data, derived from the 1970 census, suggest the existence of

> aging regions, whose elderly populations [exhibit] high degrees of consistency on a combination of social, economic, and demographic characteristics . . . [not necessarily] congruent with . . . traditional state groupings or geographical regions [p. 109].

Variability among these regions is largely accounted for by combinations of four factors: size of rural population, degree of population mobility, level of economic sufficiency of the elderly, and level of employment or institutionalization of the elderly.

Increasing concentrations of elderly persons in urban (metropolitan) centers are clearly illustrated by the geographic distribution of the aged presented in Table 10–2. In 1977, only 5 percent of the elderly lived in the smallest communities, in contrast to the 63 percent living in metropolitan areas, divided about evenly between central city (31 percent) and surburban (32 percent) communities. It is also clear from Table 10–2 that black (55 percent) and Hispanic (53 percent) elderly persons are more likely to live in central city than in suburban areas, while for white elderly individuals the converse is true.

These data tell us where elderly persons are located but do not provide any information as to why this distribution has occurred with respect to community residential patterns. Some effort has been made to account for the data on the basis of economic factors (e.g., jobs, income), social interaction patterns, availability of services, and even health and functional capacity variables (see Lawton, 1980). It should be noted that present analyses fail to support the rather commonplace view that it is "healthier" to live in the country than in the city—particularly central city areas.

As Table 10–3 suggests, the line of progression from "more impairment" to "less impairment" runs from nonmetropolitan, nonfarm locations to farm residence to urban central city to suburban living. An obvious contributor to this finding would seem to be the relative unavailability or inac-

TABLE 10–2.   Geographic Distribution of Over-Sixty-Five Population by Ethnicity, 1977

A. 65 + as Percentage of Population of Same Ethnic Group

	All Areas	Metropolitan		Nonmetropolitan[a]		
		Central City	Other	Large	Medium	Small
White	10.4	12.7	8.7	11.7	12.3	12.2
Black	7.6	7.6	4.5	9.0	10.2	9.1
Hispanic	4.1	4.4	3.7	3.6	4.5	5.9
All 65+	10.3	11.4	8.4	11.4	12.1	11.8

B. Percentage Distribution of 65+ among Geographic Areas by Ethnicity

White	101[b]	29	34	9	24	5
Black	100	55	11	8	22	4
Hispanic	101	53	31	4	11	2
All 65+	101	31	32	9	24	5

Source: U.S. Bureau of the Census. Social and economic characteristics of the metropolitan and nonmetropolitan population: 1977 and 1970. *Current Population Reports,* ser. P-23, no. 75. Washington, D.C.: Government Printing Office, 1978.

[a]*Large:* counties with largest place population of 25,000+. *Medium:* counties with largest place population 2,500–24,999. *Small:* counties with no place population ≥ 2,500.

[b]Percentages do not always add to 100 because of rounding.

TABLE 10–3.   Prevalence of Impairments Among Over-Sixty-Five Population

(Per Thousand 65+)

	Metropolitan Areas		Outside Metropolitan Areas	
	Central City	Other	Nonfarm	Farm
Limitation in mobility (percentages)	17.5	15.2	19.5	18.9
Limitation in activity (percentages)	41.3	39.6	47.5	47.8
Severe visual impairments	46.2	36.9	56.6	41.0
Hearing impairment	258.7	273.1	342.8	298.5
Speech defects	8.0	a	10.6	
Paralysis	20.2	21.1	26.7	
Impairment of back or spine	66.3	57.4	74.6	a
Impairment, upper extremity and shoulder	23.9	33.6	34.1	
Impairment, lower extremity and hip	76.2	74.3	87.9	76.9

Sources: National Center for Health Statistics. *Prevalence of selected impairments.* Ser. 10, no. 99. Rockville, Md.: USDHEW, 1975. National Center for Health Statistics. *Limitation of activity due to chronic conditions—United States, 1972.* Ser. 10, no. 96. Rockville, Md.: USDHEW, 1974.

[a]Sample size too small for reliable estimate.

cessibility of specialized or sophisticated health services in rural as opposed to urban areas. One might also speculate, given the paucity of detailed comparative data on this score, that the social support network of small communities (the "friendly small town") provides the kind of tightly knit supportive climate that allows older persons who experience greater degrees of physical impairment to maintain themselves at an acceptable level. One may further hypothesize that the environmental press is much weaker and more benign in small communities than in metropolitan areas, although the wide range of possible variations in this area must be recognized.

Availability of Services

In an extensive evaluation of communities reported by Blake, Lawton, and Lau (1978), adults of all ages were asked to describe the components of an ideal community. Eleven components were categorized along the three dimensions suggested by Insel and Moos (1974) and described earlier in this chapter. It was found that both old and young adults saw high-quality medical care and schools, availability of good jobs, and a wide variety of stores and businesses as most important in an ideal community. Possibly the most interesting finding was the high degree of consensus among younger and older persons as well as among small-town, medium-city, and large-city residents.

Schooler's (1975) national sample of older people, also described earlier in this chapter, was asked about local services. Eighty-two percent of rural elderly reported themselves to be "far" from desired services, compared to only 10 percent of urban elderly responding to this item. When asked to rate "convenience" of services, however, about 30 percent of rural and elderly persons alike rated such services as "not convenient." More surprising is the fact that more of the rural respondents (47 percent) considered such services "convenient" than did the urban respondents (33 percent).

Neighborhoods and Services

Critical distance is an important feature of environmental values and environmental satisfaction for many older persons, who usually seek such information about neighborhoods (Regnier, 1975). How distant are the bus stop, grocery or supermarket, church, post office, drugstore, department or variety store, physician's office, hospital, senior center, public park, library, laundromat? Regnier cites a study of this question by Newcomer (1973) which delineates the importance of and distances to such services and resources. The results of this study are shown in Table 10–4.

TABLE 10–4. Service Importance and Critical Distance

Service	Importance	Critical Distance	Recommended Distance
Bus stop	1	1 block	adjacent to site
Park/outdoor	2	1–3 blocks	adjacent to site
Grocery store	3	1–3 blocks	1 block
Laundromat	4	on-site	on-site
Supermarket	5	4–10 blocks	3 blocks
Post office	6	4–10 blocks	3 blocks
Bank	7	1–3 blocks	3 blocks
Service center	8	1–3 blocks	on-site
Cleaners	9	4–10 blocks	3 blocks
Department store	10	4–10 blocks	3 blocks
Social centers	11	1–3 blocks	3 blocks
Senior citizen club	12	on-site	on-site
Bingo, cards	13	1–3 blocks	on-site
Arts, crafts, hobbies	14	1–3 blocks	on-site
Movies	15	indeterminate	3 blocks
Parties, socials	16	1–3 blocks	on-site
Lectures, discussion	17	indeterminate	on-site
Organized trips	18	indeterminate	indeterminate
Church	19	indeterminate	indeterminate
Physician	20	indeterminate	indeterminate
Public library	21	indeterminate	indeterminate
Dentist	22	indeterminate	indeterminate
Luncheonette/snack bar	23	indeterminate	indeterminate
Bar	24	no importance	no importance

Source: Newcomer (1973).

Although critical distance is a useful indicator for decision making by the elderly as well as for planners, two cautions about determining critical distance should be observed. The first is that critical distance cannot be assessed solely on the basis of physical (objective) distance (e.g., number of blocks or miles). The ambience and topography of surrounding environments vary greatly. For example, as Regnier has pointed out, a distance of four city blocks up an extremely steep hill, across traffic-congested streets, through a high crime area is much more difficult for an older person to negotiate than the same physical distance on level ground, with no traffic, and through a safe, quiet neighborhood.

The second caution to be noted is that satisfaction or dissatisfaction with the location of services and resources will be strongly influenced by such factors as the competence and motivation of older individuals, the quality of their support networks, whether they own and drive a car, and the like.

Objective versus Subjective Environmental Qualities

In addition to analyses of the environments of older people on the basis of objective environmental qualities of features, subjective environmental qualities are of crucial importance in determining the behavior of the elderly. Adequate explanation, understanding, and prediction of behavior in later life must take into account the fact that behavior is interwoven with environmental contingencies. Lawton (1980, pp. 16–17) in particular has emphasized the need for information about the objective and subjective quality of older people's environments, based on systematic and careful sampling of representative environments. To understand the aging process we must search less for fixed behavioral laws and more for contingent relationships; what appear to be basic properties or behaviors of old people may in fact be behaviors largely contingent upon the environmental context.

As Proshansky (1973) has noted, we must take into account the relationship between the older person's physical and social world and the world that person "constructs" from it (i.e., the subjective environment). For example, an older person (indeed, a person of any age) might exhibit "office behavior," "church behavior," or "home behavior" as a function of differently perceived settings and behavioral contexts. The importance of subjective environmental quality is also apparent in the individual's need to be properly oriented in physical and emotional space. This pervasive need, according to E. T. Hall (1959), is ultimately linked to survival and sanity. Remove a cat's whiskers (a major orienting apparatus) and its consequent disorientation threatens survival. Similarly, a continuous input of paradoxical communications (mixed messages) from a parent can confuse and disorient a developing child to the point at which "crazy-making" occurs (Haley, 1963). To be disoriented in space, physically, cognitively, or emotionally, is to be or act psychotic or "senile."

The transition from these views to the concept of person-environment congruence is not difficult. Environmental congruence is associated with a positive mental state resulting not only from competence but also from satisfaction of personal needs. Incongruence is associated with a negative mental state (cf. Kahana, 1980, cited in Lawton, 1980, p. 15). Keeping in mind this positive-negative dimension, the environmental continuum can be said to range from overwhelmingly stressful to stimulating and challenging.

Coming back to the Lawton-Nahemow model, the adaptation level (AL) schematized in Figure 10–1 would therefore represent an approximation of total environmental congruence. Within this framework are incorporated such variables as environment, individual competence, need satisfaction, and individual expectancy. In other words, total environmental congruence is a perfect fit between the individual and the environment—an environment that is in balance with the needs, expectations, and competence of the individual.

Ths disparity between the expectations of older individuals themselves and the expectations of the general public are illustrated graphically in Figure 10–2. The discrepancy between expectations and actual experience with respect to crime, health, income, housing, and a number of other factors is

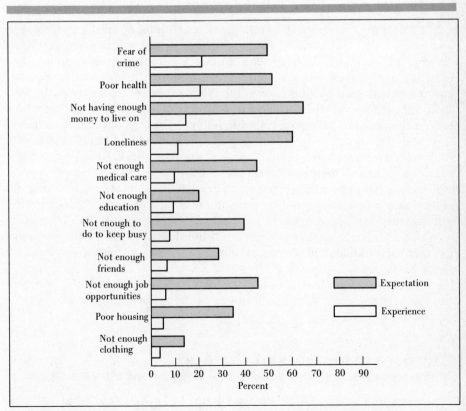

FIGURE 10–2. Problems of Older People: Public Expectations versus Personal Experience
Source: Harris et al., 1976

obvious. In parallel fashion, any disparity between the expectations of older persons and the realities of their environments provides important information about behavior. When an elderly person moves (or is moved) from an accustomed, congruent environment, where furniture, exits, entries, lights, switches, space dimensions, and scale are familiar and convenient and fit expectations, into an environment where types of noise and noise levels, furniture, controls, people, etc., are unfamiliar, strange, or unanticipated, or occur at levels of intensity or frequency which are personally intolerable, it should not be surprising if deviant or maladaptive behavior appears as a consequence.

What the ultimate effect of person-environment transactions will be in specific instances will depend in large part upon the interaction of objective and subjective environmental qualities. Neither is sufficient without the other; both must enter the equation when considering what positive or negative behaviors the environment is likely to produce or foster on the part of elderly persons.

Perception of the Environment

One can no more speak of an "ideal" environment for the elderly than one can refer to the impact of urban or rural living on elderly persons as "better" or "worse." Such generalizations are simply inappropriate. The issue is always the effects of a given environment at a given time on a particular individual. In the same (or a similar) environment experienced by Mrs. B. in our earlier case study, an elderly woman other than Mrs. B., one with a greater degree of competence and different perceptions of the environment, may well cope much more effectively. It is often observed that elderly persons may continue to experience terror at the thought of going out at night even in a crime-free neighborhood; they are still plagued by their perception of threats or dangers in the surrounding environment. By the same token, old people may refuse to use public transportation when it is perceived to present hazards (e.g., getting on or off, pushing, crowds of people) in the face of which they feel apprehensive or even helpless, in spite of the objective fact that such transportation may be demonstrated to present few or no hazards whatsoever.

These issues are particularly relevant to considerations of the microenvironment of the elderly, to be discussed in the following section.

Microenvironments of the Aged

"The environmental crisis in human dignity" (Proshansky, 1973) is a dramatic way of characterizing one of the major problems which gerontologists struggle to resolve in designing microenvironments for the elderly.

> The environmental crisis in human dignity lies not just in the overuse, the misuse, and the decay of physical settings, but far more significantly in how we conceive of the individual in relation to any such setting. [Proshansky, 1973. p. 1]

Proshansky labels this situation a crisis because spaces and places are not only improperly designed in physical terms, but because designs also overlook human needs for privacy, territoriality, and freedom of choice, and often conceive of the individual as a simple machine. Unintended consequences, once they appear, are often ignored, and no attempt is made to evaluate just how well the setting actually works. The danger is that old people will adjust, at the price of a continuing erosion of the properties that make them distinctly human—an issue to be discussed in detail shortly.

Small Units of Residency

These comments introduce our discussion of the smaller units of residency and personal space. Perceptions of environmental congruence and familiarity and the dimensions of relationship, personal development, and system maintenance (Kiritz & Moos, 1964) become much more intense in the microenvironment.

It is striking to note that about 70 percent of all elderly heads of families own their own housing. According to Struyk (1977), in 1973 about 62 percent of the elderly heads of households in large metropolitan areas owned their own homes, 74 percent in nonmetropolitan urban locations, 83 percent in rural nonfarm areas, and 90 percent on farms. Those most likely to be homeowners are white, currently married, the "young-old," and those with better education.

Housing Quality

The quality of housing for those over the age of sixty-five varies, as might be expected, on the simple basis of income. Also not surprising is the significantly greater prevalence of housing deficiencies (e.g., lack of complete kitchen or plumbing facilities, broken plaster, peeling paint, leaking roofs, holes in floors) among elderly renters than among elderly owners (Lawton, 1980). The greatest disparity in percentages of units reporting housing deficiencies is between those white suburban elderly in western states and the rural black elderly in the south, where deficiencies in some instances are as much as twenty-three times greater. In spite of these data, surveys of housing satisfaction among nationally based samples of elderly in public housing indicate a high overall degree of satisfaction with their current housing status. Whether these surveys do in fact accurately reflect real satisfaction or are artifacts remains moot. Perhaps the relatively high levels of satisfaction reported in such studies means that these elderly persons have in time learned to adapt, in the sense that they have learned to live with less.

Housing Satisfaction

Availability and accessibility of neighborhood and community services and resources comprise only one aspect of environmental congruence. Satisfaction with housing must also be considered. Although many elderly persons prefer to live in their own homes regardless of condition or location, different types of housing fitting a relatively broad spectrum have developed to accommodate those aged who either require or prefer alternative housing arrangements.

One study that addressed itself at least indirectly to environmental congruence is an extensive investigation carried out by Hamovitch, Peterson, and Larson (1976). This study provides a complex analysis of the global concept of housing "fulfillment" and of the specific ways various types of housing accommodations meet the needs of aged individuals.

An antecedent to this investigation is Francis Carp's (1966) classic study of in-movers to Victoria Plaza, which sampled a low income group of elderly. A major focus was on satisfaction with specific physical aspects of their premove housing. Carp's longitudinal design provides a wealth of data including selected personal characteristics of the elderly subjects. Some of Carp's data challenge conclusions drawn by Rosow in his earlier study of social aspects of housing for the elderly (Rosow, 1961). The Hamovitch, Peterson, and Larson study tests both the Carp and Rosow conclusions about elderly housing.

Hamovitch et al. selected samples of individuals representing a wide range of socioeconomic conditions and living in a variety of housing arrangements. Sampling was from:

1. A coastal retirement community (middle to upper middle class)
2. A desert retirement community (middle class)
3. A DPSS (Department of Public and Social Service) and urban retirement hotel (low income)
4. Denominational high-rise apartments (Anglo-Caucasian, black, and life care)
5. A trailer park (lower middle class)
6. High and low age density
7. A matched sample (matched with sample 1)
8. Out-movers.

Table 10–5 shows the results of life satisfaction by sample communities. One general conclusion to be drawn from these data is that the least satisfied are metropolitan black elderly, low-income trailer park elderly, and out-movers, who seem "still to be searching for their ideal life pattern" (Hamovitch, Peterson, & Larson, 1976).

Types of Residence for the Elderly

Elderly persons reside in a wide range of diverse residential facilities: individual homes, board-and-care residences, hotels, mobile homes, public

TABLE 10–5.   Life Satisfaction by Sample Communities

Location	Low Life Satisfaction		High Life Satisfaction	
	N	%	N	%
Coastal	231	50.2	229	49.8
Desert	58	59.8	39	40.2
Urban Hotel	35	68.6	14	27.5
DPSS	66	75.0	21	23.9
Denominational High-Rise				
A: Anglo-Caucasian	21	53.8	18	46.2
B: black	62	67.4	30	32.6
C: life care	13	40.6	19	59.4
Trailer park	49	75.4	16	24.6
High age density	134	63.8	76	36.2
Low age density	133	63.9	75	36.1
Matched sample	201	49.5	204	50.2
Out-movers	40	61.5	25	38.5

Source: Hamovitch, Peterson, & Larson (1976).

housing units, congregate retirement units, and institutions. These, in turn, vary from luxurious to impoverished and inadequate.

Increasing proportions of new public housing units have been designated for elderly individuals and persons with handicaps. At least 56 percent of public housing residents are persons aged sixty-two years old or older. Table 10–6 shows levels of occupancy for various Housing and Urban Development programs in 1976. At this writing HUD is also committed to 700,000 additional units. Prospects for these "commitments," however, are uncertain, in light of the federal government's objective to "cap" additional built units

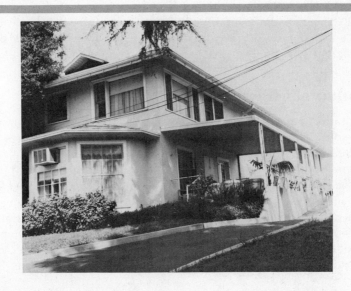

**TABLE 10–6. Elderly Occupancy in HUD-Assisted Housing
Programs, June 1976**

Program	Total Units	Number Occupied by Elderly[a]	Elderly as Percentage of Occupants
Public housing	1,035,861	455,779[b]	44
Section 236	550,000	192,000	35
Section 202	45,275	45,275	100
Section 231	54,606	54,606	100
Section 8[c]			
New construction	25,636	22,548	88
Substantial rehabilitation	4,341	3,233	75
Existing housing	232,505	110,621	48
Loan management	95,292	44,015	46

Source: Welfield, I., & Struyk, R. J. *Occasional Papers in Housing and Community Development,* no. 3, 1979. Washington, D.C.: Office of Policy Development and Research, U.S. Department of Housing and Urban Development, 1978.

[a]"Elderly" includes people 62+ and younger handicapped people.

[b]Includes elderly in both elderly-designated units and nondesignated units.

[c]Figures as of Dec. 31, 1977.

at 3.8 million (thus effectively eliminating some 300,000 additional units; Kinnard, 1982, personal communication).

It is interesting to note that of all planned public housing Section 202 facilities, as of 1980 only one, Pilgrim Tower (associated with and managed by California Lutheran Homes, Los Angeles), is devoted exclusively to the care of deaf elderly. In most other instances, deaf elders and elderly with severe hearing impairments must take their chances in residences and facilities without special design considerations geared to their special needs. An interesting example of these needs is revealed in the unexpected reply of the manager of Pilgrim Tower to the query, "What's your greatest management problem?" The answer: "Plumbing." Why plumbing? Because deaf elderly persons cannot determine the functional status of toilet and sink drains *by the sound,* which is the way that hearing persons without exception make such judgments.

Institutions for the Elderly

Institutional settings represent a major class of microenvironments for older persons. These generally are categorized as nursing homes (skilled nursing facilities, or SNFs), personal care units (intermediate care facilities), and retirement residences featuring independent living. Nursing homes are defined for state licensure as providing twenty-four-hour skilled nursing, medical, and other health services under the supervision of a registered nurse. State regulations for nursing homes vary, but federal regulations under the provision of Medicare (Title XVIII of the Social Security Act) and Medicaid ("Medi-Cal" in California; Title XIX) have introduced some standardization. Institutions are not required to accept Medicaid residents. Because

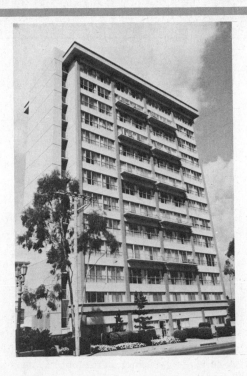

the level of reimbursement for Medicaid payments is low and does not cover the cost of comprehensive, "quality" services, many institutions limit the number of Medicaid residents to a small proportion or virtually exclude such individuals in favor of full-paying "private" residents.

Some states may license and thereby regulate intermediate care and board-and-care facilities, but the regulations and criteria vary widely. Table 10–7 shows the distribution of beds in proprietary (for profit) and nonproprietary (nonprofit) nursing homes. Table 10–8 shows some of the demographic characteristics of nursing home residents. Note that the largest proportions of elderly individuals residing in nursing homes are Caucasian, female (largely widows), and over seventy-four years of age.

Institutional Microenvironments

In 1977, the National Center for Health Statistics (1978) counted in its Master Facility Inventory 18,300 nursing homes and personal care (PC or "intermediate care") facilities, not including mental hospitals. Taken together these housed 1,300,000 residents, of whom 85 percent were sixty-five years old or older.

The question most frequently raised by researchers, planners, and families of elderly persons is, what is the quality of life for older people in institutional settings? The theoretical constructs alluded to earlier in this chapter

TABLE 10–7. Percentage Distributions of Nursing Homes by Sponsorship and Number of Beds, 1973–74

	Nonprofit (3,900 Institutions)	Proprietary (11,900 Institutions)
Number of beds		
Fewer than 50	36	42
50–99	36	35
100–199	20	21
200 or more	8	2
	100	100
Certification status		
Both Medicare and Medicaid	24	27
Skilled nursing or both skilled and intermediate	26	21
Intermediate care only	24	29
Not certified	25	22
	99	99

Source: National Center for Health Statistics. *Selected Operating and Financial Characteristics of Nursing Homes.* Vital and Health Statistics series 13, no. 22. Rockville, Md.: USDHEW, 1975.

will provide the basis for discussion of this very ambiguous term, "quality of life," with respect to institutional microenvironments. Following the Kiritz-Moos (1974) classification of environments along relationship, personal development, and system maintenance dimensions, we may operationalize Gibson's approach to ecological perception, a crucial factor in determining subjective microenvironmental quality. According to Gibson (1966, 1979), each person must actively engage in the process of "information pickup" in

TABLE 10–8. Characteristics of Nursing Home Residents and Community- Resident Elderly (Percentages)

Characteristic	Nursing Home	Community
Sex		
Male	28	41
Female	72	59
Race		
White	95	91
Nonwhite	5	9
Marital status		
Married	12	54
Widowed	69	37
Divorced or separated	3	3
Never married	15	6
Age		
65–74	17	63
74+	83	37

Source: National Center for Health Statistics. *Characteristics, Social Contacts, and Activities of Nursing Home Residents.* Vital and Health Statistics ser. 13, no. 27. Rockville, Md.: USDHEW, 1977.

order to perceive the "affordances" of the environment directly. Environmental affordances simultaneously define the structure and function of the environment and of the perceiving individual, thereby increasing the individual's knowledge of the world and his or her place in it.

Individual or environmental limitations restrict information pickup activities in various ways. In the presence of such limitations, normal interactions with (and perceptions of) objects and events are seriously impaired. Environmental limitations which are social in nature might include constraints imposed upon the activities of the institutionalized elderly by other people (for example, family members, physicians, staff members), by the institution itself, or by the sociocultural context in which the institutionalized older person lives (for instance, behavioral norms which enthusiastically encourage bingo but do not condone going to the racetrack; which encourage TV watching but prohibit hugging, kissing, and other sexual activities).

The negative effects of ageist attitudes on the part of others and of noxious actions toward aged residents (e.g., treating institutionalized older persons in a demeaning, condescending way) would seem to be obvious. Less obvious are the deleterious consequences for the aged of social environments lacking dignity, respect, and support.

Studies reported by Kiritz and Moos (1974) examine the physiological effects of social environments. Their work cites experimental evidence suggesting that cohesion or affiliation reduces susceptibility to physiological stress responses. Not only is a cohesive group less susceptible to stress but, conversely, a group member who deviates from the norms of the cohesive group may begin to experience stress response. Furthermore, additional evidence supports the hypothesis that "responsibility is a dimension of the social environment which is associated with physiological changes in its members" (namely, greater corticosteroid responses, 17 to 20 percent higher heart rates, greater incidence of coronary atherosclerosis, increased excretion of adrenalin, and the like). These physiological changes are related most persuasively by experimental evidence to such environmental dimensions as personal responsibility, involvement and interaction, work pressures, and uncertainty (that is, the clarity or ambiguity of the setting, of one's roles, or of the amount and degree of environmental change).

Privacy and Self-Esteem

Several important dimensions of person-environment transactions were examined by Aloia (1973), who studied the relationships among perceived privacy options, the sense of control over the direction of one's own life, and the degree of self-esteem in institutionalized and noninstitutionalized elderly. One general finding from the data indicates the significant influence of privacy options (or lack thereof) and control upon the level of perceived self-esteem.

The relationship between privacy and self-esteem appears to be part of a more complex interaction between individual and environment. Privacy for the older person becomes an important means of achieving competence in interaction with the environment. This is especially critical in institutional microenvironments where privacy options tend to be limited. "The [elderly] individual also maintains or establishes control physically, through the effective use of space and distance, and psychologically, by limiting and protecting personal communications" (Aloia, 1973, p. 87).

A similar study of the privacy question and institutionalized elderly found that desire for privacy correlated not at all with such demographic variables as age, sex, level of education, or marital status. Desire for (or importance of) privacy, however, was in this study closely associated with length of time in the institution (Schwartz, 1969). The findings indicated a situation analogous to time spent in a hospital. If one expects one's stay in a hospital to be of relatively short duration, then one is willing to forgo certain privacy options (including a private room, especially if cost is an important factor) because the inconvenience and undesirability are highly temporary. But if the situation is perceived as permanent, then the privacy issue assumes considerably greater personal importance.

Bayne (1971) suggests that in large measure the dependency, apathy, and withdrawal so frequently observed in elderly residents of nursing homes may be a function of their accommodation to an environment that purports to promote health but actually encourages the sick role, that provides treatment but does so through tight regulation and stifling control. The very effectiveness of such a program can endanger the institutionalized person's will to self-determination by virtue of the passivity produced through the imposition of unnecessary controls.

Further evidence strongly suggests that elderly persons tend to deteriorate physically and psychologically as fundamental needs for autonomy, self-direction, self-esteem, and functional competence are ignored or neglected (Cornbleth, 1977; Kart & Manard, 1976; Reid, Haas, and Hawkings, 1977; Schulz & Brenner, 1977; Wolk & Teleen, 1976). All of these consequences of environmental constraints or limitations are associated with the relationship dimensions of environment mentioned earlier (cf. Kiritz & Moos, 1974).

The loss of independence or autonomy, whether it occurs in institutional or extrainstitutional microenvironmental settings, may lead to overwhelming negative perceptions of helplessness (cf. discussion of "learned helplessness," Chapter 3), which are often precursors of premature death (Carp, 1977; Seligman, 1975). Such perceptions are implicated in the conceptual model developed by Kiritz and Moos (1974) describing the relationship between the social environment and physiological functioning. This model, illustrated in Figure 10–3, is complementary to the Lawton-Nahemow (1973) model of behavioral ecology in later life. At the same time, Figure 10–3 depicts the person-environment transactional perspective by indicating how the individual affects the environment, which reciprocally and in turn affects the individual.

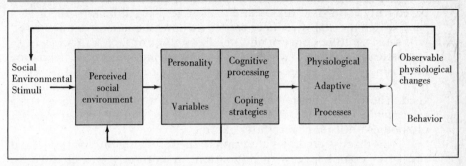

FIGURE 10–3.   Conceptual Model: Social Environment and Observable Physiological Changes
Source: Kiritz & Moos (1974).

In sum, Lawton states,

The vulnerability of this age group [the elderly] makes more compelling the search for ways of elevating behavior and experienced quality of life through environmental means. By this line of reasoning, if we could design housing with fewer barriers, neighborhoods with more enriching resources, or institutions with higher stimulating qualities, we could improve the level of functioning of many older persons more than proportionately [1980, p. 15].

CRITICAL DISCUSSION

"Nursing Home Regulations: Sense or Nonsense?"

Although the total number of older persons residing in nursing homes at any given time represents barely 4 to 5 percent of America's elderly, such institutions consume literally billions of dollars in private payments as well as Medicare and Medicaid funds. Standards and regulations for such facilities are therefore of legitimate concern.

The fundamental issue is not whether criteria and regulations should be promulgated and maintained. It would be no more feasible or reasonable to argue against regulating nursing homes than it would be to maintain the same position with respect to automobile, bedding, housing, or other product safety standards. The question is what kinds of criteria are to be used and how are they to be implemented, enforced, and evaluated.

Standards for "adequate" (or minimum) care are in fact specified in statutes and regulations covering nursing homes today in virtually all states. Inspections of nursing homes are regularly carried out on the assumption that if nursing homes conscientiously comply with such regulations, adequate care of the aged residents will thereby be assured, and public concern allayed.

Are these assumptions upon which regulations and inspections are based truly valid? Is it reasonable to assume that minimum standards of care, which inevitably reduces care to the lowest common denominator, will satisfy public concern and need? In point of fact, an increasingly sophisticated public (which is itself growing older) is becoming increasingly more aware that nursing homes can and should be more than clean, orderly, well-run, well-regulated, sterile warehouses for the aged. The public sentiment is that if life in a nursing home is not a *worthwhile* enterprise, then such facilities are merely repositories for old bodies until they mercifully expire.

This discussion draws attention to the following proposition: Total and strict compliance with regulations as currently written in most states does not insure "quality care," an impressive term for which no legal definition exists. The corollary to this is that strict adherence to and compliance with current standards tends to deter such care. It is demonstrable that such compliance in fact interferes with attempts to provide enrichment and improve quality of life for institutionalized elderly individuals, a consequence of greater moment than the economic burden of complying with irrelevant and inappropriate regulations.

A second proposition is that the preoccupation of current regulatory criteria with essentially medical and public health concerns and with management issues (such as sanitation, hygiene, drugs, temperature of water, utilization review, record keeping, linen control, laundry) tends to deflect attention from the equally (perhaps more) urgent task of providing worthwhile living for elderly nursing home residents. Many if not most such regulatory details contribute only peripherally to quality of life as perceived and defined by most gerontologists.

The third proposition is that it is inappropriate, if not irrational, to apply criteria and enforce standards and regulations that focus almost exclusively on credentialing, documentation, administrative practices, and operations, rather than on outcome criteria. The situation might be compared to determining the quality of a restaurant not by eating the food served there, but by determining where and how much the cook was trained, what types of stoves and cooking utensils are used, how clean and orderly the kitchen and eating areas are, and whether there is at least one waiter for every four customers. That may tell us *something*, but it certainly tells us nothing about how palatable the food is or what the experience of eating there is like—yet in the final analysis, that is what eating out is all about. Just so, what finally matters for the institutionalized aged is the quality of their lives.

As it becomes evident that criteria for nursing home standards of care pay major attention to the "technology" of care (i.e., factors directly concerned with biological survival) and much less attention to quality of life (i.e., factors that make surviving worthwhile), it also becomes clear that America supports a nursing home regulatory system that promulgates more nonsense than good sense. Many competent, well-intentioned nursing home administrators, overwhelmed with the demand for more and more detailed, often irrelevant documentation and impracticable administrative practices, opt for paper compliance with regulations. Others, disenchanted and demoralized by such a system, leave the field. The nursing home enterprise, a growth industry in America now and in the foreseeable future, needs *more* competent, well-meaning administrators, not fewer.

A system which produces such outcomes, no matter how efficient or well-intentioned, can fairly be described as an irrational system. It can also be characterized as failing to achieve its ostensible goal, namely, serving and protecting the consumer (the aged resident) in full measure, and satisfying public concern and need. Perhaps a better system, more rational and more appropriate, would be a system based on outcome criteria ("the proof of the pudding is in the eating"), monitored and assessed by those with the largest personal investment: elderly residents, their families, and the constituent staffs.

The Penalizing Microenvironment

Institutionalized elderly may operate at a double disadvantage when they are subject to both individual (internal) and environmental or social (external) limitations. Individual limitations include sensory, perceptual, cognitive, emotional, and psychomotor impairments or disabilities. These factors may handicap the institutionalized elder's ability to engage actively in information pickup, thus reducing the level of meaningful contact between the elder and his or her environment.

External limitations include social and environmental restrictions upon activity (see earlier discussion of social restraints on behavior). Environmental limitations are those inherent in a filtered, impoverished environment. One such limitation is a paucity of environmental cues (those items which enable one to identify and discriminate spatial areas—"landmarks") which makes it difficult to find one's way around. Another is a lack of environmental stimulation of the senses (visual, auditory, gustatory, olfactory, haptic). An ambiguous or poorly defined environmental setting (i.e., one lacking clarity, from the perspective of Kiritz and Moos, 1974), and an environment that penalizes the older person with disabilities because of its poor, inappropriate design are still other examples of limiting environments. The negative effects of such environments are well known:

> Close examination of nursing home residents . . . reveals that more than 50%
> display behavioral problems which are linked directly to inability to
> accomplish their activities of daily independent living (ADL). A number of the
> behavioral symptoms have been shown to be closely linked to isolation from
> others and environmental deprivation at any age [O'Brien & Wagner, 1980, p.
> 82; cf. Ernst et al., 1978; Ernst, Beran, & Kleinhauz, 1979; Lawton, 1974;
> McDonald, 1978; Wallach, Kelley, & Abrams, 1979].

The whole category of furniture nicely illustrates the problem. Chairs, tables, shelves, storage bins, blackboards, doorknobs, and all the accoutrements of a nursery or other school environment are almost without exception specifically designed for children so as not to penalize them with respect to their functioning in that environment. Special so-called orthopedic designs are commonly employed by persons with special motor disabilities or deficits.

Yet those who choose furniture utilized in settings for older persons tend to ignore the penalties imposed by inappropriate furniture designs. Chairs or sofas that are too low or too soft or are without arms create serious problems for those who suffer from arthritis or restricted mobility or stiffness or other deficits and find it enormously difficult to get in and out of such seating. Similar problems can readily be seen in other aspects of the environment which presume to serve the aged: poorly designed beds; storage space so low or so high as to be virtually inaccessible to the elderly; tables of inconvenient height or dimensions; indistinguishable or nonexistent visual or other orienting cues (e.g., no signs, posters, clocks, message boards, calendars, etc.); windows, elevators, water faucets, and heat controls almost impossible for stiff fingers and joints to manipulate; wheelchairs which are unstable or allow uncomfortable and even unsafe slumping by the elderly occupant; heavy doors and "blind" entry and exit portals; and eating and cooking utensils and stoves, medicine cabinets, storage bottles, and stairs that range from inconvenient and unsuitable to positively dangerous. The range of problems

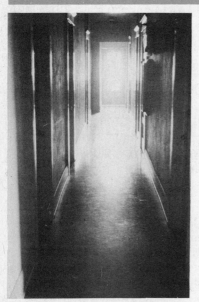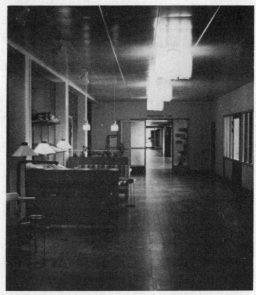

These two examples of corridors in long term facilities show the contrast between a sterile, barren environment and one that compensates and stimulates the institutionalized aged.

suggests the desirability of developing a diagnostic approach to designing the microenvironment for the elderly, one that will eliminate negative elements and establish criteria for relevant and adequate design concepts.

Infantilizing the Elderly

A special cautionary note is in order at this point. In designing microenvironments which do not penalize the older person and thus impair or minimize whatever functional capacities are available, it must be borne in mind at the same time that a very fine line often exists between the supportive, compensating, prosthetic environment and environmental inputs which either subtly or blatantly preempt the functional capacities of aged individuals and thereby infantilize them. Designers and behavioral scientists who desire to contribute to environmental design must also recognize that it is neither possible nor wise to eliminate all risks for the older person. Nor is it desirable to try to do anything more than will facilitate self-sufficiency. In person-environment transactional terms, any environment which tends to infantilize older people will subvert their sense of self-worth and self-esteem, and will ultimately defeat many of the positive effects which can be envisioned for an environment designed specifically for institutionalized older people.

A great many institutional microenvironments in which aged persons live, as well as written descriptions of such environments, suggest the persistence of the simplistic notion that humans are infinitely adaptable. This is surely an erroneous view. Both common sense and very good empirical data persuasively demonstrate that human adaptability is finite. Given the fact that our experience repeatedly shows the limits of adaptability with respect to certain modes and intensities of environmental press (and following the ecological models of aging proposed by Lawton and Nahemow, and by Kiritz and Moos), it is curious, even surprising, that relatively little attention is being paid to environments specifically designed to adapt to the special needs and requirements of the aged with disabilities.

The Prosthetic Environment

The design of microenvironments for the aged must be aimed not only at ameliorating stresses, minimizing the effects of losses, and compensating for deficits, but must do so in ways which enhance the individuals' effectiveness, support their competence, and thus help them maintain self-esteem. Design modifications and concepts which omit or underestimate these outcomes, especially for the aged, may be seen as irrelevant, if not pernicious. Proper design concepts, construction, and modifications, when effectively implemented, on the other hand, constitute the kind of prosthetic environment which compensates the elderly in large measure for their losses, and helps them maintain functional competence to a significant degree. Such

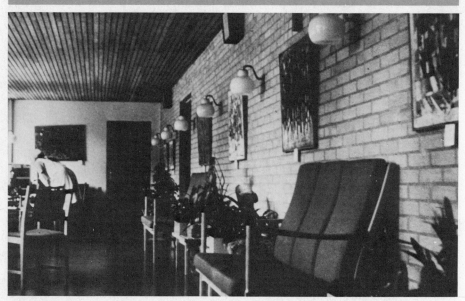

This corridor in a Swedish housing facility illustrates some of the best features in micro-design principles for the aged: high back chairs with arms, environmental stimulation, "texture" and cues, adequate and well-placed lighting.

designs can be said to sustain self-esteem, which is what the design of microenvironments for the elderly is really all about.

Other students and investigators of person-environment transactions have articulated congruent formulations which are readily adaptable to designing environments for the aged. Raymond Studer, for example, in his analysis of behavior-contingent physical systems (1970), is obviously leaning heavily on Skinnerian operant behavioral analysis when he views a designed environment as a "learning system." Such a system requires that environmental variables be arranged so as to bring about the desired state of behavioral outcomes.

This principle is one of the keys to the appropriate design of microenvironments for the aged. Alongside the list of items to be avoided, we must make note of those positive environmental aspects which enable the aged person with disabilities to continue to function reasonably competently. The environment must not penalize the aged person for his or her deficits, to be sure; it must also be reasonably barrier-free. More than that, the environment must be designed not only to make life possible but also to make life worthwhile. The environment must maintain beauty (or bring beauty back, if it has been missing); it must overcome the filtering effects of possibly declining sensory efficiency by increasing the amount and intensity of environmental stimulation and impact; it must provide real options and thus the possibility of real choice (not the least of which is the privacy option); it must provide

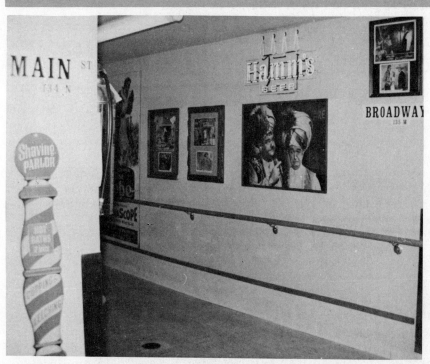

An "intersection" in a nursing home which uses street signs, old posters, and advertising signs to "normalize" life by providing the environmental cues and the visual stimulation so necessary to competent functioning.

for relatively easy negotiation of space, through clarity and extensive use of "readable" environmental cues; it must help maintain to some degree a familiar life-style and provide some incentives for modification and growth; it must provide continuing opportunities and mechanisms for activity which can be taken seriously and found personally rewarding by the individual; it must make involvement in the ebb and flow of daily living gratifying and reassuring, rather than anxiety-arousing; and finally, it must offer variety and adventure within limits that are satisfying to the individual. In other words, the goal of designing microenvironments for institutionalized elderly must be to "normalize" institutional life. The conceptualization and application of this goal have been systematically and eloquently described by Wolfensberger and his colleagues and "translated" from these researchers' Scandinavian setting to fit the Canadian and North American scene: "Normalization principles require that individuation, growth challenges, respect for rights, etc., must be recognized in and supported by a delicate interplay between programs and physical environments" (Wolfensberger et al., 1972, p. 73).

O. R. Lindsley's observation (1964) that our society is willing to spend money on the design of environments that maintain life, but not on those that maintain dignified behavior, drives home the point.

Summary

If we are to understand more fully the behaviors of older people we need to specify the dynamic, symbiotic relationships between aged individuals and their environments. These relationships are variable and complex, compounding the difficulties in defining environmental components. Heuristic schemes developed by Moos and associates and by Lawton and Nahemow provide useful ecological models of adaptation and aging. A number of investigators have added many other relevant dimensions to the picture in their efforts to specify ecological variables.

This chapter has treated the macroenvironment (states, communities, neighborhoods) with respect to location of elderly persons and availability of services to these individuals. The concept of environmental congruence becomes an important variable in establishing a fit between the adaptive capacities of the old and the environments in which they live. Microenvironments are discussed in terms of small units of residency, housing quality, satisfaction with housing, and types of residence.

Institutions for the elderly consist of nursing homes differentiated with respect to "levels of care." The design of institutional microenvironments is a critical consideration in determining the functional capability of elderly residents. Privacy, autonomy, self-esteem, and continued capacity for competent activities of daily living hinge on such dimensions of the microenvironment as environmental stimulation, environmental clues, and environmental support. Administrators, service providers, designers, and planners need to be able to distinguish between penalizing (noncongruent) and nonpenalizing (compensatory or prosthetic) environments. The environment as a behavior-modifying agent is also discussed.

References

Aloia, A. Privacy options, locus of control, and self-esteem in the aged. Doctoral dissertation, California School of Professional Psychology, 1973.

Altman, I. *The environment and social behavior.* Belmont, Cal.: Wadsworth, 1975.

Altman, I., & Lett, E. The ecology of personal relationships: A classification system and conceptual model. In I. McGrath (Ed.), *Social and psychological factors in stress.* New York: Holt, Rinehart & Winston, 1970.

Barker, R. On the nature of the environment. *Journal of Social Issues,* 1963, **19**(4), 17–38. (a)

Barker, R. *The stream of behavior.* New York: Appleton-Century-Crofts, 1963. (b)

Barker, R. G. *Ecological psychology: Concepts and methods for studying the environment of human behavior.* Stanford: Stanford University Press, 1968.

Bayne, J. R. Environmental modification for the older person. *Gerontologist,* 1971, **11**(4, part 1), 314–317.

Bevan, W. The contextual basis of behavior. *American Psychologist,* 1968, **23**(10), 701–714.

Blake, B. F., Lawton, M. P., & Lau, S. *Community resources and need satisfaction: An age comparison.* Philadelphia, Pa.: Philadelphia Geriatric Center, 1978.

Brunswik, E. Scope and aspects of the cognitive problem. In H. Gruber, R. Jessor, & K. Hammond (Eds.), *Cognition: The Colorado symposium.* Cambridge, Mass.: Harvard University Press, 1957.

Carlson, R. *The end of medicine.* New York: Wiley, 1975.

Carp, F. *A future for the aged.* Austin: University of Texas Press, 1966.

Carp, F. Impact of improved living environment on health and life expectancy. *Gerontologist,* 1977, **17**(3), 242–249.

Cornbleth, T. Effects of a protected hospital ward area on wandering and non-wandering patients. *Journal of Gerontology,* 1977, **32**(5), 573–577.

Dubos, R. *Man, medicine, and environment.* New York: Prager, 1968.

Ernst, P., Beran, B., Safford, F., & Kleinhauz, M. Isolation and the symptoms of chronic brain syndrome. *Gerontologist,* 1978, **18**(5), 468–474.

Ernst, P., Beran, B., & Kleinhauz, M. Dr. Ernst and his colleagues reply. *Gerontologist,* 1979, **19**(6), 530–533.

Fitch, J. Experiential basis for aesthetic decisions. In H. Proshansky, W. Ittelson, & L. Rivlin (Eds.), *Environmental psychology.* New York: Holt, Rinehart & Winston, 1970, Pp. 76–83.

Gibson, J. J. *The senses considered as perceptual systems.* Boston: Houghton Mifflin, 1966.

Gibson J. J. *The ecological approach to visual perception.* Boston: Houghton Mifflin, 1979.

Haley, J. *Strategies of psychotherapy.* New York: Grune & Stratton, 1963.

Hall, C., & Lindzey, G. *Theories of personality.* 2nd ed. New York: Wiley, 1970.

Hall, E. T. *The silent language.* Greenwich, Conn.: Fawcett, 1959.

Hall, E. T. *The hidden dimension.* Garden City, N.J.: Anchor Books (Doubleday), 1969.

Hamovitch, M., Peterson, J., & Larson, A. *Housing needs and satisfactions of the elderly.* NIH Monograph (mimeo report). Los Angeles: University of Southern California, Andrus Gerontology Center, 1976.

Hawley, A. *Human ecology.* New York: Ronald Press, 1950.

Insel, P. M., & Moos, R. H. (Eds.). *Health and the social environment.* Lexington, Mass.: D. C. Heath & Company, 1974.

Kahana, E. A congruence model of person/environment interaction. In M. P. Lawton, P. Windley, & T. Byerts (Eds.), *Aging and the environment: Directions and perspectives.* New York: Garland STPM Press, 1980.

Kart, C. S., & Manard, B. B. Aging regions of the United States: 1970. In C. S. Kart & B. B. Manard (Eds.), *Aging in America: Readings in social gerontology.* Port Washington, N.Y.: Alfred Publishing, 1976.

Kart, C. S, & Manard, B. B. Quality of care in old age institutions. *Gerontologist,* 1976, **16**(3): 250–256.

Kiritz, S., & Moos, R. Physiological effects of social environments. *Psychosomatic Medicine,* 1974, **36**(2), 96–114.

Lawton, M. P. Assessment, integration, and environments for older people. *Gerontologist,* 1970, **10**(1), 38–46.

Lawton, M. P. Coping behavior and the environment of older people. In A. Schwartz & I. Mensh (Eds.), *Professional obligations and approaches to the aged.* Springfield, Ill.: Charles C. Thomas, 1974. Pp. 67–93.

Lawton, M. P. *Environment and aging.* Monterey, Cal.: Brooks/Cole (Wadsworth), 1980.

Lawton, M. P., & Nahemow, L. Ecology and the aging process. In C. Eisdorfer & M. P. Lawton (Eds)., *Psychology of adult development and aging.* Washington, D.C.: American Psychological Association, 1973. Pp. 619–674.

Lewin, K. *Principles of topological and vector psychology.* New York: McGraw-Hill, 1936.

Lindsley, O. R. Geriatric behavioral prosthetics. In R. Kastenbaum (Ed.), *New thoughts on old age.* New York: Springer, 1964. Pp. 41–60.

McDonald, M. Environmental programming for the socially isolated aging. *Gerontologist,* 1978, **18**(4), 350–354.

Moos, R. H. *The human context: Environmental determinants of behavior.* New York: Wiley-Interscience, 1976.

Murray, H. *Explorations in personality.* New York: Oxford University Press, 1938.

National Center for Health Statistics. *An overview of nursing home characteristics.* Provisional data from the 1977 National Nursing Home Survey. Advance data no. 35. Hyattsville, Md.: USDHEW, 1978.

Newcomer, R. Housing services and neighborhood activities. Paper presented at the 26th annual meeting of the Gerontological Society of America, Miami, Fla., 1973.

O'Brien, J., & Wagner, D. Help-seeking by the frail elderly. *Gerontologist,* 1980, **20**(1), 78–83.

Proshansky, H. The environmental crisis in human dignity. *Journal of Social Issues,* 1973, **29**(4), 1–20.

Proshansky, H., Ittelson, W., & Rivlin, L. *Environmental psychology: Man and his physical setting.* New York: Holt, Rinehart & Winston, 1970.

Regnier, V. Neighborhood planning for the urban elderly. In D. Woodruff & J. Birren (Eds.), *Aging: Scientific perspectives and social issues.* New York: D. Van Nostrand, 1975. Pp. 295–312.

Reid, D., Haas, G., & Hawkings, D. Locus of desired control and positive self-concept of the elderly. *Journal of Gerontology,* 1977, **32**(4), 441–450.

Rosow, I. *Social integration of the aged.* New York: Free Press, 1967.

Sargent, F. Man-environment: Problems for public health. *American Journal of Public Health,* 1972, **62**, 628–833.

Schooler, K. The relationship between social interaction and morale of the elderly as a function of environmental characteristics. *Gerontologist,* 1969, **9**(1), 25–29.

Schooler, K. A comparison of rural and nonrural elderly on selected variables. In R. Atchley & T. Byerts (Eds.), *Environments and the rural aged.* Washington, D.C.: Gerontological Society of America, 1975.

Schooler, K. Response of the elderly to environment: A stress-theoretic perspective. In M. P. Lawton, P. Windley, & T. Byerts (Eds.), *Aging and the environment: Directions and perspectives.* New York: Garland STPM Press, 1981.

Schulz, R., & Brenner, G. Relocation of the aged: A review and theoretical analysis. *Journal of Gerontology,* 1977, **32**(3), 323–333.

Schwartz, A. Perception of privacy among institutionalized aged. *Proceedings,* 77th annual meeting, American Psychological Association, Washington, D.C., 1969.

Schwartz, A. A transactional view of the aging process. In A. Schwartz & I. Mensh (Eds.), *Professional obligations and approaches to the aged.* Springfield, Ill.: Charles C. Thomas, 1974. Pp. 5–29.

Schwartz, A., & Proppe, H. Toward person/environment transactional research in aging. *Gerontologist,* 1970, **10**(3), 228–232.

Seligman, M. E. P. *Helplessness: On Depression, development, and death.* San Francisco: W. H. Freeman, 1975.

Sells, S. B. An interactionist looks at the environment. *American Psychologist,* 1963, **18**(11), 696–702.

Sommer, B. *Personal space.* Englewood Cliffs, N.J.: Prentice-Hall, 1969.

Struyk, R. The housing situation of elderly Americans. *Gerontologist,* 1977, **17**(5), 130–139.

Studer, R. The dynamics of behavior-contingent physical systems. In H. Proshansky, W. Ittelson, & L. Rivlin (Eds.), *Environmental psychology.* New York: Holt, Rinehart & Winston, 1970. Pp. 56–75.

Wallach, H., Kelley, F., & Abrams, J. Psychosocial rehabilitation for chronic geriatric patients: An intergenerational approach. *Gerontologist,* 1979, **19**(5): 464–470.

Wolfensberger, W., Nirje, B., Olshansky, S., Perske, R., & Roos, P. *The principle of normalization in human services.* Toronto, Canada: National Institute on Mental Retardation, York University Campus (4700 Keefe Street, Downsview), 1972.

Wolk, S., & Teleen, S. Psychological and social correlates of life satisfaction as a function of residential constraint. *Journal of Gerontology,* 1976, **31**(1), 89–98.

For Further Reading

Bennett, R. (Ed.) *Aging, isolation, and resocialization.* New York: Van Nostrand Reinhold, 1980.

Byerts, T., Howell, S., & Pastalan, L. *The environmental context of aging.* New York: Garland STPM Press, 1979.

Fiske, D., & Maddi, S.(Eds.) *Functions of varied experience.* Homewood, Ill.: Dorsey Press, 1961.

Howell, S. Environments as hypotheses in human aging research. In L. W. Poon (Ed.), *Aging in the 1980s.* Washington, D.C.: American Psychological Association, 1980. Pp. 424–432.

Koncelik, J. *Designing the open nursing home.* Stroudsburg, Pa.: Dowden, Hutchinson, & Ross, 1976.

Liebowitz, B., Lawton, M. P., & Waldman, A. A prosthetically designed nursing home. *American Institute of Architects Journal,* 1979, **68**, 59–61.

Rowles, G. *Prisoners of space? Exploring the geographical experiences of older people.* Boulder, Colo.: Westview Press, 1978.

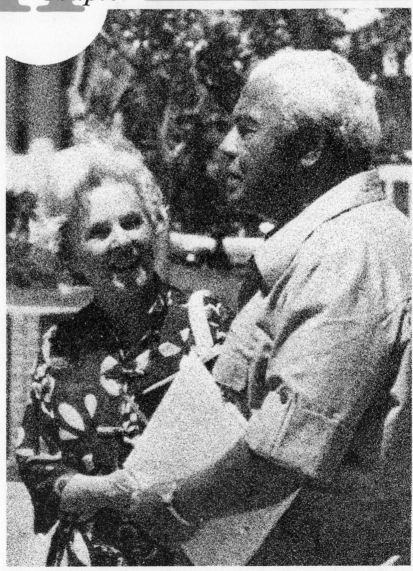

while you and i have lips and voices which
are for kissing and to sing with
who cares if some oneeyed son of a bitch
invents an instrument to measure spring with?

> *e. e. cummings*

By making imaginative use of change to channel change, we can not only
spare ourselves the trauma of future shock, we can reach out and
humanize distant tomorrows.

> *Alvin Toffler*
> *Future Shock (1971)*

Did You Know . . .

At 100, Grandma Moses was still painting?

At 94, Bertrand Russell was active in international peace drives?

At 93, George Bernard Shaw wrote the play *Farfetched Fables?*

At 91, Eamon de Valera served as president of Ireland?

At 91, Adoph Zukor was chairman of Paramount Pictures?

At 90, Pablo Picasso was producing drawings and engravings?

At 89, Mary Baker Eddy was director of the Christian Science Church?

At 89, Albert Schweitzer headed a hospital in Africa?

At 89, Arthur Rubenstein gave one of his greatest recitals in New York's Carnegie Hall?

At 88, Michelangelo did architectural plans for the Church of Santa Maria degli Angeli?

At 88, Pablo Casals was giving cello concerts?

At 88, Konrad Adenauer was chancellor of Germany?

At 85, Coco Chanel was the head of a fashion design firm?

At 84, W. Somerset Maugham wrote *Points of View?*

At 83, Alexander Kerensky wrote *Russia and History's Turning Point?*

At 82, Winston Churchill wrote *A History of the English-Speaking Peoples?*

At 82, Leo Tolstoy wrote I *Cannot Be Silent?*

At 81, Benjamin Franklin effected the compromise that led to the adoption of the U.S. Constitution?

At 81, Johann Wolfgang von Goethe finished *Faust?*

At 80, George Burns won an Academy Award for his performance in *The Sunshine Boys?* (Wallechinsky, Wallace, & Wallace, 1977).

This list is only a tiny, select sample of the varied activities and accomplishments, widely known or not, of persons in the later years of life. One might ask, in light of these examples, is gerontology exclusively a new science? Is it basically an array of varied services to the elderly? Is it merely (and fundamentally) consciousness-raising? Is it essentially an educational process? Or is it a combination of these things? Whatever it has been in the past, where is it going now? What are its future tasks?

An intriguing human interest story appeared in the *Los Angeles Times* (Rucker, 1978) under the catchy headline "OFFICE SWEETHEART IS GOING STRONG AT 91."

Bessie Lyons, the person about whom the story was written, was described as a diminutive, energetic woman who had been regularly employed since age sixteen, mostly in secretarial work. She had worked as an insurance agent at one time, and had been a member of the Internationl Machinists' Union during a World War II stint with Douglas Aircraft.

"When you work," Bessie was quoted as saying, "you don't have time for aches and pains."

Long after most people have retired, Bessie Lyons had hired on as a secretary for a property management firm and hadn't missed a day of work since. She first came to public attention on Valentine's Day 1974—her eighty-seventh birthday—when she enjoyed the honor of being chosen "office valentine" because of her tireless efforts and her persistent cheerfulness.

Her employer, a man of some seventy-five years, is very proud of Mrs. Lyons. He has boasted that she can type as well and as fast as anyone and can take dictation about as fast as he can speak.

"She keeps this place rolling and has fun at the same time," he explains.

Bessie herself admits to gulping down vitamins every day. She enjoys a mild drink now and then and goes out at least three evenings a week. Bessie obviously continues to enjoy life. She firmly believes—and will tell anyone who asks—that keeping busy is the key factor.

Successful Agers: The Other Side of the Century

Are aging individuals such as Bessie Lyons to be considered atypical— exceptions to the rule? What can gerontologists learn from such agers? What role do they play in the context of gerontological inquiry and service? Are they to be considered (and thus treated) as curiosities, a kind of social novelty?

The history of gerontology has been burdened with a preoccupation with the pathologies, deficits, and ills of a biased sample of elderly individuals. During an earlier period most attention was given to the sick aged, to aged in hospitals, and to severely impaired institutionalized older persons. The negative impressions of old age which grew from this situation were further compounded by the use of inappropriate research and measurement methods.

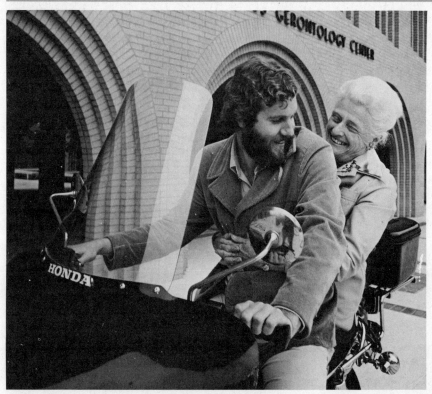

The findings of gerontology are helping to bring together the old and the young. A major contribution of gerontology is the demythologizing of the old for the young.

Many of those negative impressions will be challenged by systematic study of successful aging as increasing attention is directed toward more positive aspects of growing older: the capacities, strengths, skills, and potentials of persons in late maturity. Gerontology will be able to demonstrate that individuals such as Pablo Casals, Grandma Moses, George Burns, and Bessie Lyons, are not simply "exceptions to the rule."

A positive approach is very much encouraged by the unequivocal assertions of older individuals themselves. Ollie Randall, postoctogenarian founding member of the National Council on the Aging, has said, "If I have only one more day of life remaining, I still have a future." This was echoed by the eighty-year-old actress and model Judith Lowery. "Age," she said, "is my greatest asset. My wrinkles are what get me my jobs. . . . I never sit in a rocking chair unless I am well paid for it" (*Modern Maturity*, 1971).

This shifting of emphasis from the pathologies of aging to successful aging is a most appropriate response to Abraham Heschel's unsettling comment of over a decade ago: "Enabling us to reach old age, medical science may think it gave us a blessing; however, we continue to act as if it were a disease" (1971).

In 1973 a physician by the name of Jewett reported certain personality characteristics, traits, habit patterns, and hereditary factors that he described as common to long-living successful agers (Jewett, 1973). Jewett based these findings on a personal study of seventy-nine individuals between 87 and 103 years of age.

These "elite aged" have been characterized by Jewett and others as persons who, beyond merely surviving, are able to maintain social contacts befitting their needs and interests, pursue activities which challenge and intrigue them and are consonant with their life goals, and have a good capacity to adapt to changing life situations and events, that is, "roll with the punches." They are described as religious in the broadest sense of the word, with a well-developed sense of humor—and they enjoy life.

The vast majority of long-livers are of moderate size and body structure. Their habits and life-styles—dietary patterns, use of alcohol, coffee, drugs, smoking, exercise, working, sleeping, playing—are characterized by moderation. They enjoy relative freedom from accidents and are less plagued by anxiety.

These characteristics of successful long-livers appear to be independent of cultural constraints; they are shared by the old-old in rural and nonindustrialized places as well as by those of urban, industrialized societies, a notion corroborated by studies of the long-living Abkhasians (Benet, 1974) and a more recent study of 101 Caribbean centenarians (Snyder & Schwartz, 1981), and by reports of factors contributing to well-being or "successful" aging (Butler, 1974; Larson, 1978; Palmore, 1979).

Pursuit of the notion of successful aging will enable gerontologists to encourage others to open new doors of inquiry and to explore alternative ways of understanding and preparing for old age. Clues to successful aging, for example, are to be discovered in careful evaluation of the middle years, according to some gerontologists (Greenleigh, 1974). Enriching the dialogue between the elderly and their middle-aged children is also strongly recommended by gerontologists as a useful strategem for successful aging (Schwartz, 1977; Weinberg, 1974).

Attention to the ingredients of successful aging has also stimulated a renewed interest in the processes of creativity in the later years. The use of autobiographical journals and programmed reminiscing in the study of successful aging has uncovered the fact that these procedures also have potential therapeutic value for elderly who are depressed or have lost their zest for living. The method described by some as "guided autobiography (Reedy & Birren, 1980) is based on a systematic, written life review, which is said to lead to greater self-acceptance, lower anxiety and tension, a greater sense of energy and vigor, and greater social connectedness (cf. Allport, 1942; Butler, 1961, 1974; Lauer & Goldfield, 1970; Lickorish, 1975).

New Cohorts of Aged

Few gerontologists have failed to recognize the portents of rapidly changing societies and of a rapidly changing world. Most professional gerontologists are alert to the implications of the fact that future aged cohorts will be very different from those now living. In the three to five decades immediately ahead, all providers of services (and policymakers and researchers as well) will be dealing with elderly who presumably will be healthier than today's aged, because they will be better educated and more sophisticated about health care and health maintenance. Aged of the future for the most part will be better trained and more inclined (and will have greater opportunity) to be involved in careers on a selective, by-preference basis. As a consequence they are likely to be better off economically.

Increasing Political Clout

Because of the larger number and greater proportion of elderly persons in the population (approximately 15 to 18 percent of the population, or some 35 million people, will be sixty-five or older at the turn of the century), indications are that the future aged will be much more politically astute, articulate, and assertive. It follows that the old will therefore be more politically powerful and effective. As a special interest group (one that will include minority aged), the aged of the future can be expected to have gained considerable experience in the political arena, with their activities modeled after and sometimes linking up with the efforts of minority and women's groups. Even now organized senior citizen's groups, such as the American Association of Retired Persons (AARP), which recently merged with the National Retired Teachers Association to form an organization of 13 million members, can point to specific accomplishments: their legislative lobbying helped roll back the federal mandatory retirement age, won significant concessions on governmental proposals to reduce Social Security benefits, and strongly influenced the passage of provisions against ageism in the laws of the land. Nevertheless, in spite of changing patterns, public policy regarding the aged remains ambiguous in definition and scope and, at best, uneven and inconsistent in implementation and enforcement (Estes, 1979).

Aging Advocacy

A major task of gerontology in the past has been to generate and disseminate new information about aging. Doubtless this will remain a high priority.

Most gerontologists expect that public policy will be responsive to new data and that public policy will thus shift into ever greater congruence with current knowledge about aging. Professional gerontologists' fantasies not-

withstanding, how realistic is it to believe that public attitudes and the lucu-
brations of policymakers will readily respond to gerontologists' data and
experience with the aged, as though awarding a contract to the most intel-
lectually attractive bid? The discussions in Chapter 6 suggest that this expectation is not realistic at all.

A more practical scenario would redefine gerontology's role as a scientific, educational, and service enterprise in the society of the future. These
three aspects of professional activity are not likely to diminish. The changing
local, national, and international scene points to another, increasingly urgent
need: for gerontology to assume an advocacy role much more radical, more
persistent, and more comprehensive than has been the case to date. Cancer
research has, in the light of its findings, taken on an increasingly public and
aggressive advocacy role; aging research cannot allow itself to be far behind.

CRITICAL DISCUSSION
Advocacy for What?

A retrospective view of gerontology suggests that its traditional advocacy role may in fact be a two-edged sword. In certain respects, at least,
changes engineered by gerontology advocates for elders are sometimes
neither appropriate nor relevant (Estes, 1979; Weakland, 1981). For
example:

> When retirement became a commodity to be sold to Americans
> (Graebner, 1980), gerontologists played a supportive role by devising
> theories which stressed the need for elders' "adjustment" to the
> hardships and losses associated with aging. Because many such losses
> were socially generated, this emphasis upon individual conformity to the
> status quo must be viewed as system-sustaining and conservatively biased
> [Evans & Williamson, 1981, p. 24–25].

In a society where status and power are inextricably linked to
work, money, productivity, and ownership, mandatory retirement and
the Social Security system also are forms of social control and in certain
instances even repression of the old. They inevitably cast most elderly
into the dependent economic role of consumers instead of producers
(Evans & Williamson, 1981).

The Social Security system in effect invented "social aging" by for-
mally labeling individuals "old" as a feature of public pension eligibility. Age categorization inexorably tends to harden the lines of segregation between elderly persons and the rest of society. Aging advocates
and the categorical benefits programs supported by them have thus contributed, even if inadvertently, to the negative image of old people as
an essentially nonproductive and therefore superfluous segment of
society.

The case in point here is retirement, which in America in recent
decades has been the major mechanism for removing mature adults from
the work force. Considerable effort has been expended in assisting
(read: persuading) older workers to adjust to permanent loss of career

and remunerated work life, and of all the economic advantages and social and psychological benefits accruing thereto. At the same time, relatively little attention (certainly little public attention) has been given to consideration of an alternative: continuation of lifelong work and careers in late maturity (with attendant benefits) but at somewhat reduced levels of time and energy consistent with the interests and needs of the individual (Schwartz, 1974).

This plan has already been tried successfully elsewhere in the world. A Swedish experiment begun in mid-1976, called the partial-pension or phased retirement program, allows older workers to cut work time by as much as half while still receiving (from wages plus partial pension) income equal to about 85 percent of previous after-tax income from full-time work.

If advocacy for America's aged is truly to effect fundamental changes—in contrast to merely cosmetic changes—then it must be radical advocacy, carried out by true heroes and heroines. This will provide the antidote to at least the more explicit forms of social control and constraint of the old evident in the efforts to soft-pedal the power of the aged as a political voting bloc (Ragan & Davis, 1978), in dire predictions of a backlash against the elderly if they continue to press for age-based gains (Hudson, 1978), and in arguments that the only feasible goals for the aged are mere incremental gains (Pratt, 1976).

The question is not only advocacy for what, but also for whose benefit.

The norms of the graying society of tomorrow can only be expected to become increasingly dissonant with professional activities that are less than flexible, assertively innovative, and clearly relevant to the implicit and explicit needs of that society. The community of gerontological and geriatric researchers, scholars, and service providers will learn to communicate—because they must—not merely with each other, but in comprehensible terms with society at large at all levels. For example, a business-as-usual stance on the part of a mental health industry still clinging to outmoded clichés, arcane jargon, and inappropriate measures and rituals will do little to serve the needs of the future aged. Gerontology has the vitality, energy, imagination, and knowledge base necessary to assume an even more aggressive, dynamic advocacy and leadership role for change than heretofore. What faces gerontology is the reappraisal and redefinition of some of its roles and the reevaluation (and possibly reordering) of its priorities.

Conciousness-Raising

Although not part and parcel of gerontology's scientific and service activity, the sensitizing of the larger society to the issues and facts of aging has turned out to be an activity of major proportions and consequence. At the turn of this century the aged comprised a small percentage of the population.

Societal interest in the aged, in terms of public policy or the provision of special services or even recognition of the special needs of the old, was even smaller. There is no question but that the picture has changed.

The lessons learned from other social movements (including those of minority groups, women's liberation, and civil rights) have contributed to the growing prominence of aging as an issue in our country. The growth of research and practice in gerontology has focused national attention on this expanding segment of the population, as is quite evident from the White House Conference on Aging, for example, and government funding of age-based programs. For example, when Social Security and Medicare-Medicaid programs are taken into account, expenditures for the aged now constitute about one-third of the federal budget. None of this occurs in a vacuum. Gerontologists from academia and from public and private organizations and agencies will continue to play key roles in this rising tide of public awareness of aging.

The Media and Aging

The aging network, including such groups as AARP, the National Council of Senior Citizens, the National Council on the Aging, and the Gray Panthers, can take credit as a major influence in encouraging (and sometimes forcing!) the communications media to avoid stereotypes, myths, and negative images of aging and to pay more attention to fact and to positive images. Much stereotyping still appears in newspapers, but gerontology's continued efforts do pay off. All the public communication media—newspapers, radio, and television—are slowly but surely beginning to recognize gerontology as an important source of information. Articles on special issues concerned with aging appear with greater frequency in metropolitan dailies, such as the *New York Times* and *Los Angeles Times*. Many of these go well beyond mere listings of "senior citizens activities" and attempt to explore in some depth (or at least highlight) substantive issues, such as the economic well-being of the elderly, their housing and health, and pre- and postretirement activities. Radio stations are airing discussions by experts in the field and carrying public service announcements of particular interest to the aged.

Television continues to provide less than adequate programming for the elderly and more often than not presents older persons in an inaccurate and demeaning manner. Gerontologists must provide the major stimulus for more acceptable programming for the aged and for TV shows that do justice to older people. One pioneer in the field of TV gerontology is Richard Davis of the University of Southern California. Through negotiations with the Sears Foundation, through collaboration and production consultations with major networks and individual producers of movies and television programs, he has led the way in the successful production of such exemplary films and TV specials as "Peege," "Portrait of Grandpa Doc," the "Use It or Lose It" educational series, and the nationally syndicated series "Over Easy."

Intensive efforts, via formal and informal gerontology programs, to

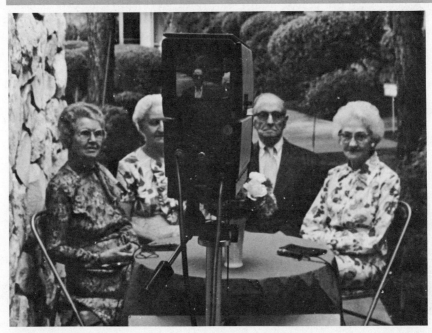

The use of television to provide information, as a motivational tool, and as a method of assessment is another "frontier" that gerontologists are beginning to explore.

increase public awareness and sensitivity to age-related issues are beginning to have an impact upon major social institutions (cf. Chapter 7) and industry. What began as an informal pilot project in preretirement preparation conducted by Virginia Boyack, California Federal Savings and Loan's vice-president for Life Planning, and Jesse Rifkind, former chief of Xerox's Advanced Development Laboratory, has now become part of Xerox's corporate policy and a continuing program. Other large corporations are following suit; Lockheed's Extension Program is one example. Two years ago the Lutheran Church in America introduced an extended session on aging as a regularly scheduled feature of its annual convocation. Most local Jewish Federations have introduced Committees on Aging into their organizational and regular activity structure. Other church groups have begun to focus significant attention on the aged segment of their constituencies. All such movements will increasingly look to gerontology in the future for data and for assistance.

Medical schools and other professional training programs are beginning to respond to the obvious need for special training in aging. Los Angeles' UCLA/USC Long Term Care Center has developed a viable program of research and training in geriatric medicine. Of the 385 Family Practice Residency training programs in the United States, approximately 10 percent are located in California. Of those training programs in Southern California, 95 percent have now incorporated at least some elements of didactic and experiential geriatric training into their resident physician curricula. The University of Southern California School of Medicine's Family Practice Program in particular has become one of the leaders in developing a well-integrated, comprehensive geriatric curriculum for physician trainees.

It will be obvious to even the most casual reader that many additional activities could be specified and much more could be said about them, and it is acknowledged that what has been presented here is only the tip of the iceberg. Additional familiarity with gerontology will inevitably reveal the rich complexity of the contributions gerontology has made and will continue to make to the aged and to the broad spectrum of society. Gerontology cuts across every dimension of life and in so doing leaves its imprint. Gerontologists find themselves within traditional, even ancient streams of human concern. Yet because they are in a very real sense pioneering in a new field of endeavor, they experience all the high drama and excitement of being on the "cutting edge."

In this manner gerontology's persistent efforts to enlarge public perspectives and raise public sensitivity to aging issues and needs have had a major, positive impact. Not every conclusion about aging presented by gerontology has been widely accepted without debate. But the process has introduced a strong element of advocacy into gerontology. And this, we believe, begins to delineate the future of gerontology within both a formal and an informal matrix of activity.

The Future of the Science of Gerontology

Whether gerontology is on its way to becoming a recognized discipline in its own right or should more appropriately be considered a specialty field within existing disciplines and professions remains uncertain. But from its past and present emerge certain indications of gerontology's future agenda and the tasks with which it must reckon.

Like the Roman god Janus, gerontology presents more than one face. Indeed, it presents many faces to the observer. Therein lies the striking paradox inherent in the study of aging. On one hand, many of the problems associated with later life are viewed not so much as age-specific problems but as human ones that occur in one form or another at all ages of life. On the other hand, older people are in significant ways different from those in other age groups. The primary question for the gerontologist is, how are they different? (Butler, 1979). In spite of the proliferation of biomedical, psychological, and social research—publications in gerontology in the 1959–75 period totaled about 50,000 (Birren, 1979)—aging remains largely unexplored territory.

There can be no doubt that the scientific focus of gerontology, the characteristic which most distinguishes it from the anecdotal approach of the past, will remain central to gerontological tasks of the future. The following is not a detailed discussion, but merely highlights some major areas of concern.

Methodology: Basic Research

A very large proportion of gerontological research to date has been heavily descriptive or empirical, with relatively little theoretical foundation. Although this may at first blush be considered a deficiency, it nevertheless reflects a normal stage in the usual progression of scientific endeavor. A thornier issue for aging research is the need to resolve methodological problems having to do with confounding factors in age-group comparisons. One of these problems is the differential representation of sexes. Experimental designs employing equal numbers of old and young males and females do not accurately reflect the true proportions of men and women in their respective age groups. Health status differences represent another confounding factor, inasmuch as even the simplest screening procedures are likely to eliminate a disproportionate number of older subjects (Krauss, 1980). The same can be said about differences in level of education.

The methodological problems inherent in differentiating generational differences from age changes have often confounded interpretations of data derived from systematic investigations of aging (see the discussion of research methods in Appendix A). Findings of "decline" in the responses or performance of older persons, for example, may not necessarily be indicative of true deficits (or at least age-caused deficits) but rather may reflect the loss of one adaptive mechanism and the emergence of a new, different, and more useful or relevant mechanism in its stead. It may also reflect a *distillation* of earlier and generally used mechanisms into a different and more integrated coping or response strategy.

Investigation of genetics is pursued as basic research in aging because at a minimum the genetic component is assumed to be implicated in the determination of the lifespan of any given species. However, conclusions about the role of heredity in lifespan development and the aging process must necessarily remain tentative. Even the best longitudinal studies of twins and siblings are complicated by external intervening variables, such as dietary and nutritional patterns, rural or urban living, marital status, exercise or the lack of it, smoking, relative presence or absence of disease, even levels of radiation to which individual's are exposed over a lifetime.

At least two tasks face basic researchers: first, to tease out the differential role of genes, inasmuch as genes are thought to perform one function early in life and another in old age; second, to resolve the difficulties in attempting to integrate biological, behavioral, and social data about aging (Birren, 1979).

Biomedical Studies

Gerontological research has produced important data on the nature and extent of cell changes associated with aging. These studies constitute important basic research simply because cells are the fundamental units of structure and function in living organisms. Information on such changes thus offers important clues about the nature and role of physiological changes in the aging process. Basic cellular research in aging is related to genetic research, since its field of inquiry includes the study of the genetic material DNA, which contains the blueprint for the organization and development of the entire organism. It is also the source of most information about the everyday maintenance and function of cells in the body. A basic research strategy is to examine closely changes in cell size and color with age. Changes in cell integrity, permeability, function, and replication across time are also studied. One perspective in such study is not so much to eliminate the aging process as to modify it in some useful way or slow it down.

Metabolic and chemical elements (endocrine control system) are also studied in conjunction with a variety of experimental conditions, for example, stress and nutritional variations. As might be expected, a substantial amount of this work is done with animals, where study of living cells can be accomplished under relatively well-defined conditions and where proper controls can be effectively maintained. For the most part, a variety of subhuman species (typically rats, mice, fruit flies, and larvae) are utilized. Such species are readily available to research laboratories; they are relatively short-lived and so age effects are more easily tested; and their cellular responses to experimental conditions are judged, within defined limits, to be applicable to human physiology.

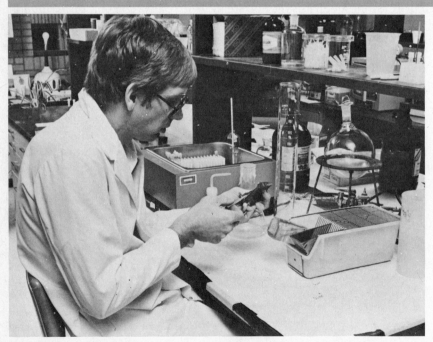

Much of the basic scientific research on aging is done with laboratory animals. Endocrinological research is one of the important directions that aging research will be taking in the future.

Biomedical strategies of research also include studies of homeostatic (state-of-equilibrium) imbalance as it relates to other aspects of the aging process. Disease and stress factors become critical considerations in such investigations. Biomedical research in aging also turns the scientific spotlight on the efficiency of various organs and organ systems (e.g., liver, kidney, circulatory system) with respect to maintenance of body temperature, blood sugar regulation, processing of drugs, waste disposal, and the like, all of which are studied in great detail.

Underlying all other agenda items for future biomedical research is the task of increasing clarification of what constitutes *normal* aging, in contrast to what may be considered atypical or pathological processes occurring in tandem with the aging process. That alone identifies a most formidable and urgent task for tomorrow's biomedical research scientists.

Multidisciplinary Emphasis

Virtually without exception, scientists agree that aging is a multidimensional and multifactored process, a view that the authors have attempted to underscore throughout this text. It follows that the key to a rigorous, vital, and fully productive gerontology as a scientific, educational, and professional pursuit lies in cultivating and enlarging its multidisciplinary approach. The fact that this ideal has hardly been realized in no way detracts from its desirability as a goal.

The authors share with others in the field of aging the view that interdisciplinary rivalries can be accommodated at several levels (Carp, 1974). Most indications are that the best hope for interdisciplinary accommodation is at the undergraduate and preprofessional levels of training. Although the multidisciplinary "team" approach exists more in the breach then in the doing, the need to achieve this goal is one of gerontology's most exciting challenges. Answering that challenge constructively and purposefully will bring together those who need to be brought together to address in concert the age-old problems of aging: the researcher and the practitioner, the clinician and the theorist; physician, psychologist, nurse, social worker, attorney, legislator, pharmacist, business person, occupational therapist, architect, designer, clergy, and expressive artist.

Essential to those collaborations will be keeping both pure and applied research workers in close touch with each other:

> Attempts to solve practical field problems without a theoretical background tend to become isolated field studies that are inefficient because it is not possible to generalize from one situation to another. At the same time, theory without application is apt to become trivial, caught up with minutiae, and liable to build conceptual structures that prove to be a house of cards, even if they sometimes take years to collapse [Welford, 1980, p. 615].

Applied Research

The graying of our society has stimulated an increasing demand for clinical services to the aged. If it is safe to assume that good practice is based upon sound theory and reliable data, then increasing emphasis upon applied research will figure prominently in gerontology's future. Applied research to develop more effective diagnostic and evaluation tools and skills, particularly for psychology, psychiatry, medicine, and social work, is certainly integral to gerontology's future course. Decisions made daily that affect elderly persons in regard to therapeutic interventions, conservatorship, counseling services, housing, work policies and programs, and the like require appropriate, relevant, valid, and reliable assessment tools and techniques.

The first task is research in testing out methods for screening cognitive and functional capacity. Work is being done along this line with such devices as the Face-Hand Test, the Graham-Kendall "Memory for Designs," the Mental-Status Questionnaire (of which there are several versions: Goldfarb, Kaplan, Pfeiffer), and the Bender Motor Gestalt Test. The purpose of such studies (Haglund & Schuckit, 1976) is to refine instruments and procedures so as to distinguish more accurately between impaired and normal elderly and to differentiate brain-damage-generated dysfunction from maladaptive behaviors that are psychogenic (caused by emotional disturbances). This work must be carefully coordinated with family and social histories, with physical and health status evaluations, and with environmental inventories, all potential contributors to the determination of clinical judgments. For example, the effects on behavior and mental functioning of impaired vision in the elderly is one instance of what is meant by applied research in the clinical area (Snyder, Pyrek & Smith, 1976).

A second aspect of clinical assessment is the reevaluation of traditional constructs and measurements and their validity with respect to gerontological applications. This is demonstrated in the seminal work of Warner Schaie and his associates on I.Q. and aging, and the complementary assessment of the Wechsler Adult Intelligence Scale (WAIS) by Martha Storandt (1977). The much-needed recapitulation of MMPI test "profiles" in examining personality changes with age (McCreary & Mensh, 1977) is another example of clinically related applied research. Insofar as most traditional and conventionally used clinical measures have been developed using younger age cohorts, their use with and application to older persons (especially in the seventy-five-and-older range) is invalid and therefore misleading. In addition, the language and formats of such evaluation tests are for the most part inappropriate to an older population. This is a task to which gerontology and geriatric medicine must address themselves in the immediate future.

A third, relatively new dimension useful for establishing clinical referents has recently been suggested: a "social indicators" index. Kaplan and Ontell (1974) have proposed the development of age-related social indicators that will furnish interpreted information about social conditions (are they getting better or worse?) and social goals (future compared to past). For example, a statistic like the mortality rate for those over seventy-five is not a social indicator. But this statistic becomes a social indicator when, for instance, it is compared to the past and when cross-geographical, cross-cultural, and cross-age comparisons are made. If the aged were regarded as a distinctive social entity, a social indicators report would include a description of how the aged population fares in each social domain (e.g., health, housing, education, economics). At the same time it should be noted that social indicators are more than descriptive statistics. In spite of some problems connected with such proposals (for example, the problem of making value judgments about social conditions), it is clear that research along these conceptual lines would have considerable relevance not only to the concerns of clinicians but also to current applied research in the arena of public policy and the aged.

Intervention Evaluation

Another important agenda item for gerontology over the next decades will be substantial investment in developing and refining techniques for assessing intervention strategies. Individual and group counseling of older persons has caught the attention of professionals and nonprofessionals alike including some with considerable training and experience with the aging, some with little or none. A diverse array of professionally run, paraprofessionally directed, and self-help programs have been springing up like mushrooms. While the variety of helping programs and the diversity of helpers may be construed as a positive factor, much more applied research must be forthcoming in the near future to establish useful criteria for selecting and training effective counselors of older people. There is, in addition, an urgent need for effective impact (outcome) evaluation of counseling, self-help, and community programs for the aged (O'Brien & Streib, 1977).

Because so much of clinical geropsychology and geropsychiatry has focused narrowly on the psychogenic (cognitive and emotional) origins of behavior—especially maladaptive behavior—clinical research will in the future need to follow the lead of studies such as the ones undertaken at the University of Bonn in West Germany to identify normal patterns of aging (Thomae, 1976). As with studies using autobiographies of older persons, these psychological investigations cover a variety of configurations of aging patterns, particularly successful agers. Such programs of applied research will address themselves also to the development of tools to assess continuity and change in coping strategies in later life.

Environmental Assessment

As was already indicated in Chapter 10, person-environment transactions specific to old age will assume greater importance and demand much more in the way of systematic investigations than they have in the past.

Research strategies need to be designed that will identify salient elements of prosthetic (compensating) environments for the elderly and how such factors contribute to or detract from the life satisfaction, health, and well-being of elderly persons. A sturdy case can be made for prosthetic environments as a free-operant conditioning mode and for the applicability of operant techniques to behavior modification in the old (Hoyer, 1973; Lindsley, 1964).

One strong stimulus for addressing this task is the anticipated growth in number of long-term-care institutions in America and other industrialized countries around the world. As the role of long-term-care facilities slowly evolves, the need to better understand and more concretely specify the nature of quality of life and environmental contingencies will become all the more critical to gerontological theory and practice.

Minorities

We can expect gerontology to give increased attention in the years ahead to the varied groups of ethnic aged, those "invisible" elderly who are a minority within a minority. Samoan, Pilipino, Korean, Japanese, Puerto Rican, and native American elderly are among those who fall within this group. We can expect gerontologists, especially social gerontologists, to help us learn more about and understand better whatever variations in the aging process exist within such minority groups. We can also expect to learn more about the commonalities of aging that cut across ethnic and cultural lines, about what is culture-specific and what is not. To some extent this can be learned from the minority aged embedded within our own society. More valid answers are most likely to be found in cross-national studies of aging.

International Gerontology

Although scientific gerontological research has proliferated and flourished rather dramatically in America, with its principal base in universities, the scientific study of aging has become increasingly international in scope. For example, a review, of scientific reports appearing in the journal *Mechanisms of Aging and Development* (published in the Netherlands) between 1973 and 1977 indicates that out of 177 scientific articles, 84 reported work conducted in twenty-two foreign countries, including Denmark, Czechoslovakia, France, Hungary, Rumania, Italy, Japan, Israel, India, Sweden, Great Britain, and the USSR. For additional research studies on the international scene, see the international issue of the *Gerontologist,* 1975, **15**, (3). Another indication of gerontology's international scope is the participation at the International Congress of Gerontology, which convenes every three years. The 1981 congress in Hamburg, West Germany, reported some 1,790 participants representing gerontological research and practice in fifty-three countries.

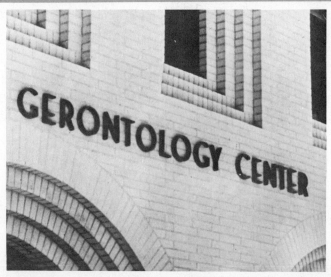

Centers for the study of aging, virtually non-existant a generation ago, have proliferated and now occupy positions of prominence in cities and on campuses across the nation.

The Future of Gerontological Education

Advocacy and *consciousness-raising* and their impact on public policy depend ultimately on the relevance of core concepts to basic social-economic realities. Slogans, no matter how attractive, are never substantial enough to have lasting impact. The fiasco of the McClain movement in California (for old age public pensions) is witness to this. If a vital senior consensus is finally marshaled, it will be because a growing number of elders have become aware of the social and political realities that affect their wellbeing.

The growing educational opportunities for older persons seem to promise an expanding base of informed seniors. It is important to visualize the substantial increase in adult education for seniors. For example, in 1960 there were fewer than ten universities that had any programs for or about the aged. Today there are over 2,000 higher education programs focusing on aging. Hundreds of thousands of older persons attend classes or seminars with curricula that center on improving their life satisfaction or on understanding their roles in our society. The American Association of Retired Persons, senior citizen centers around the nation, retirement communities, and other groups all act as part of an informal educational structure that adds to the impact of the more formal educational institutions. What is emerging is an informed and vital aging cohort. But those persons have more than political sophistication. Education enriches their lives by introducing new skills, new vistas, new aesthetic horizons and new, enriched interests. Education helps to shape a larger, more creative life in old age; it needs to be viewed as a major item on gerontology's future agenda.

Gerontology's Future: Science Wedded to Practice and Art

While the roots of gerontology as we know it today grow from seeds buried deeply in rich scientific soil, much of the richness of gerontology is fed by a vast and complex network of direct as well as indirect services provided for the elderly. The practitioner, the planner, the administrator, the policymaker, and the philosopher, the poet, and the artist, too, take their stand right alongside the scientists within the domain of gerontology. Rightly understood, these all constitute necessary elements and a source of strength for the study of aging. In order to understand what aging is all about for human beings, we need more than mere facts about aging. We need to remember the dictum of the gestaltists: the whole is more than the mere sum of its parts. Victor Weisskopf, former head of the Department of Physics at MIT, has put the matter congently and eloquently:

> A Beethoven sonata is a natural phenomenon that can be analyzed physically by studying the vibrations in the air; it can also be analyzed chemically, physiologically, and psychologically by studying the processes at work in the brain of the listener. However, even if these processes are completely understood in scientific terms, this kind of analysis does not touch what we consider relevant and essential in a Beethoven sonata—the immediate and direct impression of the music. In the same way, we can understand a sunset or the stars in the night sky in a scientific way, but there is something about experiencing these phenomena that lies outside science. . . . There cannot be a scientific definition of . . . concepts like the quality of life or happiness. While it is certainly possible to analyze the nervous and physiological reactions that occur during the process of experiencing such ideas, there remains an important part of the experience that is not touched by this analysis. . . . scientific results may not be the most relevant ones for human social problems and may even be counterproductive for the solution of these problems [1977, p. 208].

So while gerontology lays legitimate claim to its scientific conceptualizations and methodological approaches, the intrinsic value of its science will be considerably enhanced if its scientists, professional service providers, and nonscientists continue to recognize and give credence to other ways of dealing with and understanding the aging process, such as art, poetry, literature, and other forms of expression and impression, including the research strategy known as participant observation. The newcomer to gerontology needs to be assured that there are many roads to the understanding of aging and that the scientific mode should not be considered the only "serious" way of comprehending the behavior of those who survive to the end of their allotted lifespan.

Epilogue

Although no claim to unique wisdom is made by the authors, we have thought it useful to describe for the newcomer to gerontology what we believe gerontology's future directions and prospects to be.

An introduction to gerontology, as to any discipline or body of knowledge, requires a reasonably comprehensive as well as accurate portrayal of the field. At the same time it is necessary to avoid getting bogged down in details and technicalities so specific as to be of interest primarily to the more advanced student or experienced specialist. Any person fairly new to this field, having gone through the contents of this text, will surely appreciate that our excursion into gerontology can very well be likened to that of the novice traveler who visits as many foreign countries as possible on the first time-limited journey. First impressions no doubt reveal that there is much to be seen and heard, much to be learned, and much to be savored and understood. The novice traveler who has an adequate guide is likely to come away with some new perspectives, some sense of the size, shape, boundaries, climate, and flavor of the places visited. But a first-time visitor cannot yet have the same sense of nuance or familiarity with the nooks and crannies of those places as the experienced traveler.

The analogy is appropriate to this text. Just as with most professions or disciplines, the study of gerontology encompasses much more than a mere archeological exercise, although digging up bits of information about aging does have its rewards. The study of gerontology, like the study of law, social work, medicine, engineering, or psychology, has what are essentially very pragmatic goals. Built into it is the assumption that what we learn about aging through research and practice will be translated into further research on the frontiers of aging. What we come to learn and understand about aging will also be applied to practice which serves the needs of society and betters the lives of those in their middle and later years. The assumption is also that what we learn will directly and indirectly improve the prospects for life satisfaction for a growing number of those who will survive into late maturity in the immediate and distant future.

Summary

We can learn much about aging from the special characteristics and life-style contributors to longevity. As gerontology faces an increasingly aged world it will pay more attention to successful aging and the so-called elite aged than it has in the past. New directions for research can be expected which will focus on the study of aging patterns. Confronted with new cohorts of aged who can be expected to be better educated, healthier, more involved with work, and more politically "savvy" and effective than their forebears, gerontology will need to reassess its traditional roles and priorities in order to be relevant. Its advocacy role particularly needs reevaluation.

Among the future tasks envisioned for gerontology is the need to maintain persistent efforts to enlarge public perspectives and raise public sensitivity to issues of aging. The various communications media and the institutions of society (religion, education, business institutions, etc.), which are already responding, will increasingly look to gerontology as an information source.

Gerontologists as scientists and clinicians have their work cut out for them. Scientific methodological problems in biomedical and clinical research that have confounded many prior investigators and have contaminated assessment procedures need careful study and resolution.

The continued multidisciplinary emphasis of gerontology will insure its vitality as a scientific and service endeavor. The fragmentation sometimes evident in gerontology requires a greater emphasis on synthesis and integration of theoretical concepts and the growing volumes of empirical data. Mainstream gerontological activities in the future will be the development of appropriate, valid, and reliable clinical tools, intervention assessment techniques, and environmental assessment and manipulation criteria, and the facilitation of the "visibility" of minority elderly.

References

Allport, G. *The use of personal documents in psychological science.* New York: Social Science Research Council, 1942.

Benet, S. *Abkhasians: The long-living people of the Caucasus.* New York: Holt, Rinehart, & Winston, 1974.

Birren, J. Progress in research on aging in the behavioral and social sciences. In Orimo, H., Shimada, K., Iriki, M., & Maeda, D. (Eds.), *Recent advances in gerontology: Proceedings of the 11th International Congress of Gerontology, Tokyo, August 20–25, 1978.* Amsterdam-Oxford-Princeton: Excerpta Medica, 1979. Pp. 49–58.

Buhler, C. Meaningful living in the mature years. In R. Kleemier (Ed.), *Aging and leisure.* New York: Oxford University Press, 1963. Pp. 345–387.

Butler, R. The life review: An interpretation of reminiscence in the aged. *Psychiatry,* 1963, **26**, 65–76.

Butler, R. Successful aging and the role of the life review. *Journal of the American Geriatric Society,* 1974, **22**, 529–535.

Butler, R. Man and aging: Philosophical bases of gerontology from the perspective of clinical medicine. In Orimo, H., Shimada, K., Iriki, M., & Maeda, D. (Eds.), *Recent advances in gerontology: Proceedings of the 11th International Congress of Gerontology, Tokyo, August 20–25, 1978.* Amsterdam-Oxford-Princeton: Excerpta Medica, 1979. Pp. 10–17.

Carp, F. The realities of the interdisciplinary approach: Can the disciplines work together to help the aged? In A. Schwartz & I. Mensh (Eds.), *Professional obligations and approaches to the aged.* Springfield, Ill.: Charles C. Thomas, 1974.

Estes, C. *The aging enterprise.* San Francisco: Jossey-Bass, 1979.

Evans, L., & Williamson, J. Social security and social control. *Generations,* 1981, **6**(2), 18–20.

Graebner, W. *A history of retirement.* New Haven: Yale University Press, 1980.

Greenleigh, L. Facing the challenge of change in middle age. *Geriatrics,* 1974, **29**(11), 61–68.

Haglund, R., & Schuckit, M. A clinical comparison of tests of organicity in elderly patients. *Journal of Gerontology,* 1976, **31**(6), 654–659.

Heschel, A. J. *To grow in wisdom.* New York: Synagogue Council of America, 1971.

Hoyer, W. Application of operant techniques to the modification of elderly behavior. *Gerontologist,* 1973, **13**(1), 18–21.

Hudson, R. Emerging pressures on public policy for the aging. *Society,* 1978, **15**, 30–33.

Jewett, S. Longevity and the longevity syndrome. *Gerontologist,* 1973, **13**(1), 91–99.

Kaplan, O., & Ontell, R. Social indicators and the aging. In A. Schwartz & I. Mensh (eds.), *Professional obligations and approaches to the aged.* Springfield, Ill.: Charles C. Thomas, 1974.

Krauss, I. Between- and within-group comparisons in aging research. In L. Poon (Ed.), *Aging in the 1980s.* Washington, D.C.: American Psychological Association, 1980. Pp. 542–551.

Larson, R. Thirty years of research on the subjective well-being of older Americans. *Journal of Gerontology,* 1978, **33**(1), 109–125.

Lauer, R., & Goldfield, M. Creative writing in group therapy. *Psychotherapy: Theory, Research, and Practice,* 1970, **7**(4), 248–251.

Lickorish, J. The therapeutic use of literature. *Psychotherapy: Theory, Research, and Practice,* 1975, **12**(1), 105–109.

Lindsley, O. R. Geriatric behavioral prosthetics. In R. Kastenbaum (Ed.), *New thoughts on old age.* New York: Springer, 1964. Pp. 41–60.

McCreary, C., & Mensh, I. Personality differences associated with age in law offenders. *Journal of Gerontology,* 1977, **32**(2), 164–167.

O'Brien, J., & Streib, G. *Evaluative research on social programs for the elderly.* Washington, D.C.: Administration on Aging, DHEW Publication No. (ODH)77-20120, 1977.

Palmore, E. Predictors of successful aging. *Gerontologist,* 1979, **19**(5), 427–431.

Pratt, H. *The gray lobby.* Chicago: University of Chicago Press, 1976.

Ragan, R., & Davis, W. The diversity of older voters. *Society,* 1978, **15**, 50–53.

Reedy, M., & Birren, J. Life review through guided autobiography. Paper presented at annual meeting of the American Psychological Association, Montreal, Canada, Sept. 3, 1980.

Rosenbaum, H. Age is my greatest asset. *Modern Maturity,* June–July 1971, **14**(3), 32–33.

Rucker, S. Office sweetheart is going strong at 91. *Los Angeles Times,* Feb. 13, 1978.

Schwartz, A. Retirement: Termination or transition? *Geriatrics,* 1974, **29**(5), 190–198.

Schwartz, A. *Survival handbook for children of aging parents.* Chicago: Follett, 1977.

Snyder, C. L., & Schwartz, A. N. Physiological, psychological, and social aspects of longevity among 101 Caribbean centenarians. Paper presented at the 12th International Congress of Gerontology, Hamburg, Germany, 1981.

Snyder, L., Pyrek, J., & Smith, C. Vision and mental functioning of the elderly. *Gerontologist,* 1976, **16**(6), 491–495.

Storandt, M. Age, ability level, and method of administration and scoring the WAIS. *Journal of Gerontology,* 1977, **32**(2), 175–178.

Thomae, H. (Ed.). *Patterns of aging.* (Vol. 3, Contributions to Human Development Series; K. Riegel & H. Thomae, Eds.) Basel, Switzerland: S. Karger, 1976.

Wallechinsky, D., Wallace, I., & Wallace, A. *The book of lists.* New York: William Morrow, 1977.

Weakland, J. Radical changes in gerontology: Semblance and substance. *Generations,* 1981, 6(2), 24–25.

Weisskopf, V. The frontiers and limits of science. *American Scientist,* 1977, **65**, 201–210.

Weinberg, J. What do I say to my mother when I have nothing to say? *Geriatrics,* Nov. 1974.

Welford, A. Where do we go from here? In L. Poon (Ed.), *Aging in the 1980s.* Washington, D.C.: American Psychological Association, 1980. Pp. 615–621.

For Further Reading

Butler, R. *Successful aging.* Arlington, VA: Mental Health Association, 1974.

Elders respond to the humanities. *Aging,* US Department of Health and Human Services, Jan–Feb, 1982.

Knopf, O. *Successful aging.* New York: Viking Press, 1975.

Linn, M., & Carmichael, L. Introducing pre-professionals to gerontology. *Gerontologist,* 1974, *14*(6): 476–478.

Perry, P. The night of ageism. In H. Cox (Ed.), *Focus: aging.* Gilford, CN: Publishing Group, 1978.

Peterson, D., Lowell, C., & Robertson, L. Aging in America: toward the year 2000 *Gerontologist,* 1976, *16*(3): 264–270.

Pressey, S., & Pressey, A. Genius at 80 and other oldsters. *Gerontologist,* 1967, *7*(3): 183–187.

Thomas, L. Sexuality and aging: essential vitamin or popcorn? *Gerontologist,* 1982, *22*(3): 240–243.

Alternative Approaches to the Study of Aging

Appendix A

With the increased interest in and emphasis on the study of aging, gerontologists are reevaluating the appropriateness of existing research methods, strategies, and designs and developing new approaches to investigation in order to provide valid, reliable information about the aging process. Because aging is described as a time-related process it is tempting to assume that the passage of time "causes" aging. Yet time itself is but an abstract representational system employed to describe and reference sequences of events and their durations; it is of little if any value in explaining variability in characteristics and behavior across the lifespan. Of greater salience is knowledge about the events in the lives of individuals or groups, and how these events contribute in part or in whole to the experience of growing older.

In Chapter 1, reference was made to cross-sectional and longitudinal approaches to the study of aging. These, along with the time-lag approach, represent the most widely adopted methods employed to investigate aging and older persons to date. To review, cross-sectional strategies permit comparisons of the dynamic and static aspects of existence between different birth-groups (cohorts) at a given point in time. In Figure A–1, this approach is represented by the columns A_1-B_2-C_3 and B_1-C_2-D_1 and is designed to yield information about *age differences*. The longitudinal approach, represented in Figure A-1 by the rows B_1-B_2-B_3 and C_1-C_2-C_3, allows for multiple assessments over time of behavior or characteristics of individuals from within the same cohort. Adoption of this research strategy allows the investigator to learn about *age changes*. Finally, the time-lag approach examines *cohort differences* by means of sampling various aspects of behavior or characteristic qualities of individuals from different cohorts measured at different points in time such that the ages of all persons sampled are the same. This approach is represented by the diagonals A_1-B_1-C_1 and B_3-C_3-D_1 in Figure A–1.

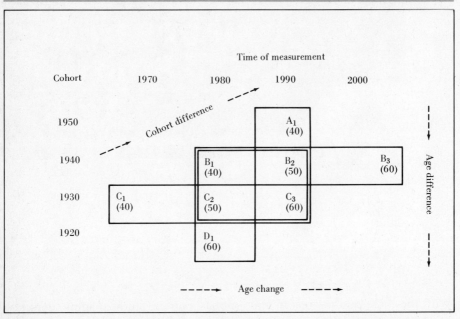

FIGURE A-1.   Comparison of Developmental Research Designs Based on Age, Cohort, and Time of Measurement
Source: Elias, M. F., Elias, P. K., & Elias, J. W. *Basic processes in adult development.* St. Louis: C. V. Mosby, 1977, p. 33.

While the preponderance of research in the field of gerontology has been conducted with the use of cross-sectional, longitudinal, or time-lag designs, of these, certainly cross-sectional research has been foremost, no doubt due to its economy with respect to frequency of measurement (the "one-shot" study), financial considerations, and other factors which contribute to its administrative simplicity, as described in Table 1–4 (see Chapter 1). Longitudinal and time-lag research are more time-consuming, and may ultimately become problematic as the result of participant attrition, inconsistency in record keeping, research staff turnover, investigator disenchantment, and the potential inability to secure continued funding over extended periods of time. While practical considerations are certainly important in the choice of an appropriate strategy for gerontological investigation, opting for a particular method or strategy simply because of its administrative simplicity, cost-time effectiveness, or other similar features can seriously affect the quality of information which results and the way in which it may be evaluated and interpreted. Indeed, when selecting the optimal approach to any investigation of aging or older persons, the types of questions the investigator hopes to answer should be the most important factors in the decision to accept or reject a given strategy as valid and appropriate.

Reexamination of the three research approaches just mentioned—

cross-sectional, longitudinal, and time-lag—may serve to illustrate this point. While these designs have been employed to investigate age differences, age changes, and cohort differences, respectively, as shown in Figure A–1, Table A–1 suggests that (1) cross-sectional studies cannot provide evaluation of age differences independent of the effects of age change; (2) longitudinal studies yield no independent assessment of age change and cohort difference; (3) time-lag studies are inadequate for the independent analyses of the effects of age differences and cohort differences. In other words, of the three main effects of age, cohort, and time of measurement, each approach is capable of holding one effect constant while confounding the effects of the other two. Thus, despite their widespread use in the study of aging and older persons, these designs are essentially invalid and misleading. This observation should be kept in mind as the student examines the literature on aging: the inappropriate choice of an approach to the study of aging can have disastrous consequences for the elderly and for our understanding of their lives.

Fortunately, there are other approaches to research which hold great promise. Each of these alternative approaches is in fact founded upon the more fundamental designs of the aforementioned strategies, as can be seen in Figure A–1. In essence, to avoid the confounded effects of cross-sectional, longitudinal, and time-lag studies, the investigator simply (at least from a theoretical point of view) increases the scope of study to encompass an additional level of inquiry. For example, the cross-sectional design can be expanded to a cohort-sequential design by investigating (at least) columns A_1-B_2-C_3 and B_1-C_2-D_1 of Figure A–1. This additional sophistication permits the investigator to determine independently the effects of age and cohort, and thus to distinguish between age changes and age differences. Evaluation of more than one row (e.g., at least B_1-B_2-B_3 and C_1-C_2-C_3) transforms a longitudinal study into a time-sequential investigation, and enables the investigator to evaluate the independent effects of age (i.e., age change) and time of measurement (i.e., cohort differences). Finally, elaboration of the time-lag approach is achieved by evaluating the positive *and* negative diagonals,

TABLE A–1. Potential Confounded Effects and Isolated Effects in Developmental Research Designs

	Confounded Effects			Isolated Effects		
Design	Age	Cohort	Time of Measurement	Age	Cohort	Time of Measurement
Cross-sectional	X	X				
Longitudinal	X		X			
Time-lag		X	X			
Cohort sequential			X*	X	X	
Time sequential		X*		X		X
Cross-sequential	X*				X	X

Source: Elias, M. F., Elias, P. K., & Elias, J. W. *Basic processes in adult development.* St. Louis: C.V. Mosby, 1977, p. 35.

*Effects are assumed to be insignificant

B_1–C_3 and B_2–C_2, of Figure A–1, thus yielding the cross-sequential design. This latter design allows the gerontologist to discriminate between the independent effects of age difference and of cohort difference. While an elaborate statistical justification and proof of the utility and appropriateness of these sequential research strategies is well beyond the scope of this volume, the student should be aware of the significant advantages that each of these offers over the more popular univalent designs which continue to dominate the field of developmental research and aging and, once again, should bear in mind when evaluating the gerontological literature the importance of a congruent fit between the nature of the problem to be investigated and the means of investigation.

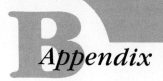

Can You Live to Be 100?

*B*Appendix

BY Diana S. Woodruff

We have the biological capacity to live to be 100. There are documented records of people surviving to at least 120 years of age. In fact, biologists currently set the upper limit for the human life at 120 years.

The following questionnaire is designed to make you more fully aware of the factors contributing to long life although this test has not been validated and, of course, there is no test that can tell you with absolute certainty how long you actually will live.

Begin by looking through the actuarial table on page 370 for the average life expectancy of persons of your sex, age and race. After finding your life expectancy on the table, add and subtract years according to how you answer the following questions.

ADD OR SUBTRACT YEARS: ±

1. Have any of your grandparents lived to age 80 or beyond? If so, add one year for each grandparent living beyond that age. Add one-half year for each grandparent surviving beyond the age of 70.
2. If your mother lived beyond the age of 80, add four years. Add two years if your father lived beyond 80. You benefit more if your mother lived a long time than if your father did.

1 _____

3. If any parent, grandparent, sister or brother died of a heart attack, stroke or arteriosclerosis before the age of 50, subtract four years for each incidence. If any of those close relatives died of the above before the age of 60, subtract two years for each incidence.

2 _____

3 _____

4. Have any grandparents, par-

ADD ALL PLUSES: _____
ADD ALL MINUSES: _____
SUBTOTAL (Subtract all minuses from the pluses): _____

369

Average Life Expectancy Table

Age	Caucasian Male	Caucasian Female	Black Male	Black Female	Oriental Male	Oriental Female
10	70.9	78.4	65.8	74.4	72.9	80.4
11	70.9	78.4	65.8	74.4	72.9	80.4
12	70.9	78.4	65.8	74.4	72.9	80.4
13	70.9	78.4	65.9	74.4	72.9	80.4
14	71.0	78.5	65.9	74.4	73.0	80.5
15	71.0	78.5	65.9	74.5	73.0	80.5
16	71.1	78.5	66.0	74.5	73.1	80.5
17	71.1	78.5	66.1	74.5	73.1	80.5
18	71.2	78.6	66.1	74.6	73.2	80.6
19	71.3	78.6	66.2	74.6	73.3	80.6
20	71.4	78.6	66.3	74.7	73.4	80.6
21	71.5	78.7	66.5	74.7	73.5	80.7
22	71.6	78.7	66.6	74.8	73.6	80.7
23	71.7	78.7	66.8	74.8	73.7	80.7
24	71.8	78.8	66.9	74.9	73.8	80.8
25	71.9	78.8	67.1	74.9	73.9	80.8
26	71.9	78.8	67.3	75.0	73.9	80.8
27	72.0	78.9	67.4	75.1	74.0	80.9
28	72.1	78.9	67.6	75.1	74.1	80.9
29	72.2	78.9	67.8	75.2	74.2	80.9
30	72.2	79.0	68.0	75.3	74.2	81.0
31	72.3	79.0	68.1	75.4	74.3	81.0
32	72.4	79.0	68.3	75.4	74.4	81.0
33	72.4	79.1	68.5	75.5	74.4	81.1
34	72.5	79.1	68.6	75.6	74.5	8.11
35	72.6	79.2	68.8	75.7	74.6	81.2
36	72.6	79.2	69.0	75.8	74.6	81.2
37	72.7	79.3	69.2	75.9	74.7	81.3
38	72.8	79.3	69.4	76.0	74.8	81.3
39	72.9	79.4	69.6	76.1	74.9	81.4
40	73.0	79.4	69.8	76.2	75.0	81.4
41	73.1	79.5	70.0	76.4	75.1	81.5
42	73.2	79.6	70.3	76.5	75.2	81.6
43	73.3	79.6	70.5	76.6	75.3	81.6
44	73.4	79.7	70.8	76.8	75.4	81.7
45	73.5	79.8	71.0	77.0	75.5	81.8
46	73.7	79.9	71.3	77.1	75.7	81.9
47	73.8	80.0	71.5	77.3	75.8	82.0
48	74.0	80.1	71.8	77.5	76.0	82.1
49	74.1	80.2	72.1	77.7	76.1	82.2
50	74.3	80.3	72.4	77.9	76.3	82.3
51	74.5	80.5	72.7	78.2	76.5	82.5
52	74.7	80.6	73.1	78.4	76.7	82.6
53	74.9	80.7	73.4	78.6	76.9	82.7
54	75.2	80.9	73.8	78.9	77.2	82.9
55	75.4	81.0	74.2	79.1	77.4	83.0
56	75.7	82.1	74.6	79.4	77.7	83.2
57	75.9	81.4	75.0	79.7	77.9	83.4
58	76.2	81.5	75.4	80.0	78.2	83.5
59	76.5	81.7	75.8	80.3	78.5	83.7
60	76.8	81.9	76.3	80.7	78.8	83.9
61	77.2	82.2	76.8	81.0	79.2	84.2
62	77.5	82.4	77.2	81.4	79.5	84.4
63	77.9	82.6	77.7	81.8	79.9	84.6
64	78.3	82.8	78.2	82.2	80.3	84.8
65	78.7	83.1	78.7	82.5	80.7	85.1
66	79.1	83.3	79.2	82.9	81.1	85.3
67	79.5	83.6	79.7	83.2	81.5	85.6
68	80.0	83.9	80.2	83.5	82.0	85.9
69	80.4	84.1	80.7	83.9	82.4	86.1
70	80.9	84.4	81.3	84.4	82.9	86.4
71	81.4	84.7	81.9	84.9	83.4	86.7
72	81.9	85.1	82.5	85.5	83.9	87.1
73	82.4	85.4	83.2	86.2	84.4	87.4
74	83.0	85.8	84.0	86.8	35.0	87.8
75	83.5	86.2	84.7	87.5	85.5	88.2
76	84.1	86.6	85.5	88.2	86.1	88.6
77	84.7	87.1	86.2	88.9	86.7	89.1
78	85.4	87.6	87.0	89.6	87.4	89.6
79	86.0	88.1	87.7	90.3	88.0	90.1
80	86.7	88.6	88.5	91.0	88.7	90.6
81	87.4	89.1	89.3	91.7	89.4	91.1
82	88.1	89.7	90.1	92.4	90.1	91.7
83	88.8	90.3	90.8	93.1	90.8	92.3
84	89.5	90.9	91.5	93.6	91.5	92.9
85	90.2	91.5	92.1	94.1	92.2	93.5

Source: *Can You Live to be 100?* by Diana S. Woodruff, Ph.D. © 1977 by Diana S. Woodruff. Reprinted by permission of Chatham Square Press, Inc.

ents, sisters or brothers died before the age of 60 of diabetes mellitus or peptic ulcer? Subtract three years for each incidence. If any of these close relatives died before 60 of stomach cancer, subtract two years. Women whose close relatives have died before 60 of breast cancer should also subtract two years. Finally, if any close relatives have died before the age of 60 of any cause except accidents or homicide, subtract one year for each incidence.

5. Women who have never had children are more likely to be in poor health and they are at a greater risk for breast cancer. Therefore, if you can't or don't plan to have children, or if you are over 40 and have never had children, subtract one-half year. Women who have had a large number of children tax their bodies. If you've had over seven children, or plan to, subtract one year.

6. Was your mother over the age of 35 or under the age of 18, when you were born? If so, subtract one year.

7. Are you the first born in your family? If so, add one year.

8. How intelligent are you? Is your intelligence below average, average, above average or superior? If you feel that your intelligence is superior, that is, if you feel that you are smarter than almost anyone you know, add two years.

9. Are you currently overweight? Find your ideal weight on the table on page 372. If you weigh

more than the figure on the table, calculate the percentage by which you are overweight and subtract the appropriate number of years shown on the table on page 373. If you have been overweight at any point in your life, or if your weight has periodically fluctuated by more than ten pounds since high school, subtract two years.

10. Do you prefer vegetables, fruits and simple foods to foods high in fat and sugar and do you always stop eating before you feel really full? If the honest answer to both questions is yes, add one year.

11. How much do you smoke? If you smoke two or more packs of cigarettes a day, subtract 12 years. If you smoke between one and two packs a day, subtract seven years. If you smoke less than a pack a day, subtract two years.

12. If you are a moderate drinker, that is, if you never drink to the point of intoxication and have one or two drinks of whiskey, or half a liter of wine, or up to four glasses of beer per day, add three years. If you are a light drinker, that is, if you have an occasional drink, but do not drink almost every day, add 1½ years. If you are an abstainer who never uses alcohol in any form, do not add or subtract any years. Finally, if you are a heavy drinker or an alcoholic, subtract eight years.

13. How much do you exercise? If you exercise at least three times a week at one of the

4 _____

5 _____

6 _____

7 _____

8 _____

9 _____

10 _____

11 _____

12 _____

ADD ALL PLUSES: _____
ADD ALL MINUSES: _____
SUBTOTAL (Subtract all minuses from the pluses): _____

"Ideal" Weights for Men

Height (in Shoes, 1-Inch Heels)		Weight in Pounds (In Indoor Clothing)		
Feet	Inches	Small Frame	Medium Frame	Large Frame
5	2	112–120	118–129	126–141
5	3	115–123	121–133	129–144
5	4	118–126	124–136	132–148
5	5	121–129	127–139	135–152
5	6	124–133	130–143	138–156
5	7	128–137	134–147	142–161
5	8	132–141	138–152	147–166
5	9	136–145	142–156	151–170
5	10	140–150	146–160	155–174
5	11	144–154	150–165	159–179
6	0	148–158	154–170	164–184
6	1	152–162	158–175	168–189
6	2	156–167	162–180	173–194
6	3	160–171	167–185	178–199
6	4	164–175	172–190	182–204

. . . and For Women

Height (In Shoes, 2-Inch Heels)		Weight In Pounds (In Indoor Clothing)		
Feet	Inches	Small Frame	Medium Frame	Large Frame
4	10	92–98	96–107	104–119
4	11	94–101	98–110	106–122
5	0	96–104	101–113	109–125
5	1	99–107	104–116	112–128
5	2	102–110	107–119	115–131
5	3	105–113	110–122	118–134
5	4	108–116	113–126	121–138
5	5	111–119	116–130	125–142
5	6	114–123	120–135	129–146
5	7	118–127	124–139	133–150
5	8	122–131	128–143	137–154
5	9	126–135	132–147	141–158
5	10	130–140	136–151	145–163
5	11	134–144	140–155	149–168
6	0	138–148	144–159	153–173

Source: Metropolitan Life Insurance Co.

The Risk to Life of Being Overweight

| Age | Markedly Overweight (More Than 30 Percent) | | Moderately Overweight (10 to 30 Percent) | |
---	Men	Women	Men	Women
20	−15.8	−7.2	−13.8	−4.8
25	−10.6	−6.1	−9.6	−4.9
30	−7.9	−5.5	−5.5	−3.6
35	−6.1	−4.9	−4.2	−4.0
40	−5.1	−4.6	−3.3	−3.5
45	−4.3	−5.1	−2.4	−3.8
50	−4.6	−4.1	−2.4	−2.8
55	−5.4	−3.2	−2.0	−2.2

Source: Metropolitan Life Insurance Co.

ADD OR MINUS YEARS: ±

following: jogging, bike riding, swimming, taking long, brisk walks, dancing or skating, add three years.

14. If you generally fall asleep right away and get six to eight hours of sleep per night, you're average and should neither add nor subtract years. However, if you sleep excessively (ten or more hours per night), or if you sleep very little (five or fewer hours per night), you probably have problems. Subtract two years.

15. If you enjoy regular sexual activity, having intimate sexual relations once or twice a week, add two years.

16. Do you have an annual physical examination by your physician which includes a breast examination and Pap smear for women and a proctoscoptic examination every other year for men? If so, add two years.

17. Are you in poor health? Do you have a chronic health condition (for example, heart disease, high blood pressure, cancer, diabetes, ulcer) or are you

frequently ill? If so, subtract five years.

18. How much education have you had? Add or subtract the number of years shown in table below.

13 _____

14 _____

15 _____

Level of Education — Years of Life

Level of Education	Years of Life	
Four or more years of college	add 3.0	**16** _____
One to three years of college	add 2.0	**17** _____
Four years of high school	add 1.0	
One to three years of high school	0.0	**18** _____
Elementary school (eight years)	subtract 0.5	
Less than eighth grade	subtract 2.0	

19. If you are working, what is the socioeconomic level of your occupation? If you do not work, what is your spouse's occupation? If you are retired, what is your former occupation? If you are a student, what is your parents' occupation level? Add or subtract the

ADD ALL PLUSES: _____
ADD ALL MINUSES: _____
SUBTOTAL (Subtract all minuses from the pluses): _____

number of years shown in table below.

Occupational Level	Years of Life
Class I—Professional	add 1.5
Class II—Technical, administrative, and managerial. Also agricultural workers.	add 1.0
Class III—Proprietors, clerical, sales, and skilled workers	0.0
Class IV—Semiskilled workers	subtract 0.5
Class V—Laborers	subtract 4.0

20. If your family income is above average for your education and occupation, add one year. If it's below average for your education and occupation, subtract one year.
21. If your job involves a lot of physical activity, add two years. On the other hand, if you sit all day on the job, subtract two years.
22. If you are over the age of sixty and still on the job, add two years. If you are over the age of sixty-five and have not retired, add three years.
23. If you live in an urban area and have lived in or near the city for most of your life, subtract one year. If you have spent most of your life in a rural area, add one year.
24. If you are married and living with your spouse, add one year.

Formerly married men: If you are a separated or divorced man living alone, subtract nine years, and if you are a widowed man living alone, subtract seven years. If, as a separated, divorced, or widowed man you live with other people, such as family members, subtract only half the years given above. Living with others is beneficial for formerly married men.

Formerly married women: Women who are separated or divorced should subtract four years, and widowed women should subtract 3½ years. The loss of a spouse through divorce or death is not as life-shortening to women, and they live about as long whether they live alone or with family, except for those who are heads of households. Divorced or widowed women who live with family as the head of their household should subtract only two years for the formerly married status.

25. If you are a woman who has never married, subtract one year for each unmarried decade past the age of twenty-five. If you are a single male living with a family or friends, you should also subtract one year for each unmarried decade past the age of twenty-five. However, if you are a man who has never married and are living alone, subtract two years for each unmarried decade past the age of twenty-five.
26. Are you always changing things in your life, changing jobs, changing residences, changing friends and/or spouses, changing your appearance? If so, subtract two years. Too much change is stressful.

19 _____

20 _____

21 _____

22 _____

23 _____

24 _____

25 _____

26 _____

27. Do you generally like people and have at least two close friends in whom you can confide almost all the details of your life? Is so, add one year.
28. Do you always feel that you are under time pressure? Are you aggressive and sometimes hostile, paying little attention to the feelings of others? Subtract two to five years depending on how well you fit this description.
29. Are you a calm, reasonable, relaxed person? Are you easy-going and adaptable, taking life pretty much as it comes? Depending upon the degree to which you fit this description, add one to three years. If you are rigid, dogmatic, and set in your ways, subtract two years.
30. Do you take a lot of risk, including driving without seat belts, exceeding the speed limit and taking any dare that is made? Do you live in a high crime rate neighborhood? If you are vulnerable to accidents and homicide in this way, subtract two years. If you use seat belts regularly, drive infrequently, and generally avoid risks and dangerous parts of town, add one year.
31. Have you been depressed, tense, worried or guilty for more than a period of a year or two? If so, subtract one to three years depending upon how seriously you are affected by these feelings.
32. Are you basically happy and content, and have you had a lot of fun in life? If so, add two years. People with feelings like this are the ones who live to be 100.

27 _____

28 _____

29 _____

30 _____

31 _____

32 _____

ADD ALL PLUSES: _____

ADD ALL MINUSES: _____

SUBTOTAL (Subtract all minuses from the pluses): _____

Calculation of Your Longevity

From page 370, write your life expectancy based on your present age:

SUBTOTAL from page 369: _____

SUBTOTAL from page 371: _____

SUBTOTAL from page 373: _____

SUBTOTAL from page 374: _____

SUBTOTAL from page 375: _____

TOTAL AGE EXPECTED TO LIVE: (Add) _____

Information Retrieval in Gerontology: The Literature Search

Appendix C

BY Jean Mueller

This appendix is intended to help both the student and the lecturer prepare a working bibliography for term papers, lectures, master's thesis research projects, etc. Because gerontology encompasses such a wide array of social as well as individual problems and issues, with biomedical, psychosocial, and demographic dimensions, the opportunities for research, demonstration projects, and the acquisition of basic knowledge in gerontology are vast. These problems and issues are evident in all areas of life affecting the older population: housing, health, education, recreation, finances, and communication, to name but a few. As a result, the literature of gerontology is scattered across many academic disciplines.

Although efforts have been made to implement a systematic and accessible information system focusing on gerontology bibliography, in the main inadequate funding will account for their very limited success to date. As a consequence, the very multidisciplinary nature of the field presents the researcher with a much more complex task in information retrieval than might have been previously encountered in library research. This means that the researcher in gerontology, when initiating a literature search, should be prepared to spend some time at either a large public library or a university library that supports a gerontology program.

The "Shape" of the Literature

It has generally been assumed that the literature of gerontology could adequately be represented by a core list of fewer than 100 journals. This notion was supported by Administration on Aging contracts designed to collect and analyze the available literature in this field. The results of a study undertaken by an independent contractor and an analysis of on-line searching conducted at the Universtity of Southern California Andrus Gerontological Information Center over a two-year period demonstrated the existence of a core list of perhaps 45 primary journals. While this finding was consistent with expectations at that time, the same investigations also identified another 900 journals that reported on *some aspect of multidisciplinary gerontology* as well.

In addition to the journal literature, there are many government documents available, including congressional reports and hearings, agency reports, demonstration projects, final reports of grants, and from the past fifteen years, a growing number of books. Full access to this multidepository literature is often essential to the success of a project.

The student should be aware of the characteristics of books as compared to journals in the preparation of a subject bibliography. Journal literature is basic to the reporting and dissemination of pure as well as applied research. It takes on the average five years for research to enter the literature in book form; the period for reporting the same research in a journal is approximately 2½ years.

On the other hand, the nature of book literature is to summarize, evaluate, compare, interpret, and review previously reported literature, primarily from journals. The scope and perspective of books are usually broad. Because of the need to treat the interrelatedness of the problems and issues they address, books are usually lengthy treatises. When a problem is identified as multifaceted and multidisciplinary in nature, books become an ideal format for discussion, comparison, and evaluation.

The more focused and timely journal is more appropriate, then, for reporting "state of the art" research and practice, while books are often better when making a comparative "review of the literature," developing a thesis or perspective, or attempting a historical analysis of a topic. Most research projects will—and should—include both types of literature.

The Sources

Although many libraries may not have a number of the sources listed below, articles published in these journals are most likely to be identified during a manual or on-line search of the literature. Only the larger libraries are likely to have direct (or indirect) access to many of the titles indicated here. This list is by no means exhaustive, but will provide the researcher with a valuable introduction to the literature contained in journals:

Activities, Adaptation, and Aging
Aging and Work
Aging News/Research and Training
Current Literature on Aging
Death Education

Educational Gerontology
Experimental Aging Research
Gerontologist
Gerontology and Geriatrics Education
International Journal of Aging and Human Development
Journal of the American Geriatrics Society
Journal of Gerontological Nursing
Journal of Gerontological Social Work
Journal of Gerontology
Journal of Minority Aging
Journal of Nutrition for the Elderly
Older American Reports
Social Security Bulletin

Monographs

The books available in a given library are listed in the card catalog, by subject, author, title, or series. There is also considerable information in books of collected readings, that is, books which contain chapters or articles by several authors, each writing in his or her subject specialty. Many monographs in gerontology are currently available in this form. Because individual chapters are not listed by subject in the card catalog or in most indexes, this body of literature is hidden except to those who take the time to peruse the tables of content or indexes of such works. Prior to 1981, the "Bibliography of Current Literature in Gerontology and Geriatrics" published in each issue of the *Journal of Gerontology* by Nathan Shock included subject listings for many chapters in collected readings, texts, and handbooks on gerontology. The index was not continued after 1981, however, and now each issue must be consulted for information about a given subject area.

Bibliographies and references lists in many books and journal articles are often a good source of additional material.

The Literature Search: Online Access

The researcher in gerontology will quickly discover that identifying relevant journal literature through indexes can be a tedious chore. A manual search of such useful indexes as *ERIC, Psychological Abstracts, Science Citation Index, Social Science Citation Index, U.S. Monthly Catalog to Government Publications, PAIS, Index Medicus,* and *Dissertation Abstracts International,* for example, can take considerable time and effort. In addition, it is often difficult to combine several concepts without having to look under all the relevant main subject headings (e.g., "burnout of professional employees in long-term-care facilities").

Efficient information retrieval in gerontology has improved exponentially with recent advances in computer technology. Most indexes now find their way into machine-readable form early in the production process. Vastly enlarged storage capabilities, reduced costs, the development of cost-efficient telecommunication networks, and the writing of search programs to interact with the data in the computer—the mechanisms are finally in place to make computer bibliographic searching a cost- and time-effective approach to library research.

Considerations in On-Line Literature Searching

On-line searching as a research tool is now available in many libraries and should be considered a viable research method, along with the card catalog or the Wilson indexes to journal literature, for example.

In essence, on-line searching is the use of a computer to access the same (or additional) indexes that formerly were only available to the researcher in printed form. The difference is that the librarian or information seeker will conduct the search after a reference interview to ascertain the specific subject matter desired.

As indicated, on-line searching has proved to be an especially valuable research tool in gerontology. The computer allows the searcher, in conjunction with the researcher, to carefully formulate a search strategy—that is, to identify key words or phrases, enter them into a terminal, and qualify the limits of the search. For example, a search of a relevant data base might be restricted to the retrieval of articles published within the previous two years.

There are two basic approaches to subject searching using on-line methods. One pertains to "free-text searching." When a subject area is so new or so limited that standard subject headings or index terms have not been determined and applied by an indexer-abstractor, any applicable word or phrase can be entered into the computer to facilitate retrieval of relevant citations. If the terms appears in the title, the abstract, or anywhere in the citation, the bibliographic reference will be retrieved.

The second approach is the use of index terms or descriptors. Most indexes and data bases have a subject authority list or thesaurus that indexers consult when applying subject terms or descriptors to newly included references. However, descriptors vary from data base to data base, and can play a vital role in the successful retrieval of relevant information. For example, in one data base, "nursing homes" may be indexed under "long-term care," while in another they might be found under "extended care." Entering "nursing homes" in a data base for which "long-term care" is the standard index term will result in the omission of many relevant citations from the final product. Care must also be taken not to enter a term in a "free-text" search as a subject that could be misread by the computer as the name of an author. For example, the term "housing" is very obviously a subject heading, and might be commonly found in titles. It is also, however, an integral part of the name of a very prolific corporate author, namely, the U.S. Department of Housing and Urban Development (HUD). In this case, the searcher should limit "housing" to an index term or a term which might be included in a title, to prevent retrieval of irrelevant information. Almost infinite combinations are possible in an on-line search, and in gerontology, particularly, the creative use of several search terms and qualifiers can greatly enhance the effectiveness of the literature search.

Another consideration in the request of an on-line search focuses on the frequent need to conduct "cross-data base searching," that is, to run a search strategy against more than one data base. If the topic is limited to an academic discipline (e.g., adult education), a single data base search might be sufficient for most needs. Further, if the topic can be identified by a single subject heading, then a manual search of the corresponding printed index would generally be faster.

Most researchers, nonetheless, discover that their information needs are more complex, necessitating access to several disciplinary data bases. A search, once formulated in a single data base within a single discipline, can be run against selected other data bases in minutes, thus saving considerable time.

Conducting the On-Line Search

Once the decision is made to conduct an on-line search, it is important to take a very pragmatic approach. The user should identify a library that has access to several on-line vendors (e.g., Bibliographic Retrieval Service, Dialog Information Services, System Development Corporation, and New York Times Information Bank). Some highly valuable data bases can be accessed only through one vendor, so several vendors may have to be queried in order to complete a search. Those not affiliated with an institution which conducts on-line searching may have to obtain special permission in order to make use of this service.

The user should be prepared to pay a fee in addition to computer costs—on-line reference services place an additional demand on the time and resources of library staffs, and most will charge from $10 to $25 for this service in addition to direct computer costs.

Some libraries will request that the researcher make an appointment to discuss information needs prior to contracting for an on-line search. Other libraries will accept search requests without appointments and may even, in some cases, take requests by telephone.

Generally, there are a few format and logistical questions to consider when requesting an on-line search. A search can be limited to a specific time frame, for example, so that all relevant references in the data base will be identified for only the year or years indicated. Retrieved references can be limited to certain languages of publication as well.

Searchers can be tailored so as to be very broad, retrieving almost all relevant references—but will then include many irrelevant references, given the nature of computer searching. A search may also be structured with a very narrow focus, retrieving a higher proportion of very useful materials but missing some relevant information as well. The decision about the breadth of any on-line search should be based on the purpose of the search. Both broad and narrow configurations are appropriate and desirable at one time or another.

The last two decisions which must be made relate to the output format and when to expect the output. Sometimes the urgency of the search will determine the output format. A search can be printed with or without abstracts, and can also be printed "on-line" for immediate availability. Searching can also be conducted "off-line": case printing is done by the host computer and mailed to the requesting library from three to seven days later. Often the deciding factors are cost and time. Printing "on-line" requires computer-connect time, and a search of non-government-produced data bases can often be more expensive. If the search results are needed immediately, cost for "on-line" printing can be reduced by printing only short citations and no abstracts. If time permits, abstracts should be printed and an "off-line" search mailed. A judgment can often be made from the abstract about the appropriateness of an article for the intended purpose of the user, a judgment that cannot be made on the basis of the title alone.

The Data Bases

The data bases which appear below are especially useful in gerontology. All have a corresponding printed index, unless otherwise noted. Names of corresponding print indexes are noted only if they are different from the names of their associated data bases. One major publisher of indexes is *not* available on-line, and is so indicated.

*ABI/Inform
*AGEX Andrus Gerontological Exchange, University of Southern California
    (check library for availability)
ASI American Statistics Index
BIOSIS (print index: *Biological Abstracts*)
Books in Print
Comprehensive Dissertation Abstracts
CIS Index
ERIC (print equivalents: *Resources in Education and Current Index to Journals in Education*)
**Index to Legal Periodicals
*Magazine Index (available on microfilm in many libraries)
Management Contents
Medline (print index: *Index Medicus*)
*NIMH National Institute of Mental Health
*NTIS National Technical Information Service
New York Times Information Bank (print index: *New York Times Index*)
Psychological Abstracts
PAIS Public Affairs Information Service Bulletin
**Readers' Guide to Periodical Literature

SCI Science Citation Index
SCAN National Clearinghouse on Aging (check library for availability)
SSCI Social Science Citation Index
**Social Sciences Index
Sociological Abstracts
USGPO (print index: *Monthly Catalog of U.S. Government Publications*)

*No corresponding printed index
**Not available on-line

Other Information Sources

Although not absolutely essential for the completion of a working bibliography, the following list of resources has been included to help provide
ready reference to many areas in the field of aging. It is by no means a comprehensive list, for these materials are continuously being updated as new
information is published. Thus care should be taken to identify the most current reference sources when seeking specific information, statistics, or other
data in order to be assured of up-to-date accuracy.

Association for Gerontology in Higher Education. *National directory of educational programs in gerontology.* 3rd ed. Washington, D.C.: Association for Gerontology in Higher Education, 1982.

Edwards, W. M., & Flynn, F. *Gerontology: A core list of significant works.*
Resources in Aging Series. Ann Arbor: University of Michigan and
Wayne State University, Institute of Gerontology, 1978.

Harris, L., & Associates. *The myth and reality of aging in America.* Washington, D.C.: National Council on the Aging, 1975.

Harris, L., & Associates. *Aging in the eighties: America in transition.* Washington, D.C.: National Council on the Aging, 1981.

Missinne, L., & Seern, B. *Comparative gerontology: A selected annotated bibliography.* Washington, D.C.: International Federation on Aging, 1979.

McIlvanie, B., & Mundkur, M. *Aging: A guide to reference sources, journals,
and government publications.* Bibliography Series no. 11. Storrs: University of Connecticut, 1978.

National Council on the Aging. *Factbook on aging: A profile of America's
older population.* Washington, D.C.: National Council on the Aging,
1978.

Place, L. F., Parker, L., & Berghorn, F. J. *Aging and the aged: An annotated
bibliography and library research guide.* Westview Guides to Library
Research. Boulder, Colo.: Westview, 1981.

Rook, M. L., & Wingrove, C. R. *Gerontology: An annotated bibliography.*
Washington, D.C.: University Press of America, 1978.

Sourcebook on aging. 2nd ed. Chicago, Marquis Who's Who, 1979.

U.S. Bureau of the Census. *Demographic aspects of aging and the older pop-*

ulation in the United States. (Current Population Reports, ser. P-23, no. 59.) Washington, D.C.: Government Printing Office, 1976.

U.S. Bureau of the Census. *Social and economic characteristics of the elderly.* Current Population Reports, ser. P-23, no. 85. Washington, D.C.: Government Printing Office, 1979.

U.S. Congress. Special Senate Committee on Aging. *Development in aging.* (Annual in two parts.) Washington, D.C.: Government Printing Office, 1959–.

U.S. Library of Congress. Congressional Research Service. *Federal responsiblity to the elderly: Executive programs and legislative jurisdiction.* (Rev. ed.) Washington, D.C.: Government Printing Office, 1979.

Name Index

Estes, W. K., 78, 91, 114
Evans, L., 17, 26, 347, 363

Falek, A., 90, 115
Farrimond, T., 80, 114
Faun, W. E., 50, 65
Feifel, H., 284, 289, 305
Feldman, A., 115
Feldman, R. M., 80, 114, 225, 226, 242
Fichter, J., 230, 242
Finch, C., 65, 66, 67
Fisher, J., 94, 114
Fiske, D., 341
Fitch, J., 339
Flanagan, J. C., 297, 298, 299, 305
Flanagan, J. M., 184
Flynn, F., 382
Fogarty, John E., 200
Foner, A., 238, 243
Fox, C., 80, 113
Fozard, J., 46, 66
Frankfather, D., 244
Franklin, Benjamin, 343
Freeman, A. D., 184
Freeman, J. T., 9, 25
Freese, A., 306
Freud, S., 17, 20, 268
Friedman, R. J., 117
Fujii, S. M., 257, 258, 259, 264, 274
Fuller, M. M., 275, 276
Fulton, J., 287, 305, 306
Fulton, R., 287, 305, 306
Furry, C., 89, 114

Gaitz, C. M., 118
Gajo, F. D., 81, 114
Gallagher, D., 232, 233, 244, 299, 300
Galton, Francis, 8–9
Gans, H., 254, 274
Garber, J., 117
Garn, S., 56, 66
Gatz, M., 105, 114
Geiselhart, R., 84, 113
Gelfand, D., 248, 273, 274, 275, 276, 277
George, L. K., 118
Geschwind, N., 106, 114
Gesell, A., 20
Gibson, D., 66
Gibson, J. J., 78, 93, 114, 328–329, 339
Gilbert, J. G., 82, 114
Gitman, L., 48, 65
Glees, P., 31, 67
Glock, C. Y., 230, 235, 242, 243
Goethe, Johann Wolfgang von, 343

Goldfarb, A., 100, 106, 114, 356
Goldfield, M., 7, 25, 346, 363
Goldman, R., 66
Gompertz, Samuel, 139
Goode, W. J., 226, 242
Goodell, H., 68
Gordon, M., 247, 256, 274
Gordon, P., 55, 66
Gornick, V., 274
Graebner, W., 347, 363
Greenhouse, S., 65
Greenleigh, L., 346, 363
Griffith, 106
Gruber, H., 339
Gunderson, E. K., 68
Gutmann, D., 99, 114, 221, 243, 251,
    252, 274, 276

Haas, G., 330, 340
Haber, D. A., 153
Hadwen, T., 132, 153, 215, 225, 243
Haglund, R., 356, 363
Haley, J., 320, 339
Hall, C., 308, 312, 339
Hall, E. T., 320, 339
Hall, G. Stanley, 9
Hamilton, M., 306
Hammond, K., 339
Hamovitch, M., 324, 325, 339
Harman, D., 30, 66
Haroff, P., 223–224, 242
Harootyan, R., 138, 140, 152
Harris, L., & Associates, 12, 14–15, 25,
    42, 59, 136, 152, 164–165, 166,
    167, 168, 170, 172, 173, 175, 178,
    179, 180, 181, 184, 207, 234, 235,
    239, 242, 247, 274, 321, 382
Harris, R., 66
Hauser, P., 157, 184
Havighurst, R., 17, 25, 127, 130, 133,
    152, 208, 233, 242, 247, 275, 276
Hawkes, G. R., 182, 185, 214, 243
Hawkings, D., 330, 340
Hawley, A., 308, 339
Hayflick, L., 65, 66, 67
Heaney, R., 55, 66
Hendricks, C. D., 9, 25, 126, 140, 152,
    274
Hendricks, J., 9, 25, 126, 140, 152, 274
Henry, W. E., 127, 128, 129, 130, 152
Herr, J., 109, 114
Herrnstein, R. J., 92, 113
Heschel, A., 345, 363
Hildreth, J. M., 170, 174, 185

Subject Index